Practice and Service Lear
Occupational Therapy

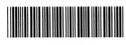

Practice and Service Learning in Occupational Therapy

Enhancing potential in context

Edited by

THERESA LORENZO
University of Cape Town, South Africa

MADELEINE DUNCAN
University of Cape Town, South Africa

HELEN BUCHANAN
University of Cape Town, South Africa

AULDEEN ALSOP
Sheffield Hallam University, UK

John Wiley & Sons, Ltd

Chichester · New York · Weinham · Brisbane · Toronto · Singapore

Other Wiley Editorial Offices

John Wiley & Sons Inc., 111 River Street, Hoboken, NJ 07030, USA

Jossey-Bass, 989 Market Street, San Francisco, CA 94103-1741, USA

Wiley-VCH Verlag GmbH, Boschstr. 12, D-69469 Weinheim, Germany

John Wiley & Sons Australia Ltd, 42 McDougall Street, Milton, Queensland 4064, Australia

John Wiley & Sons (Asia) Pte Ltd, 2 Clementi Loop #02-01, Jin Xing Distripark, Singapore
129809

John Wiley & Sons Canada Ltd, 22 Worcester Road, Etobicoke, Ontario, Canada M9W 1L1

Wiley also publishes its books in a variety of electronic formats. Some content that appears in
print may not be available in electronic books.

Library of Congress Cataloging-in-Publication Data
    Practice and service learning in occupational therapy : enhancing potential
in context / editors Lorenzo, Theresa . . . [et al.].
        p. ; cm.
    Includes bibliographical references and index.
    ISBN-13: 978-0-470-01969-6 (pbk. : alk. paper)
    ISBN-10: 0-470-01969-7 (pbk. : alk. paper)
    1. Occupational therapy—Study and teaching. [DNLM: 1. Occupational Therapy—
education. 2. Education, Professional—methods. WB 18 P895 2006] I. Lorenzo, Theresa.
  RC735.42.P73 2006
  615.8'515—dc22
                                                                    2006005572

A catalogue record for this book is available from the British Library

ISBN-13   978-0-470-01969-6
ISBN-10   0-470-01969-7

Printed and bound in Great Britain by TJ International Ltd, Padstow, Cornwall

This book is printed on acid-free paper responsibly manufactured from sustainable forestry in
which at least two trees are planted for each one used for paper production.

Contents

List of Contributors

Fasloen Adams *MSc OT, BSc OT*
Fasloen Adams is an occupational therapy lecturer in the School of Therapeutic Sciences at the University of the Witwatersrand, Johannesburg. Her areas of interest include: psychosocial rehabilitation, mental health, community development and how culture is viewed within occupational therapy. Her MSc research focused on how the social, cultural and political environment impacts on women's occupations and roles within a support and self-help group.

Auldeen Alsop *Ed D, MPhil, BA DipCOT, FCOT*
Auldeen Alsop is Professor of Occupational Therapy in the Faculty of Health and Wellbeing at Sheffield Hallam University in the United Kingdom. She has a particular interest in work-based and practice learning and has been involved in research, curriculum design and in implementing a range of innovative approaches related to learning in the workplace. She is interested in career and professional development and has published widely on the topics.

Helen Buchanan *MSc OT, BSc OT*
Helen Buchanan is a lecturer in occupational therapy in the School of Health and Rehabilitation Sciences at the University of Cape Town. She is a PhD student researching the implementation of evidence-based practice in occupational therapy. Her practice interests and publications include adult physical rehabilitation (particularly hand therapy) and clinical reasoning.

Lizahn Cloete *MSc OT, BSc OT*
Lizahn Cloete is an occupational therapy lecturer in the School of Health and Rehabilitation Sciences at the University of Cape Town. She teaches in the areas of economic empowerment, inclusive employment and paediatric occupational therapy. Her research interests include foetal alcohol syndrome.

Madeleine Duncan *MSc OT, BA Hons (Psychology)*
Madeleine Duncan is senior occupational therapy lecturer in the School of Health and Rehabilitation Sciences at the University of Cape Town. She is currently a DPhil (Psychology) candidate researching psychiatric disability, chronic poverty and livelihood occupations. Her practice interests and publi-

cations include mental health, curriculum design, ethics and the development of professional practice theory.

Roshan Galvaan *MSc OT, BSc OT*
Roshan Galvaan is a senior lecturer at the University of Cape Town Occupational Therapy department. Her current area of research and practice is health promotion and promoting social justice with youth at risk. Her PhD explores the influences on occupational choices for young adolescents living in impoverished communities. She is the director of Facing Up, a community organization that creates opportunities through occupation for marginalized youth.

Elke Hagedorn *B OT*
Elke Hagedorn is a part-time occupational therapy lecturer in the area of adult mental health at the University of Cape Town. She also supervises practice placements. Prior to this, she worked in the United Kingdom in all areas of mental health, acute rehabilitation and community mental health. She is currently studying for a diploma in shiatsu.

Lucia Hess-April *MPH, BSc OT*
Lucia Hess-April is a lecturer in the Occupational Therapy Department, Faculty of Community & Health Sciences, University of the Western Cape. Her practice interests are focused in community-based rehabilitation and disability studies. Her research interests focus on the psychodynamic dimensions of disability and community development.

Robin Joubert *MOT, BA, Nat. Dip OT*
Robin Joubert is a senior lecturer and Head of Department of Occupational Therapy at the University of KwaZulu-Natal. Her practice interests include the physical field and she is particularly passionate about community-based rehabilitation. As an educationalist she is currently involved with Africanizing the South African occupational therapy curriculum. She is in the final stages of completing a Doctorate in Education.

Theresa Lorenzo *PhD (Public Health), MSc (Disability Studies), BSc OT*
Theresa Lorenzo is a senior lecturer in the Division of Occupational Therapy in the School of Health and Rehabilitation Sciences at the University of Cape Town. She is also programme convenor for the Masters in Philosophy in Disability Studies programme offered by the School. She has been responsible for service learning placement coordination and currently, coordinates the professional development programme for university practice educators and learning facilitators. She has worked and published in the disability and development field, as an advocate for the implementation of rural and urban community-based rehabilitation programmes. Her PhD focused specifically on

the experiences of disabled women in poverty alleviation and development in Khayelitsha, Cape Town, South Africa.

Alice Mackenzie *MSc, BSc OT(C), DipCOT*

Alice Mackenzie is a lecturer in the School of Health Sciences and Social Care at Brunel University, London. Her clinical experience is in the field of working with older people in mental health and physical health services, and she has a keen interest in facilitating student learning and understanding in working with older people. She currently leads the practice placement modules for the undergraduate occupational therapy programme.

Janice McMillan *MPhil, BSoc Sci Hons*

Janice McMillan is a senior lecturer in the Centre for Higher Education Development (CHED) at the University of Cape Town. Her background is in adult education, training and development, with a particular interest in adult learning, and curriculum development. Her current interests are in the field of higher education and social change, focusing specifically on the area of service learning, or community-based learning, curriculum and social change. She is currently registered for a PhD.

Lindsey Nicholls *MA, BSc OT*

Lindsey Nicholls is a senior lecturer in the occupational therapy department, Faculty of Community and Health Sciences, University of the Western Cape. She has worked as a clinician and lecturer in both the United Kingdom (London) and South Africa (Cape Town) over the past 24 years. She has an MA in psychoanalytic approaches to organizations (Tavistock Clinic, London) and has an interest in re-establishing psychoanalytic thinking within an occupational therapy discourse.

Karen Prakke *BSc OT*

Karen Prakke completed her Bachelors degree at the University of Cape Town. She has recently completed her compulsory community service year managing an occupational therapy department at Hillcrest Hospital, a chronic care facility. Karen has been actively involved in occupational therapy and occupational therapy assistant training and supervision for the University of KwaZulu-Natal. Her interest area is vocational rehabilitation and the integration of people with disabilities into the workplace.

Elelwani Ramugondo *MSc OT, BSc OT*

Elelwani Ramugondo is a senior lecturer in the Division of Occupational Therapy, School of Health and Rehabilitation Sciences at the University of Cape Town. She has registered for a PhD that explores the evolution of play across three generations within one indigenous South African group.

Her research interests include cultural relevance in occupational therapy, indigenous play, spirituality and play within practice in the context of HIV/AIDS.

Lana van Niekerk *PhD, M Occ Ther, B Occ Ther*
Lana van Niekerk completed her Bachelors and Masters degrees in occupational therapy at the University of the Free State. After working in Mental Health services at several hospitals and in private practice, she joined the staff at the University of Cape Town, Division of Occupational Therapy, where she was appointed Associate Professor and Head of the Occupational Therapy Division in 2002. She completed her doctorate in 2005.

Heather Wonnacott *MSc OT BSc OT*
Heather Wonnacott was programme manager and deputy director of Facing Up, a community-based occupational therapy programme working with youth at risk. She also supervises occupational therapy students at the University of Cape Town. Areas of interest include occupational enrichment, health promotion and community development. Her research interests focus on the occupational experiences of young adolescent girls living in impoverished communities.

Foreword I

The editors and contributors of this book need to be commended for putting together ideas that address one of the central themes of practice and service learning in the education and training of occupational therapy students and other health professionals. Going beyond addressing 'what' students need to learn, the authors explore 'where', 'why' and 'how' learning takes place across a range of practice domains. Emphasis on the challenges related to diverse contexts in which practice learning takes place is made, together with recommendations on best practice education models to address them. Practice and service learning is central to the education and training of students in most health-related professions. Therefore, one cannot possibly become an efficient or sufficiently trained occupational therapist unless one has undergone some practice and service learning experiences.

The main context of the book, South Africa, brings with it both present and the historical realities. While the present realities create opportunities for most citizens, the disadvantages created by the Apartheid Government still exist for the majority of the people in many areas of life. These realities impact on professional practice education in that students have to contend with challenges such as limited resources, poverty, cultural or language differences, inadequate academic and technological infrastructures, as well as practising in both classical first and third world health facilities. Lessons learned from such contexts in developing countries could be easily applied in any country that faces similar changes.

The book has put forward very strong arguments on the importance and value of defining and using terms such as practice and service learning in a particular context. The definitions of these terms in the introduction of the book aid the reader's understanding of the context in which these terms are used. This further assists the reader's understanding of the arguments and discussions in each chapter. The reader should also take note of terms that are used interchangeably.

Practice and service learning gives students the opportunity to practise, to experiment, put theory into practice, to render services to individuals or communities, to gain experience as well as to observe the practice of occupational therapy in real life situations. Certainly this gives students the opportunity to develop the ability to integrate what is learned in the lecture halls or seminar rooms with realities that confront them during practical experiences. Hence the title of this book, *Practice and service learning in occupational therapy* in my view is very relevant and appropriate in that it advocates for enhancement of potential which, in turn, will foster personal and professional growth and independence.

The reader will be challenged to embark on a paradigm shift regarding key principles of practice education and learning. The main argument presented in here asserts that 'professional education should expose students to a range of practice paradigms'. This poses a challenge to both practice educators and practice learning coordinators who need in-depth experience in those practice paradigms themselves to be able to supervise students. The need to create a variety of learning opportunities that expose students to service contexts similar to those that they will work in after graduating is also emphasized. The book advocates for approaches to training that go beyond the medical model, in order to produce graduates that are capable of acting as 'agents of social change'. This, however, can only be achieved if those responsible for training strive to make practice and service learning a positive experience for students.

Possible curriculum content and structure, principles of students' supervision and assessment that could be implemented in a range of practice paradigms as well as the responsibilities of each role player in practice education and learning are offered for the reader to grapple with. The authors present how learning could be promoted through feedback as well as how the students could benefit from understanding how the assessment process works. Considerable reflection on the arguments and messages conveyed in each chapter may be helpful before the reader draws any conclusions on the relevance and applicability of such information. Some of the recommended measures may have to be put into practice before conclusions are drawn regarding their effectiveness on enhancing the potential of students during practice and service learning. The idea of 'lifelong learning' is advocated to enable each practitioner to be responsible for their own continuous professional development, so as to remain efficient professional practitioners, updating their knowledge and skills in professional and healthcare practice. As the practice context changes, occupational therapists need to modify their profession's philosophy to be in line with national and international trends, practices and policies.

The ideas expressed will provide 'food for thought' for those who have a role to play in practice and service learning, as well as those who are eager to make a positive and progressive difference irrespective of the challenges across different contexts. In my view, the challenge lies in the preparedness of the reader to 'think outside the box' and to 'do things differently'.

Alfred Ramukumba
Head of Occupational Therapy Department
University of Limpopo-MEDUNSA and
President of Occupational Therapy
African Regional Group (OTARG)

Foreword II

The profession of occupational therapy has survived and thrived for 100 years because it has always adapted its practice to the needs of the people it serves. In the early years of the twentieth century, occupational therapists worked in long-stay wards in psychiatric institutions and, from the time of the First World War, in rehabilitation centres or 'curative workshops' for injured servicemen (Haworth & MacDonald, 1948, p. 7). Of necessity, intervention focused on the individual patient, removed from his everyday life to the context of the treatment setting. The first occupational therapists worked 'on prescription from the Medical Officer only. No case should be dealt with without this prescription' (Haworth & MacDonald, 1948, p. 6).

By the second half of the twentieth century, occupational therapy had expanded into many new areas of practice (Gullberg & Henriksson, 1988) and begun to develop a knowledge base for working without the direction of a doctor. For some years, the focus continued to be on the individual patient, or on a particular part of the body, even in community settings where 'the work of the community occupational therapist is the same as that of any other occupational therapist except that the contact with the patient is through his home' (MacDonald, 1976, p. 412).

Gradually, occupational therapists began to acknowledge the broader social and physical environments in which their clients lived, or to which they would return from hospital, and the influence that these contexts had on how people were able to cope with health conditions or disability (Wheeler, 1990). This necessitated the development of new theories to explain and direct occupational therapy intervention. Occupational therapy education was organized so that students were taught formal theory in educational institutions and learned their practical skills in practice settings.

The processes of learning theory and learning to practise can become detached from each other, especially when lecturers are teaching theory that they have never personally applied in practice. In some countries, the theory that is taught in universities now lags behind practice, which is changing rapidly due to social and demographic changes.

At the University of Cape Town, the occupational therapy faculty have had the courage to change their curriculum radically to reflect developments in practice. The approach described in this book moves the focus away from the individual, as in the traditional Western medical model, towards the group, whether family, community or society. It is designed to ensure that formal theory is integrated with practice and that theorizing keeps pace with developments in the field. This approach will help students to understand the power and potential of occupational therapy and give them ways of working with communities and organizations. Perhaps most importantly, it will instil in them the confidence to go into new situations and listen without feeling the need to take control.

Although the content of this book is rooted in South African culture and society, it has relevance and value for the European context, where cultural and linguistic diversity is also the norm. The text can provide useful guidance for educators and practice coordinators in countries where occupational therapy is not yet an established profession. But it can also offer ideas to the faculty of occupational therapy programmes in countries that have comprehensive health and social care services, where occupational therapy is long-established. It provides a model for preparing students more effectively for practice in the twenty-first century.

For me, one of the most exciting professional developments in the past few years was the publication of a South African textbook that described a different type of occupational therapy, oriented to meet the needs of communities and populations living with the multiple problems of poverty, displacement and rapid social change (Watson & Swartz, 2004). In this book, the editors and authors identified and articulated new opportunities for occupational therapy to continue to fulfil its professional purpose. *Practice and service learning in occupational therapy*, which shares some of the same contributors, is equally exciting in its descriptions of ways in which we can prepare a different kind of occupational therapy practitioner, fit for the future.

Jennifer Creek
Freelance Occupational Therapist UK

REFERENCES

Gullberg, M. & Henriksson, C. (1988). *Overview of the practice of the profession 1987/88*. Linköping, Sweden: World Federation of Occupational Therapists.

Haworth, N.A. & MacDonald, E.M. (1948). *Theory of occupational therapy, 3rd edn*. London: Balliere, Tindall & Cox.

MacDonald, E.M. (Editor) (1976). *Occupational therapy in rehabilitation: a handbook for occupational therapists, students and others interested in this aspect of reablement, 4th edn*. London: Balliere Tindall.

Watson, R. & Swartz, L. (2004). *Transformation through occupation*. London: Whurr.

Wheeler, P. (1990). Community. In J. Creek (Ed.), *Occupational therapy and mental health: principles, skills and practice*. Edinburgh: Churchill Livingstone, pp. 411–430.

Preface

The most fruitful development in human thinking frequently takes place at those points where two different lines of thought meet. The idea for this book germinated during a visit by Auldeen to the University of Cape Town (UCT) in 2003. As an established author interested in professional education, she was particularly intrigued by the differences between the British and South African students' experiences in practice education. Auldeen recognized that, while other books relating to practice education had addressed practical issues for students (Alsop & Ryan, 1996) and the practice of teaching and clinical supervision (Stengelhofen, 1993; Shardlow & Doel, 1996; Fish & Twinn, 1997; McAllister, Lincoln, McClead & Maloney, 1997), there were no known texts that examined how engagement in diverse and challenging practice contexts could (1) enhance students' learning through investigating new forms of practice; (2) confirm their contribution to comprehensive service delivery; and (3) promote the implementation of the minimum standards for the education of occupational therapists (Hocking & Ness, 2002) in locally and culturally relevant ways. Auldeen challenged the staff in the Division of Occupational Therapy at UCT to consider documenting some of the experiences in practice education in view of the potential contribution that these could make to the academic theory base of the profession.

We discussed ideas ranging from articles in selected professional journals to a 'special edition' of the *South Africa Journal of Occupational Therapy* but finally decided that a book would provide the best medium for opening up debate about current professional practice education challenges. At the time, some of the UCT staff were contributing to an edited text (Watson & Swartz, 2004) about emerging forms of occupational therapy practice aimed at transforming the health and development potential of individuals, groups and communities through occupation. Following the release of this edited volume we felt that a logical follow-up publication could be an exploration of how undergraduate practice learning may be used to prepare future practitioners for working effectively in previously uncharted territories such as those envisioned by other authors (Whiteford & Wright-St Clair, 2005; Kronenberg, Simo-Algado & Pollard, 2005). At the same time, the concept of service learning was gaining momentum within South Africa, although not in the UK. Educational activities associated with civic responsibility as the driver of service learning were beginning to be influential and were providing challenges for both staff and students. There were many lessons to be learned but as effective strategies evolved, it was realized that the educational value of these strategies could be relevant internationally. Thus, it was thought that this book could not only make a particular contribution to occupational therapy education but that it could also be used to inform education programmes for other professionals such as social workers, engineers, architects, lawyers, teachers, scientists, as well as other health professions.

Initially, we had no idea how the writing project would unfold but we were excited about what the intersection of thinking might yield through such a 'south–north' collaboration. Awareness of the richness and depth of practice learning that had to be captured became increasingly more apparent as the writing progressed. The process provided the editors with opportunities to debate similarities and differences between the two practice contexts. In this respect, the glossary describing some of the terms used in this book provides a jointly agreed understanding of usage across continents. We have resisted using definitions as these vary so much and because definitions tend to be more finite. Context has also been a feature of wide discussion through which much shared learning has occurred. The nature of context, particularly in the realm of practice education, influences the way in which educational processes impact on role-players, but the consequences of learning in different contexts enhance the potential of all. We hope that this book will stimulate debate and critical response to the emerging needs for social change.

In coordinating this book, the editorial team would like to thank the many communities, service providers, organizations, university practice educators and students who have contributed to our learning. The work of contributors is also acknowledged. Apart from the chapters they produced, they also gave generously of their time to engage in the educational debates at different stages of the process. We hope that those efforts reap just rewards for all concerned.

We have also benefited greatly from financial support from two sources: Speechmark, who initially funded Auldeen's travel to Cape Town to engage in early discussions about the book; and the University of Cape Town Research Committee's Visiting Scholar's Fund Committee for also helping the project come to fruition.

Additional thanks are extended to numerous people for their unflagging support and understanding about the time demands required to complete the book: Kyla and Sarah Duncan; James, Murray and Kirsty Buchanan; Ruth Katzman; and the Alsop family. Thanks also go to Gill O'Caroll for contributing freely of her graphic skills and to Alfred Ramukumba and Jennifer Creek for willingly agreeing to write the Forewords of the book. Thanks to one and all.

To all who read this book, we hope you enjoy the diversity of stories and experiences that are offered here.

Theresa Lorenzo, Madeleine Duncan, Helen Buchanan,
Auldeen Alsop *Cape Town, 2005*

REFERENCES

Alsop, A. & Ryan, S. (1996). *Making the most of fieldwork education.* Cheltenham: Stanley Thornes.

Fish, D. & Twinn, S. (1997). *Quality clinical supervision.* Oxford: Butterworth-Heinemann.

Kronenberg, F., Simo-Algado, S. & Pollard, N. (Eds.). (2005). *Occupational therapy without borders: learning from the spirit of survivors.* Edinburgh: Elsevier Churchill.

McAllister, L., Lincoln, M., McCleod, S. & Maloney, D. (1997). *Facilitating learning in clinical settings.* Cheltenham: Stanley Thornes.

Shardlow, S. & Doel, M. (1996). *Practice learning and teaching.* Basingstoke: Macmillan Press.

Stengelhofen, J. (1993). *Teaching students in clinical settings.* London: Chapman & Hall.

Watson, R. & Swartz, L. (Eds.). (2004). *Transformation through occupation.* London: Whurr.

Whiteford, G. & Wright-St Clair, V. (2005). *Occupation and practice in context.* Sydney: Elsevier.

I The Context of Practice and Service Learning

Introduction

FIELDWORK EDUCATION UNDER DEBATE

For many years, the profession of occupational therapy has used a set of terms that has universally described that component of the education curriculum through which students learn to practise occupational therapy in the field. A number of placements are organized for students that enable them to gain experience of working with patients, clients and service users of different ages and who experience different functional limitations as a result of various health conditions, and whose situation is managed in organizations across the spectrum of health and social care. The requirement set in past times by the World Federation of Occupational Therapists is for students to have practised their profession for a minimum 1000 hours in a variety of settings before they qualify as occupational therapists.

The new standards of the World Federation of Occupational Therapists (Hocking & Ness, 2002, p. 31) define fieldwork as:

> the time students spend interpreting specific person-occupation-environment relationships and their relationship to health and well-being, establishing and evaluating therapeutic and professional relationships, implementing an occupational therapy process (or some aspect of it), demonstrating professional reasoning and behaviours, and generating or using knowledge of the contexts of professional practice with and for real live people

This definition is helpful, encapsulating clearly and concisely the necessary features of what the global fraternity of occupational therapists understand as fieldwork. Increasingly, however, 'fieldwork' as a term is being challenged as no longer reflecting the nature of the learning that is undertaken by students. It is understood informally that the term fieldwork may also be under review in other parts of the world. In parts of South Africa, fieldwork refers to a time-limited, project-based form of experiential learning in the field, for example, factory visits to learn about ergonomics and occupational health; a fieldtrip to a rural area to learn about occupation, disability and poverty alleviation projects; or a period of data collection and implementation of a research project. It is clear that context influences practice education and the terms that are used to describe the processes of professional socialization in the field. In

Practice and Service Learning in Occupational Therapy. Edited by Theresa Lorenzo, Madeleine Duncan, Helen Buchanan, Auldeen Alsop
© 2006 John Wiley & Sons Ltd

the UK, a decision was taken by the College of Occupational Therapists to use the term 'practice placements' to replace fieldwork, and practice placement is currently the preferred term used in the national standards for pre-registration education (College of Occupational Therapists, 2004).

Furthermore, in the UK, the term 'placement' is now under debate. Placement has come to denote a 'place' where a student goes to practise the art and science of occupational therapy. But this term arguably limits the conceptualization of other possible learning experiences that students might have in order to develop competence to practise. Practice learning experiences may better describe the nature of learning opportunities now available to students that enable them to understand and practise occupational therapy in its broadest sense.

This book is about practice learning that provides students with opportunities to develop their skills and competence in occupational therapy, largely (but perhaps not exclusively) within some organizational framework. This book is also about service learning where students enter communities and negotiate the nature of their involvement with representatives of that community based on pre-existing, formal agreements between the higher education institution, civic organizations and other significant stakeholders. Practice involves partnership working to achieve mutually agreed goals, and learning derives from the benefits gained from the experience by both the student and the community. Different groups of students provide an ongoing service throughout the year by making their professional expertise available as a resource to the community, their contributions being directed and monitored by community representatives in consultation with university practice educators and site learning facilitators.

This book, therefore, takes risks in introducing the reader to a range of concepts, strategies and processes that support new ideas in practice and service learning and that perhaps challenge some of the traditional thinking about fieldwork. New ways of presenting learning experiences to students as service learning have been adopted in selected areas of South Africa, whilst some of the new terms concerned with practice learning and practice experiences may have been adopted in the UK. This book serves to bridge the continents and introduce the reader to some of the strategies adopted in South Africa that support and promote student learning and that are likely to be of particular interest to those involved with professional education worldwide.

PRACTICE LEARNING

The practice experiences of occupational therapy students in South Africa may not be unique but they do take place in some of the most poverty-stricken areas that remain post-apartheid. The commonly accepted view of occupational therapy practice must necessarily be broadened to encapsulate the diversity of what the profession has to offer in these situations. Here, collective efforts between health professionals and communities are directed towards equity and social development rather than primarily towards individual therapeutic or rehabilitative intervention for the impairments and activity limitations associated with health conditions. Whilst being equipped to execute the latter through clinical practice in hospital settings, the efforts of health professional students in a developing society are also directed at being socially responsive through service learning aimed at the prevention of ill-health, the promotion of public health and the full participation of disabled people in the mainstream of society. Practice learning, framed within the primary health care philosophy, is therefore expanded to include clinical practice, fieldwork and service learning.

Much has been written about clinical practice and fieldwork. This book, therefore, presents information to substantiate practice and service learning as relevant constructs for guiding contemporary occupational therapy education in developing and developed contexts. Various aspects of practice learning are discussed, including: establishing and maintaining learning opportunities in complex environments through building partnerships with diverse stakeholders; enabling students to set priorities and maximize the impact of their efforts in situations where resources are scarce; and innovative methods of supporting students in acquiring competence in comprehensive forms of practice. Relevant professional and educational theories are thus discussed and applied within the text. Above all, the book highlights how occupational therapy practice education and research can enhance potential in context, whether it is the capacity of students to become agents of change, or the capacity of individuals, groups and communities with whom students collaborate to discover answers to their own challenges.

ORGANIZATION OF THE BOOK

The book is divided into three parts. Part I provides the backdrop against which Parts II and III are written. The reader may thus want to engage with Part I before moving on to other chapters in Parts II and III. These are concerned respectively with 'Developing Professional Identity' and 'Enhancing Potential' and are introduced separately. In the various parts, this book aims to open up debates around the future development of practice and service learning as these modes of learning evolve to reflect new drivers and opportunities within professional education. It is hoped that many people from various disciplines, not only occupational therapy, will join the debate about practice and service learning by engaging with the experiences of professional educators shared in this book.

Part I deals with the philosophical, theoretical and policy dimensions of practice and service learning. Chapter 1 introduces the rationale for the book;

the terminology that is used; and the distinctions between practice and service learning. It describes the context of the book, highlighting the socioeconomic, cultural and political backdrop against which most of the chapters are written. Using South African higher education benchmarks and international occupational therapy professional standards as a point of departure, Chapter 2 discusses some of the current drivers that are shaping professional practice education curricula. The competencies that new graduates may require in a primary healthcare-led society are identified and suggestions are made for possible curriculum content and outcomes that are aligned with locally relevant practice education objectives. A series of practice narratives are presented in Chapter 3, highlighting the historical challenges and pragmatic realities faced by individuals, groups and communities with whom student health professionals collaborate. By drawing attention to the contexts within which citizens live and students work, the challenges for professional practice education are highlighted and principles for prioritizing the content of a practice-learning curriculum are identified. Chapter 4 presents a quality framework for professional practice education. It describes critical dimensions for consideration including stakeholders and how the dynamics of practice education operate between their respective roles and responsibilities. Issues of quality assurance and ethics in practice and service learning are addressed, and mechanisms for promoting accountability are suggested.

REFERENCES

College of Occupational Therapists (2004). *College of Occupational Therapists Standards for Education: pre-registration education standards, revised August 2004.* London: College of Occupational Therapists.

Hocking, C. & Ness, N.E. (2002). *Revised minimum standards for the education of occupational therapists.* Perth: World Federation of Occupational Therapists.

1 Practice and Service Learning in Context

MADELEINE DUNCAN and AULDEEN ALSOP

OBJECTIVES

This chapter discusses:

- the sociopolitical, economic and cultural context that forms the backdrop for most chapters in this book
- the professional philosophy that may inform practice in a developing country such as South Africa
- the rationale for, and the nature of practice and service learning
- the use of terminology that is aligned with new forms of practice.

INTRODUCTION

Recent international changes in how health is viewed have impacted on the 'where', 'why', 'how', 'what' and 'with whom' of health services and subsequently on the role, scope and education of health professions (Whiteford and Wright-St Clair, 2005). Greater emphasis is being placed on prevention and public health promotion through equity in the distribution of scarce financial and human resources. By making the resources of health professionals more widely accessible, the health and social development needs of diverse groups of people are being addressed and not primarily the functional and rehabilitation needs of people with impairments, as has been the case in the recent past.

Health professions, including occupational therapy, are poised to move beyond the medical model towards increased social relevance through alternative forms of service delivery (Kathard, 2005; Seifer, Hermans & Lewis, 2000). A review of the current international occupational therapy literature has revealed that role-emerging forms of practice education are currently being explored to open up new learning opportunities across a spectrum of

Practice and Service Learning in Occupational Therapy. Edited by Theresa Lorenzo, Madeleine Duncan, Helen Buchanan, Auldeen Alsop
© 2006 John Wiley & Sons Ltd

service sectors, such as health, social development, education, welfare, labour and community-based civic organizations (Banks & Head, 2004; Bonello, 2001; Thomas, Penman & Williamson, 2005; Wood, 2005). Professional education, in preparing students for these shifts in the scope of practice, is exposing them to learning experiences where biomedical, social and occupational practice paradigms are being operationalized (Hocking & Ness, 2002). All three practice paradigms are indicated in primary healthcare-led societies, such as South Africa and the UK, however the challenges are numerous and complex. This chapter introduces the reader to these complexities since they form the backdrop for most chapters in this book. It frames the various social and pragmatic influences on practice education and on the practice-learning environments within which prospective occupational therapists are trained. The chapter concludes with a rationale for the terminology that is used throughout the book.

THE SOCIAL CONTEXT OF THE BOOK

South Africa has 11 official languages and a population of 48 million. In per capita terms, South Africa is an upper-middle-income country, yet despite this relative wealth, most South African households live in poverty. The distribution of income and wealth is amongst the most unequal in the world, and many households still have unsatisfactory access to education, healthcare, energy and clean water (May, 1998). An estimated 30% of economically active adults are unemployed; 11.4–15% are living with HIV/Aids; 48% are living in poverty (monthly expenditure of R358/£29/USD55 per adult equivalent) and 58% of adults are semi-literate (Statistics South Africa, 2005). South Africa is also amongst the most violent societies in the world, third only to Brazil and Guatamala in reported violent deaths and abuse of women and children. While inequity, violence and chronic poverty occur in pockets (prevalence is unevenly distributed within regions), they nevertheless influence the development rate of the country and, by implication, the inclusion of social responsiveness within its higher education agenda (Favish, 2003).

South Africa is well resourced with health professionals compared with other African and developing countries (Watson & Swartz, 2004). Although significant progress has been made in meeting the health needs of society through the introduction of the primary healthcare approach, comprehensive health care is not yet readily accessible to the majority of the population. To address this situation, all health professional graduates in South Africa have to do a year of compulsory community service in under-served areas of South Africa before they may register their qualification with the Health Professions Council of South Africa (HPCSA) (2002). During their public service year, graduates may have to function with minimal supervision from experienced health practitioners in remote rural or under-resourced areas. They may be placed at health clinics, hospitals or special schools where no previous reha-bilitation services have been offered or where the implementation of health promotion and prevention initiatives has been marginalized due to the volume of acute cases requiring therapeutic intervention.

To engage with the job requirements of their compulsory community service year and beyond, graduates need be able to plan and administrate com-prehensive health programmes with individuals, groups and communities. Working collaboratively with a range of health workers such as traditional healers, community representatives and rehabilitation assistants, health ther-apists need a strong professional identity, skills in evidence-based practice and astute critical thinking. Their resilience, effectiveness and efficiency is closely linked to their commitment, not only to making a difference in individual lives but also within the communities where they work. While these outcomes are not unique to South Africa, they do indicate that the scope of occupational therapy practice is changing and that corresponding changes are required in practice education.

IMPACT OF CONTEXT ON PRACTICE EDUCATION

Local practice and, by implication, the evolving practice epistemology used in developed and developing countries varies substantially because of dif-ferent national healthcare and social development histories. Nevertheless, the processes of curriculum design, the principles of learning and the strategies for professional socialization are likely to be similar, thereby providing a common frame of reference for appreciating and learning from different com-munities of practice (Wenger, 1998). To attain the proposed purposes and exit outcomes of health professional education programmes, practice learning cur-ricula need to offer students graded exposure to a range of service contexts that mirror those in which they will ultimately need to work independently after graduating.

The following pragmatic factors currently influence the implementation and management of practice education, and are applicable across various chapters in the book.

- *Limited professional resources*: health professional posts in the public sector have either been abolished, frozen or redistributed to pre-viously under-served geographical areas making it difficult to find suitable, accessible practice learning opportunities for students in metropolitan regions where training centres are situated. Expert practitioners have left the public sector to seek jobs elsewhere with the result that students have access to fewer role models and expe-rienced supervisors.
- *Under-resourced infrastructures*: budget cuts have either resulted in the closure or downsizing of established occupational therapy

services. Basic equipment, materials, libraries and computers and other resources for effective practice are limited, especially in rural areas.

- *Rapid de-hospitalization and de-institutionalization* of patients from public sector hospitals has reduced the amount of time available for comprehensive intervention at tertiary and secondary levels of care in the public health sector. Patients may, for example, be sent home following a stroke, spinal cord injury or psychotic episode to wait indefinitely for access to some form of rehabilitation.

- *Stark distinctions* exist between affluent health facilities (for example, state-of-the-art private health clinics) and poorly resourced public sector amenities (for example, overcrowded health clinics in rural areas). Students find it difficult to process the emotional dissonance that arises when they are exposed to the impact of privilege and historical disadvantage on the quality of life that people are able to enjoy.

- *Cultural or language differences*: whilst attempts are made to recruit students from various racial groups to represent the diversity of the South African population, many students may still, at some time or another, be unable to communicate effectively with their clients in practice situations due to language and cultural differences.

The logistical difficulties and ethical dilemmas that education institutions face in accessing and monitoring suitable learning experiences matched to the emerging competence of undergraduates are obvious. Given the fluid service platform and the changing face of practice in a primary healthcare-led society, the traditional apprenticeship model of fieldwork (Hocking & Ness, 2005), in which students are individually linked to an experienced clinician in an established service, has become the exception rather than the rule. The few available, well-established and staffed services are earmarked for junior (first to third year) students to ensure that they gain optimal grounding through coaching and supervision from expert practitioners in the core practice processes; principles and methods of individual biopsychosocial practice. With this foundation, senior students (fourth year) are considered to have the basic competence to engage in community-based practice learning with groups and communities.

LOCALLY RELEVANT PRACTICE EDUCATION

Practice and education shape each other. The scope of occupational therapy practice in South Africa changed with the adoption of the primary healthcare philosophy (World Health Organization, 1978) as lead approach of the National Department of Health in 1994. Occupational therapists in the past tended to focus on the treatment of individuals within the medical model. As public service providers in a primary healthcare-led society through district health systems (McCoy & Engelbrecht, 1999), their current focus is on the efficient delivery of comprehensive occupational therapy that is appropriate, accessible and affordable to citizens close to where they live and work. In the context of public health (Wilcock, 1998), comprehensive occupational therapy refers to the role and scope of the profession with groups and communities addressing locally identified health promotion, prevention and community-based rehabilitation needs and social development objectives through occupation-based programmes that are implemented within health districts.

For graduates to be effective and relevant in their work, there needs to be a good match between prevalent national and local health needs, emerging paradigms of practice and what they are taught and how they learn. UNESCO (1998), in a document entitled *World Declaration on Higher Education for the Twenty-First Century: Vision and Action*, emphasized that higher education should be locally relevant, of a high quality and constantly drawing on and contributing to global knowledge production. The declaration also emphasized the social responsibilities of higher education graduates. To this end, health professions are seen to play a prominent role in promoting 'public good' through comprehensive health services based on the primary healthcare philosophy. Traditional approaches to health professional training that occur almost exclusively within the medical model are no longer considered sufficient or appropriate.

According to Hocking and Ness (2005, p. 74) occupational therapy practices and education curricula generally have tended to mirror developments in Britain, North America and Europe 'rather than developing ways of practice and education tailored to the culture and climate in which it is embedded'. Global higher education and public health service imperatives require graduates who, as citizens, act not only as facilitators of health but also as agents of social change in the contexts where they work. Walker (2000, p. 13) poses the following question against the backdrop of educational reform in post-apartheid South Africa, 'if universities are places where "citizen" identities are formed, with effects for society in which we live now and in the future and for our understanding of diversity in local and global contexts in an interlocking world, what should a "good citizen" of the present day be and know, and in the context of higher education, what might education for "democratic sensibility" look like?'. Although not directed at occupational therapy, current literature suggests that the profession is critically engaged with the socio-political concerns that this question raises about practice and education (Kronenberg, Simo-Algado & Pollard, 2005; Watson & Swartz, 2004).

RESPONDING TO SOCIO-POLITICAL IMPERATIVES

Educating prospective health practitioners in a developing country provides an ideal context for exploring new methods of practice education and theories of practice as these evolve through the work that students undertake with marginalized groups of people. Cognisant of environmental and social influences on the well-being and development of individuals, groups and communities, therapists are exploring the contribution that the profession can make towards the emancipation of people who live on the margins of society due to poverty and other oppressive socio-political influences (Kronenberg et al., 2005; Watson & Swartz, 2004). Responsive to socio-political pressures for increased democratic, equitable participation of all citizens in building cohesive societies, occupational therapy practitioners and theorists have begun to develop constructs such as *occupational apartheid* (Kronenberg & Pollard, 2005, pp. 58–86) and *occupational justice* (Townsend & Whiteford, 2005) as areas of critical concern to therapists working as agents of social change (Thibeault, 2005; Whiteford, 2004). They see their contribution towards social redress as being the creation of an occupationally just world; one that is governed in such a way as to enable individuals to flourish by doing what they decide is most meaningful and useful to themselves, their families and communities (Townsend & Wilcock, 2004; Wilcock & Hocking, 2004).

While practice education is informed by evolving professional theories, attention also needs to be paid to international and national policy frameworks for the implementation of health services. For example, the World Health Organization's (WHO) *International Classification of Functioning, Disability and Health* (ICF) (WHO, 2001) has been instrumental in precipitating practice paradigm shifts by capturing the interface between the medical and social models of disability; the continuum between body functions and structures; activity functioning; social participation and the impact of the environment on individual and public health. Used in conjunction with other seminal international health and social development policy documents, such as: the *Ottawa Charter for Health Promotion* (WHO, 1986); the *Declaration of Alma-Ata* (WHO, 1978); the Resolution on the *Standard Rules of the Equalisation of Opportunities for Persons with Disabilities* (United Nations, 1994); and the World Federation of Occupational Therapists (WFOT) *Position Paper on Community-based Rehabilitation* (Kronenberg, 2003), the ICF is also seen as providing a conceptual framework for integrated, comprehensive professional actions, such as: programmes aimed at the prevention of public ill-health; health promotion initiatives; remediation and therapeutic interventions; and various forms of rehabilitation (for example, medical, vocational, psychosocial and community-based rehabilitation).

The ICF has assumed prominence as a framework for directing the work of governments, health professions and policy makers and is seen as providing direction for national associations in the member countries of the World Federation of Occupational Therapists because, according to Wilcock and Hocking (2004, p. 226), it provides 'a language and terminology that reflects current occupational therapy knowledge'. While the ICF is a useful organizing framework for professional communication, its definition of functioning is not aligned with occupational therapy philosophy and theory about humans as meaning-making beings (Duncan, 2005). Complementary frameworks for understanding poverty, human needs and social change, therefore, also need to inform the content and structure of practice education curricula (Max-Neef, 1991; Watson & Swartz, 2004).

TERMINOLOGY

The various conceptualizations of teaching, service and research, the three pillars of higher education, are ultimately ideological. Terminology and language are important because they convey information about the assumptions, world-views and values on which higher education and learning is based. In discussing the power of dominant discourses in teaching and learning, van Wyk (2004, p. 309) suggests that the meta-language involved in the use of certain terms points to the fact that 'different discourses seek to produce and situate students, institutions and communities in particular ideologies'. Disability activists have argued that, while international policy documents such as the ICF have pre-empted significant social advances for disabled and other marginalized groups of people, there is still a long way to go in shifting the hegemonic attitudes of health professionals (Marks, 1999). Of critical concern in practice education is the deconstruction of the disabling use of language by educators, students and practitioners. Equally important is the political will on the part of the higher education institution to include the voice of communities in decisions pertaining to their involvement in student training.

The terminology that is used to describe what students are doing in different practice contexts will reflect a particular ideology or mode of working. Is what students are doing: fieldwork, clinical practice, service learning, practice learning, or all of these depending on where, with whom and why students are situated in a particular context? In this book we contend that occupational therapy has come of age as a profession in its concern with improving the human condition in its broadest sense through the focused use of occupation. Its discourses and, therefore, the terminology used to describe practice education and learning should be inclusive of positivist, interpretivist and critical emancipatory ideologies. The positivist discourse of the medical model views impairment and disability as a problem of the person that is caused directly by some health condition, disease or trauma (WHO, 2001, p. 28). The impairment(s) or activity limitation(s) require medical care provided in the form of individual treatment and/or rehabilitation by a range of health professionals. Therapeutic management of the impairment occurs in 'clinical' settings (for example hospital wards or outpatient clinics), and is aimed at cure or remediation, the adjustment of the person's capacities to perform functional activities, or at enabling participation in his or her social environment. Professional practice education in this model may quite appropriately be referred to as 'clinical practice' with the primary learning occurring through 'clinical' reasoning about the precipitating, predisposing and perpetuating influences on an individual's health and functional status. The individuals being 'treated' by students may be referred to as 'patients' or 'clients', although disabled people view the latter term as 'a euphemism that disguises the lack of choice regarding services being offered to them' (Marks, 1999, p. 149).

The social model of disability sees disability as a socially constructed identity, which requires social action to reduce the marginalizing effects of prejudice against people with impairments. Practice education in this model could assume a critical-emancipatory stance with students joining forces with disabled people and 'at-risk' persons in seeking alternative social conditions for their full participation in society. As novice health practitioners, students may collaborate with disabled people, parents of disabled children, teachers, trainees, learners, community representatives, community rehabilitation workers or employers. Depending on the purpose and ideology of the organization or agency, students may refer to the persons they are collaborating with as 'client', 'service user', or 'consumer' (terms indicating a managerial or economic purpose), or as 'participant' or 'community member' (terms indicating an equal power relationship). Ideally no distinguishing descriptor should be needed; simply the use of names distinguishing either role (for example, learner or teacher) or identity (for example, Mr X). This would signal a deliberate deconstruction of the power relationship that inevitably exists when health professionals and disabled people, self-help groups and/or community representatives work together in addressing mutually identified areas of concern (Marks, 1999; van Wyk, 2004).

DESCRIPTIONS OF TERMS

Figure 1.1 depicts the interface between the various terms used in this book. Practice education refers to the educational theory and pedagogy supporting the practical curriculum of a professional degree. Practice learning is used as an overarching, inclusive term for the shifts in knowledge, skills and attitudes that occur in students as a result of participating in a range of practical experiences in the 'real world' of work. Used interchangeably with the term 'fieldwork', practice learning is defined as:

> The time students spend interpreting specific person-occupation-environment relationships and their relationship to health and well-being, establishing and evaluating therapeutic and professional relationships, implementing an occupational therapy process (or some aspect of it), demonstrating professional reasoning and behaviours, and generating or using knowledge of the contexts of professional practice with and for real live people.
>
> (Hocking & Ness, 2002, p. 31)

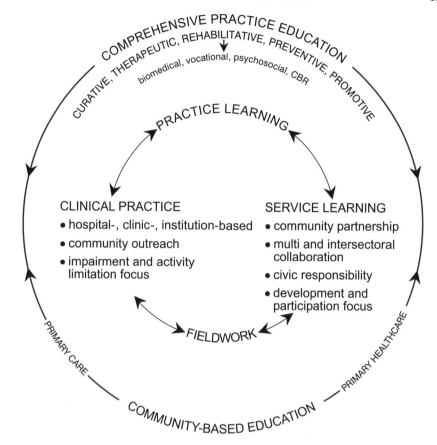

Figure 1.1 Interface of terms

In fieldwork, the emphasis has largely been on what the student gains and must do in order to meet professional standards and on what the educational institution/practice learning site will provide to ensure that professional socialization occurs, such as, suitable patients/clients and a professional role model. Although the intended emphasis in the above definition is on the traditional interpretation of students' professional development within established, well-resourced health service (or other) structures, the definition does not necessarily exclude other forms of practice learning. There is growing evidence of support for new kinds of educational practice in higher education with the growth of the 'service learning' or the community-based accredited learning movement, which acknowledges various ideologies for placing students in the field of work (Favish, 2003; Waghid, 1999). For this reason, we differentiate between fieldwork and service learning, even though both may be separately understood within a broader definition of practice learning. However, most of the occupational therapy literature refers to community-based practice education and not to service learning. Only one reference could be traced on service learning and occupational therapy (Waskiewicz, 2002). Service learning is therefore presented here as an emerging educational approach in the profession, although it has been well-established since the early 1980s in medical education in the United States (Stanton, Giles & Cruz, 1999).

Service learning may be defined as a method under which students learn and develop through thoughtfully organised service that is conducted in, and meets the needs of, the community, and is coordinated with an institution of higher education and with the community, helps foster civic responsibility, is integrated into and enhances the academic curriculum of the students enrolled, and includes structured time for the students (and community) to reflect on the service experience and outcomes (adapted from American Association for Higher Education, 1999). This definition links professional development to social responsibility through collaboration with socio-political and community-based civic structures. Service learning is sometimes confused with community service, since it does in effect, serve the community. However, service learning connects the classroom curriculum or theory to a community need and then uses the input to create an action project in collaboration with community members. Theoretically, service learning is driven by the agenda of a community and not by the curriculum agenda of the learning institution. The parameters, purpose and goals of the service are clarified and regularly monitored in consultation with community representatives. Whilst learning and change occur for both parties, the university academic requirements are always secondary to the rights, autonomy and dignity of the community which students have the privilege of serving. Whilst students bring fresh ideas and professional expertise, the form in which it is offered to the community must be such that it is never exploitative. The community in turn brings a wealth of indigenous knowledge and expertise that can be mobilized, in collaboration with higher education structures, for self-empowerment and knowledge production by the community that is integrated into curricula. Service learning is based on participatory ethics. It offers the community access to a range of academic skills and resources whilst teaching students affirmative values, leadership, citizenship and responsibility. It empowers both parties as learners, educators, facilitators and achievers. The aim of service learning is, in other words, to balance the provision of valid and valuable learning opportunities for the student, whilst at the same time assisting the community to meet its own development needs (Fourie, 2003).

CONCLUSION

A new model of excellence in higher education is emerging where universities celebrate teaching and research, whilst also taking pride in their capacity to connect thought to action and theory to practice through civil service (Boyer, 1994). By organizing cross-disciplinary programmes around pressing social issues, universities become 'connected institutions', committed to improving, in a very intentional way, the human condition. In this book, we suggest that occupational therapy education programmes may become connected to a range of social development agencies and that students, as human resources, may contribute to the delivery of services within their scope of competence. This book, therefore, extends the notion of practice learning to embrace service learning as an evolving feature of occupational therapy education.

REFERENCES

American Association for Higher Education (1999). *Writing the community: concepts and models for service learning. Service Learning in the Disciplines.* American Association for Higher Education Series. Corporation for National Service. Retrieved 10 October, 2005, from http://www.aahe.org

Banks, S. & Head, B. (2004). Partnering occupational therapy and community development. *Canadian Journal of Occupational therapy, 71*(1), 5–8.

Bonello, M. (2001). Fieldwork within the context of higher education: a literature review. *British Journal of Occupational Therapy, 64*(2), 93–99.

Boyer, E. (1994). Creating the New American College. *Chronicle of Higher Education, March,* A48.

Duncan, M. (2005). Approaches and processes in occupational therapy with mood disorders. In R. Crouch & V. Alers (Eds.), *Occupational Therapy in psychiatry and mental health.* London: Whurr, 459–479.

Favish, J. (2003). A new contract between higher education and society. *South African Journal of Higher Education, 17*(1), 24–30.

Fourie, M. (2003). Beyond the ivory tower: service learning for sustainable community development. *South African Journal of Higher Education, 17*(1), 31–38.

Health Professions Council of South Africa (2002). Regulations relating to the performance of community service by persons registering in terms of the Health Professions Act of 1974 Amendment. *South African Government Gazette, 439*(23047), 22 January.

Hocking, C. & Ness, N.E. (2002). *Revised minimum standards for the education of occupational therapists.* Perth: World Federation of Occupational Therapists.

Hocking, C. & Ness, N.E. (2005). Professional education in context. In G. Whiteford & V. Wright-St Clair (Eds.), *Occupation and practice in context.* Sydney: Churchill Livingstone Elsevier, pp. 72–85.

Kathard, H. (2005). Clinical education in transition: creating viable futures. *Advances in Speech-Language Pathology, 7*(3), 149–152.

Kronenberg, F. (2003). *Position paper on community-based rehabilitation.* Forrestfield, Western Australia: World Federation of Occupational Therapists. Available at www.wfot.org

Kronenberg, F. & Pollard, N. (2005). Overcoming occupational apartheid: a preliminary exploration of the political nature of occupational therapy. In F. Kronenberg, S. Simo-Algado & N. Pollard (Eds.), *Occupational therapy without borders: learning from the spirit of survivors.* Edinburgh: Elsevier Churchill Livingstone, pp. 58–86.

Kronenberg, F., Simo-Algado, S. & Pollard, N. (Eds.). (2005). *Occupational therapy without borders: learning from the spirit of survivors.* Edinburgh: Elsevier Churchill Livingstone.

Marks, D. (1999). *Disability: controversial debates and psychosocial perspectives.* London: Routledge.

May, J. (1998). *Poverty and inequality in South Africa: meeting the challenge.* Cape Town: David Phillip Publishers.

Max-Neef, M. (1991). *Human scale development: conception, application and further reflections.* London: Apex Press.

McCoy, D. & Engelbrecht, B. (1999). Establishing the District Health System. *South African Health Review.* Health Systems Trust, pp. 131–146.

Seifer, S.D., Hermans, K. & Lewis, J. (Eds.). (2000). *Creating community-responsive physicians: concepts and models for service learning in medical education.* Washington DC: American Association for Higher Education. Published in co-operation with Community Campus Partnerships for Health.

Stanton, T., Giles, D.E. & Cruz, N.I. (1999). *Service learning: a movement's pioneers reflect on its origins, practice and future.* San Francisco, CA: Jossey Bass.

Statistics South Africa (2005). Retrieved 21 August, 2005, from www.statssa.gov.za

Thibeault, R. (2005). Connecting health and social justice: A Lebanese experience. In F. Kronenberg, S. Simo-Algado & N. Pollard (Eds.), *Occupational therapy without borders: learning from the spirit of survivors.* Edinburgh: Elsevier Churchill Livingstone, pp. 232–244.

Thomas, Y., Penman, M. & Williamson, P. (2005). Australian and New Zealand fieldwork: charting the territory for future practice. *Australian Occupational Therapy Journal, 52,* 78–81.

Townsend, E. & Whiteford, G. (2005). A participatory occupational justice framework. Population based processes of practice. In F. Kronenberg, S. Simo-Algado & N. Pollard (Eds.), *Occupational therapy without borders: learning from the spirit of survivors.* Edinburgh: Elsevier Churchill Livingstone, pp. 110–126.

Townsend, E. & Wilcock, A. (2004). Occupational justice. In C.H. Christiansen & E.A. Townsend (Eds.), *Introduction to occupation: the art and science of living.* New Jersey: Prentice Hall, pp. 243–273.

UNESCO (1998). *World declaration on higher education for the twenty-first century: vision and action.* Retrieved 22 August, 2005, from http://www.unesco.org/eduprog/wche/declaration_eng.htm

United Nations (1994). *United Nations Standard Rules On The Equalisation Of Opportunities For Persons With Disabilities. Resolution 48/96.* Vienna: United Nations Publications. Available at: http://www.un.org/esa/socdev/enable/dissre00.htm

Van Wyk, J.-A. (2004). The role of discourse analysis in the conceptualisation of service learning in higher education. *South African Journal of Higher Education, 18*(1), 303–321.

Waghid, Y. (1999). Engaging universities and society through research, teaching and service. *South Africa Journal of Higher Education, 13*(2), 109–117.

Walker, M. (2000). Higher education and a democratic learning society: professionalism, identities and educational action research. In M. Mostert & A. Dison (Eds.), *Academic development: changes and challenges*. Grahamstown: Rhodes University.

Waskiewicz, R. (2002). Impact of service learning on occupational therapy students' awareness and sense of responsibility towards communities. In S.H. Billig & A. Furco (Eds.), *Service learning through a multidisciplinary lens: A volume in advances in service learning research*. Greenwich, CT: Information Age Publishing, pp. 123–129.

Watson, R. & Swartz, L. (Eds.). (2004). *Transformation through occupation*. London. Whurr.

Wenger, E. (1998). *Communites of practice: learning, meaning and identity*. Cambridge: Cambridge University Press.

Whiteford, G. (2004). Occupational issues of refugees. In M. Molineux (Ed.), *Occupation for occupational therapists*. Oxford: Blackwell Publishing, pp. 183–200.

Whiteford, G. & Wright-St Clair, V. (Eds.). (2005). *Occupation and practice in context*. Sydney: Churchill Livingstone Elsevier.

Wilcock, A.A. (1998). *An occupational perspective of health*. Thorofare, NJ: Slack Inc.

Wilcock, A.A. & Hocking, C. (2004). Occupation, population and policy development. In M. Molineux (Ed.), *Occupation for occupational therapists*. Oxford: Blackwell Publishing, pp. 219–230.

Wood, A. (2005). Student practice contexts: changing face, changing place. *British Journal of Occupational Therapy*, 68(8), 375–378.

World Health Organization (1978). *Declaration of Alma-Ata*. Geneva: World Health Organization. Available at http://www.who.int/hpr/archive/docs/almaata.html

World Health Organization (1986). *Ottawa Charter on Health Promotion*. Geneva: World Health Organization. Available at http://www.who.int/hpr/archives/docs/ottawal

World Health Organization (2001). *International Classification of Functioning, Disability and Health: ICF Short version*. Geneva: World Health Organization. Available at http://www.who.int/icidh

2 A Responsive Curriculum for New Forms of Practice Education and Learning

MADELEINE DUNCAN and JANICE McMILLAN

OBJECTIVES

This chapter discusses:

- pertinent educational and professional drivers currently influencing the reform of professional practice education in South Africa
- the graduate profile of a curriculum that is responsive to the health and development needs of a society in transition
- the tensions and dynamics of designing a locally relevant practice-learning curriculum that is aligned with international professional standards.

INTRODUCTION

The globalization of information and communication technology is shifting the ways in which knowledge is produced, recorded, disseminated and applied. Higher education institutions are concerned with the international currency of knowledge and aim to prepare sound 'knowledge workers', that is, skilled individuals who are able to apply theoretical knowledge to localized problems and contexts by working as members of teams or systems (Gibbons, 1998; Zwarenstein et al., 2002). In this new knowledge economy, health profession graduates will require lifelong learning skills demonstrated in their ability to produce, apply and disseminate knowledge in their local contexts (Higgs, Andresen & Fish, 2004a). Changing definitions of functioning, health and disability (World Health Organization, 2001) suggest that health professions will provide different forms of service to those who may have defined their scope of practice in the past. Regular realignment of practice and education with local and international trends in approaches to health and development needs

Practice and Service Learning in Occupational Therapy. Edited by Theresa Lorenzo, Madeleine Duncan, Helen Buchanan, Auldeen Alsop
© 2006 John Wiley & Sons Ltd

ensures the effectiveness and relevance of professions in an ever-changing socio-political, economic and technological climate (Eve & Hodgkin, 1997; UNESCO, 1998).

Cognizant of these and other drivers impacting on occupational therapy professional education in context, Hocking and Ness (2005, p. 84) suggest that 'we might recognise and articulate commonalities that unite the profession, as knowledge, skills and modes of practice diverge'. They argue that while curricula may differ in how they articulate their philosophies about occupation and occupational therapy, similarities do exist in the aspirations of the profession internationally.

This chapter describes the factors shaping, and the pedagogical principles supporting, locally tailored occupational therapy practice education in South Africa. It suggests ways in which the curriculum may be designed 'in response to contextual issues and cultural understandings to embed professional practices within local perspectives of health rather than taking a strictly biomedical stance' (Hocking and Ness, 2005, p. 83). It discusses the role of indigenous knowledge systems in locally responsive practice education and describes critical success factors for designing a practice and service learning curriculum. It identifies the profile of a graduate who is able to work within the primary healthcare approach and concludes with recommendations for the role of research in promoting the competence of future practitioners.

DEFINING A RESPONSIVE CURRICULUM

Notions of 'curriculum responsiveness' are reflected in higher education debates in South Africa. According to Moore and Lewis (2004), higher education policies reflect two broad imperatives: on the one hand, a response to developments in the global economy and the changing role of higher education internationally; and, on the other hand, a local concern for social reconstruction, economic development and equitable distribution of resources. The South African National Commission on Higher Education (NCHE) Report (NCHE, 1996), drafted soon after the advent of democracy in 1994, expresses 'responsiveness' in the following way:

> It can be described as a shift from a closed to a more open and interactive higher education system, responding to social, cultural, political and economic changes in its environment . . . There will also be greater social accountability towards the taxpayer and the client/consumer regarding the cost-effectiveness, quality and relevance of teaching and research programmes. In essence, increased responsiveness and accountability express the greater impact of the market and civil society on higher education and the consequent need for appropriate forms of regulation . . . Overall, greater responsiveness will require new forms of management and assessment of knowledge production and dissemination.
>
> (NCHE, 1996, pp. 6–7, cited in Moore & Lewis 2004, p. 32)

Social responsiveness means that the content, form and delivery of the curriculum changes so that it promotes reciprocal learning for all stakeholders in locally relevant ways. A responsive curriculum may therefore be defined as a programme of higher educational activities that advances the development and transformation of learners, the profession/discipline of which the learner is a member and, through socially relevant activities, the society that they serve.

Occupational therapy education is increasingly preparing future practitioners to work as agents of change in addressing the occupational needs of not only individuals but also of communities. This orientation has come about as the profession has started to theorize the contribution it can make in public health and social development (Watson & Swartz, 2004; Wilcock & Hocking, 2004). The challenge currently facing educators is how to operationalize these paradigm shifts through the practice education curriculum in ways that affirm the identities, needs and aspirations of local communities. The inclusion of historically disadvantaged or socially marginalized people, including disabled persons and those from ethnic minorities, into professional training is one way of shaping the profession from within. The social and cultural relevance of practice education may be achieved by creating space for the identities of various cultures within the undergraduate cohort of students to inform the way in which professional knowledge is generated and applied.

PURPOSE OF A RESPONSIVE CURRICULUM

The education of health professionals is particularly challenged by egalitarian goals in contexts where the gap between the 'have's (highly privileged) and the 'have not's (under privileged) is widening. The under privileged are unlikely to gain access to tertiary education and professional training due to inadequate secondary education and limited access to financial resources. They are also unlikely to have equal access to comprehensive healthcare and development opportunities. The purpose of a responsive curriculum in such contexts is to provide a broad training platform in keeping with the principles of primary healthcare. These principles ensure the provision of equitable, affordable, accessible, effective and efficient services close to where people live and work (World Health Organization, 1978).

Socially responsive practice education views students as a potential human resource for reaching a larger proportion of the population by expanding the work that they do through service learning. Additionally, the purpose of a socially responsive curriculum is to recruit and support future practitioners who represent the diversity of means (for example, finance, transport and personal capacity), ethnicity, race and educational preparedness within the general population. A changing, socially representative demography of students entering health professional education suggests that a responsive curriculum will be able to pay attention to the prior knowledge, skills and world-views that students bring. Such a curriculum aims to liberate students in applying their innate capacity and indigenous knowledge, thereby changing the way in which the profession is practised from within. Graduates will be finely attuned, not only to the rigours of their discipline, but also to the cultural nuances of the communities they come from and will ultimately serve.

Ntuli (1999), in speaking about culture, education and the African Renaissance writes the following:

> I would like to draw up a scenario with which many black people are familiar. I was one of nine children living in a four bedroomed house. In our house the movement between the bedroom and the kitchen or bathroom required traffic lights, especially in the mornings. We were seven boys with only three pairs of shoes. Whoever woke up earliest walked away with shoes! We had to negotiate at every stage . . . and for all scarce resources in the house. We came to understand human nature. We learned to be good negotiators. Many of the students we teach come from such backgrounds. What happens to them when they come into our institutions? Do we recognize their collective problem-solving skills and utilize them for effective teaching and learning, or do we force them into a mould created for us by Europe? Let me venture another example. African people and people of African descent generally are participatory. In African churches, worshippers do not just sit and say 'amen' and depart. They respond to the words of the preacher. They urge him on! . . . there is a call-and-response. Rap, kwaito, scathmiya, maskanda . . . all marked by the antipodal, or participatory ethos. How does this square up with our teaching methods where we require students to sit for 45 minutes listening to us without interruption in a vertically orientated learning environment? The students bring with them these skills, knowledge and experience, as well as analytic abilities, but are not given the opportunities to use or demonstrate them. We 'disadvantage' them compared to students from more affluent societies. This denial of their abilities reinforces their sense of inadequacy derived from the broader societal environment. It is these we should be building on.
>
> (Ntuli, 1999, p. 196)

A responsive curriculum widens access to tertiary study and health professional education to differently prepared students, including those with disabilities. It requires a radically revised pedagogy than that used in the past with academically well-prepared students from elite educational backgrounds (Goduka, 1996). Notions of 'under preparedness' or 'disadvantage' have historically been attributed to lack of study skills or language literacy and been remedied through 'add-on' provision of academic 'support'. Students who enter university with a conception that learning involves the quantitative accumulation of bits of knowledge that have to be rote learned and reproduced have difficulty in 'finding their own voice'. They struggle to interpret theory and explain professional practice using their indigenous and cultural heritage as valid frames of reference. A responsive curriculum liberates new forms of professional knowledge by building the personal autonomy, self-confidence and study behaviours of learners from diverse cultural and ethnic groups. It pays as much attention to the indigenous knowledge background of the student as it does to their academic and professional development.

Stated differently, a responsive curriculum is cognizant of and overtly addresses the socio-political precursors to academic performance. It achieves its purpose, amongst others, by attending on a regular basis to teachers' and students' conceptions of learning and teaching (Cliff, Parsons, Sharwood, Radloff & Samuelowicz, 1996). Remedial or 'academic support' approaches to differently prepared students are likely to be perceived as 'add-on' or 'marginalizing'. Adult education methods that affirm alternative learning styles are therefore indicated. A responsive curriculum provides students with conceptual 'tools' for understanding their own study behaviour and for identifying alternative interpretations of Eurocentric professional knowledge. These may include topical workshops and training in study skills, learning strategies and critical thinking that legitimizes culturally nuanced interpretations of documented professional theory and methods. The spin-off from this approach to practice education is the shaping of locally relevant forms of professional practice by indigenous practitioners. Creating a definitive African space for reformulating prescribed modes of working is likely to lead to locally relevant practice.

LOCAL IDENTITY OF A RESPONSIVE CURRICULUM

The central argument thus far has been that the professional socialization process should affirm indigenous cultural strengths, values and practices. Applied to Africa, this means that submerged heritages need to surface through the content and form of practice education (Higgs, Higgs & Venter, 2003). Existing professional epistemology needs to be filtered through African people's way of seeing and being (Makgoba, 1999; Shutte, 1993). This calls for a concerted effort at 'decolonizing' professional knowledge from ingrained Western thought patterns. Unlike Western thought that puts the individual at the centre of life, African thought puts the community at the centre of life. This community shares the earth with the unborn, the living spirits of the dead, nature and the universe beyond. Life is based on anti-materialistic, cohesive values that recognize humans as only existing and developing in relationships with other persons. Indigenous knowledge is also a key element of the social capital of the poor. It is one of the main assets that chronically poor people use to gain control of their lives and therefore deserves particular attention in practice education in developing contexts (Higgs & van Niekerk, 2002; Higgs et al., 2003). Indigenous knowledge, for example, forms the basis for decision making in agriculture, healthcare, food preparation, education, natural resource management and other livelihood occupations. Knowing more about indigenous knowledge will therefore inform how the 'person–occupation–

environment' relationship is understood and applied as an organizing framework for occupational therapy.

OCCUPATION AND INDIGENOUS KNOWLEDGE

wa Thionga (1990) places language, gender, class and culture as key elements in the struggle for identity and dignity in Africa. These elements deserve to be explicitly addressed in a responsive curriculum by deconstructing Eurocentrism, which, according to Samir Amin (1988, cited in Ntuli, 1999, p. 186), is 'a culturalist phenomenon in the sense that it assumes the existence of irreducibly distinct cultural invariants that shape the historical paths of different peoples'. Applied to occupational therapy, this means that existing theory about the subjectivity, identity, and agency of the occupational human may need to be revised in the construction of practice education curricula in Africa.

Different practice learning environments, clients and systems shape the expression of a profession in context (Whiteford and Wright-St Clair, 2005). The nature of the professional relationship, the processes followed during occupational therapy to effect change, or the reasoning used by occupational therapists should be informed by the culture within which they practice. A locally relevant and responsive curriculum will therefore encourage complementarity between existing Eurocentric, Western and emerging African, indigenous professional theory (Higgs, Richardson & Dahlgren, 2004b).

FACTORS SHAPING A RESPONSIVE CURRICULUM

A curriculum aimed at the development of culturally relevant forms of practice and at redress, equity and social justice is underpinned by values that affirm social responsiveness. Responsive forms of curriculum strive to make a social contribution; reflect the directives of national and international higher education policies and operate within the constraints of the local sociopolitical context. Some pertinent factors shaping practice education in the current South African context are briefly discussed.

NATIONAL EDUCATION POLICY

The South African National Plan for Higher Education (Council for Higher Education, 2001; Ministry of Education, 2001) and the Education White Paper 3 of the National Qualifications Framework (Ministry of Education, 1997) put forward the following arguments about the role of higher education in contributing to social justice, economic reform and social life more generally:

> Higher education, and public higher education especially, has immense potential to contribute to the consolidation of democracy and social justice, and the growth and development of the economy . . . These contributions are complementary. The enhancement of democracy lays the basis for greater participation in economic and social life more generally. Higher levels of employment and work contribute to political and social stability and the capacity of citizens to exercise and enforce democratic rights and participate effectively in decision-making. The overall well-being of nations is vitally dependent on the contribution of higher education to the social, cultural, political and economic development of its citizens.
>
> (Council for Higher Education, 2001, pp. 25–26)

Translating these directives into educational practice on the ground suggests that prospective health professionals should be socialized not only into their particular discipline but also into their role as citizens working towards the consolidation of democracy and social justice. Here, practice and service learning connect. On the one hand, the prospective health professional learns to operationalize the theory and methods of their particular discipline and, on the other hand, they learn what citizenship means through serving as a resource in contexts of need.

TRANSDISCIPLINARY FORMS OF CURRICULUM

The following section provides an example of a responsive first-year multi-professional course, based on theory and fieldwork that aims to consolidate learning about primary healthcare. It demonstrates how, at a first-year level, the directives of the national education policy may be operationalized in curriculum theory and practice using transdisciplinary modes of curriculum design.

The Health Sciences Faculty at the University of Cape Town developed the following five principles for guiding the content and structure of a socially responsive, multi-professional course at first-year level. The course is compulsory for all registered first-year students in medicine, nursing, physiotherapy, speech and language therapy, audiology and occupational therapy. The principles were developed following an extensive process of deliberation between representative academics and students from all participating professions as well as from medical anthropology, sociology, psychology and education (Duncan, Alperstein, Mayers, Olckers & Gibbs, 2005; Mayers, Alperstein, Duncan, Olckers & Gibbs, 2005). Using a problem-based learning approach, the course unfolds through small group activities, including fieldtrips, weekly seminars and tutorials. The principles, summarized below, are reinforced throughout all learning activities both in the course and in profession specific courses, thereby laying a theoretical and attitudinal foundation, at first-year level, that affirms the values of social responsiveness.

Commitment to Promoting Health and Well-being in the Context of the Individual, Family/group and Community

This principle ensures that the course prepares students to recognize and address the links between individual health needs and behaviours and the social development of the family/household/group and the community. Values such as interdependence, equality, equity and the affirmation of diversity are explored and affirmed as adding quality to life. Students come to appreciate that the individual cannot be considered as separate from his or her social reality.

Commitment to Practising 'Whole Person Care'

The second principle ensures that course content focuses on comprehensive care of the whole person within a human-scale development framework that also reinforces the primary healthcare approach (Max-Neef, 1991). Human-scale development moves beyond the traditional biopsychosocial approach to whole-person care. It recognizes a range of human needs and satisfiers inherent in doing, having, being and interacting. Whole-person care, through the lens of human-scale development, ensures sociocultural sensitivity and vigilance about participatory ethics in contexts where structural poverty and inequality exits. Students come to appreciate the importance of looking beyond the impairment or immediate need to the whole person within a development framework.

Commitment to Being a Reflective Practitioner

The third principle ensures that course content equips the student with a reflective approach to learning and developing practice knowledge and skills (Dahlgren, Richardson & Kalman, 2004). Students come to appreciate how personal assumptions, values and beliefs impact on professional interactions and knowledge generation. The content always starts from the self and moves outwards via experiential learning and back again to the self with the aim of asking 'what does this experience mean for me as a future health professional and how does what I think, do and feel affect the people I work with?'. Integrating reflexivity as a way of academic life lays a foundation for the affirmation of diversity, accommodation of indigenous ways of knowing and sensitivity to issues of power in the professional role.

Commitment to Health, Human Rights and Social Responsibility

Central to the fourth principle is curriculum content aimed at promoting a basic understanding of the history, concepts, philosophy and principles of primary healthcare with due consideration of participatory and biomedical ethics, professionalism and human rights. For example, disability is not an attribute of an individual but a complex set of conditions created by society for and by those of its members who are living with impairment (Marks, 1999). The issue is an 'attitudinal or ideological one requiring social change, which at a political level becomes a question of human rights' (World Health Organization, 2001, p. 28). The disability movement is becoming a global force for change, with increased collaboration among disability groups, between the disability community and governments, and between the disability community and the human rights community. This global force is challenging the hegemony of health professions and existing social structures that are based on the medicalization of disability. As consumers increasingly take responsibility for advancing their own health and development agendas and disabled people claim their rightful place in society, so health professionals have to grapple with the dominance of their attitudes, methods and epistemology. By alerting first-year students to these and other issues of power and rights, their commitment to social responsiveness is awakened.

Commitment to Practice Within a Health and Social Development Team

The fifth principle reinforces a multi-disciplinary approach to healthcare and community development through collaborative teamwork. The team may include consumers, public representatives, indigenous healers and a range of other role-players depending on the sector within which practice education is occurring. While appreciating the contribution of their own discipline, students learn to think 'beyond the box' and find ways of working with existing capacities and structures in finding new solutions to old problems.

NATIONAL QUALIFICATIONS FRAMEWORK

A driving force behind curriculum reform in South Africa has been the adoption of the National Qualification Framework (NQF) Bill of 1996 (NQF, 1997). The NQF legalizes a programme-based higher education system in South Africa. All sequential learning activities leading to the award of a particular qualification are referred to as a 'programme'; the curriculum content of which is regulated by the South African Qualifications Authority (SAQA) and professional (or sectoral) Standards Generating Bodies (SGBs). According to the South African Universities Vice Chancellors' Association (SAUVCA) (1999, p. 27) 'outcomes have to be linked to the demands of disciplines as well as those of the economy and society in general'. Qualifications need to deliver on these outcomes in terms of the quality assurance system contained in the SAQA Regulations issued in 1998.

Health professional education programmes aim to produce graduates who are able to work effectively and efficiently within the comprehensive primary healthcare approach. 'Comprehensive' here refers to multi-sectoral collaboration in delivering preventative, promotive, curative and rehabilitative health services. Whilst there has to be congruence between the purposes and aims of the respective educational centres in the country, their professional ideology and educational philosophy may differ substantially (Hocking & Ness, 2005). Difference is to be fostered as it accounts for the distinctive qualities and strengths of graduates from respective educational centres, each meeting one or more niches in the South African context.

MINIMUM STANDARDS OF PROFESSIONAL EDUCATION

The newly adopted 2002 World Federation of Occupational Therapists (WFOT) Minimum Standards pave the way for innovative alignment of educational programmes with constantly changing national and international trends (Hocking & Ness, 2004, 2005). These Standards suggest that the educational process within programmes may focus on one or more of three orientations: biomedical, occupational or social orientation (Hocking & Ness, 2002, p. 10):

- Biomedical orientation deals with existing/at-risk health conditions.
- Occupational orientation deals with occupational risk, disruption, deprivation.
- Social orientation deals with populations at occupational risk due to socio-political forces, such as war, homelessness, etc.

The complexities of a primary healthcare-led society such as South Africa requires occupational therapy graduates who are able to work flexibly and competently within all three orientations. Adopting a broader perspective on health, the primary healthcare approach requires health practitioners to work preventatively, in collaboration with individuals, groups and communities, in developing health promoting environments and social conditions (World Health Organization, 1986). Each of the three proposed orientations is therefore indicated if contextually relevant educational programmes for occupational therapists in developing countries are to be developed (Galgeigo, 2004; Wilcock & Hocking, 2004).

Of particular significance is the potential role that each of these orientations play in community-based rehabilitation (CBR) as a strategy for community development. The call is for occupational therapists to develop a critical awareness of the political nature of CBR and their potential contribution, as experts in occupation, to the equalization of opportunities for optimal living (Kronenberg, 2003). Practice education should equip prospective practitioners not only with basic biomedical, but also with social and occupational, competence. Intra-professional models and interdisciplinary frames of reference, particularly those informing an occupational view of public health (Wilcock & Hocking, 2004), poverty alleviation and social development (Kronenberg, Simo-Algado & Pollard, 2005; Watson & Swartz, 2004) need to take equal precedence with individualistic, medical and bio-psychosocial models of practice (Christiansen & Baum, 1997).

Table 2.1 portrays a possible progression of an undergraduate occupational therapy curriculum, from first through to fourth year, that accommodates the three practice orientations recommended by WFOT (Hocking & Ness, 2002).

Objectives for each year of study should reflect the progressive integration of biomedical, occupational and social constructs suggested by WFOT Minimum Standards. As students apply these against the backdrop of local historical, social, economic, political, cultural and scientific information, they gain confidence not only in clinical but also in population reasoning. Both these

Table 2.1 A responsive curriculum based on WFOT minimum standards

Year of training	Theoretical focus of curriculum	Practical professional development
1st	The well-being and development of the occupational human across the life-cycle Occupation as means and as end Introduction to an occupational perspective of primary healthcare	Macro and micro occupational analysis of indigenous occupations Understanding impact of poverty, violence, HIV/Aids and politics on well-being, development and occupational participation
2nd	Disability studies Occupational performance and performance component assessment and remediation principles International Classification of Functioning (WHO, 2001) Health promotion and prevention Poverty alleviation and social development Occupational therapy theory, models and processes	Assessment of performance component, occupational performance dysfunction and context Projects that apply: United Nations Standard Rules for Equalization of Opportunities for Disabled Persons (UN, 1994) Health promotion through occupation
3rd	Preventative, curative and rehabilitative occupational therapy programmes for individuals and groups	Applied clinical reasoning: in-depth case studies of and services with individuals and groups
4th	Interpretation of National Policies Occupational justice and primary healthcare CBR and comprehensive occupational therapy programmes and generalist services in multi-sectoral contexts.	Applied population reasoning: in-depth study of and services in collaboration with groups, communities or organizations OT programme development and implementation.

forms of reasoning are required to develop comprehensive occupational therapy programmes. Professional development should, in particular, address the exploration of personal values and beliefs about social justice, occupational justice and an occupational perspective of public health (Wilcock, 1998). Graded practical challenges (at a level appropriate to the year of study) and professional growth experiences should be available representing the scope of the profession in different service/practice domains (see Chapter 4, Table 4.2).

CRITICAL SUCCESS FACTORS OF A RESPONSIVE CURRICULUM

A responsive curriculum may be guided by a number of critical success factors that broadly summarize what is expected of a graduate, both with respect to being a health professional (generic) and an occupational therapist (specific) (Table 2.2).

The graduate profile of a socially responsive curriculum may contain some of the following features:

- A lifelong learner and reflective practitioner who applies scientific methodology as well as inductive, naturalistic enquiry to generate understanding about the health of humans as occupational beings.
- A health service provider who endorses the theoretical and philosophical base of occupational therapy through appropriate actions aimed at meeting the health and occupational needs of individuals, groups and communities in the local context with due consideration of indigenous knowledge systems.
- A skilled, entry grade practitioner who is able to apply an occupational therapy process in a variety of settings and in different sectors of the public service with clients across the lifespan according to the primary healthcare philosophy.
- An effective team worker who has the ability to create, nurture and optimize opportunities for the development of human potential through occupation, particularly people with disabilities and persons who are occupationally at risk.
- A self-motivated individual who is committed to working with others in a spirit of collegiality, social justice and collaboration.
- A professional who is compliant with the ethics, norms, values and standards of the occupational therapy profession.
- A conscientised[1] citizen who is committed to the affirmation of diversity and transformation of society through addressing occupational justice with due consideration of indigenous African (or other) worldviews.

[1] 'Conscientisation' refers to learning to perceive social, political and economic contradictions, and to take action against the oppressive elements of reality (Freire, 1972, p. 15).

Table 2.2 Critical success factors of a responsive curriculum

Generic critical success factors	Specific critical success factors
Commitment to health, human rights and social justice	Study and use human occupation for the therapeutic, developmental, vocational and social benefit of individuals, groups and communities
A positive attitude to education and reflective practice, and the transformation of experience into learning	Collect, evaluate, analyse and use specific and context-related information pertaining to the occupational needs and capacities of individuals, groups and communities
Enthusiasm for development and the capacity to facilitate this in others	
Accountability for own opinions, actions and decisions	
Willingness to engage in and respect issues of diversity	Practise the principles and methods of research as an adjunct to occupational therapy services
Appreciation of the value and importance of health and the impact that health has on social development	Appreciate the parameters, behaviours and responsibilities that mark professionalism
Effectiveness in all forms of communication	Apply clinical and population reasoning in promotion of occupational enrichment, enablement and empowerment of individuals, groups and communities
A commitment to and appreciation of the primary healthcare approach	
Ability to undertake the tasks and responsibilities of management and organizational development	Display expertise in the development and maintenance of strategic alliances and beneficial partnerships with all role players for the advancement of occupational justice
Commitment to teamwork and an active contribution to inter-, multi- and transdisciplinary liaison	Promote occupational participation and fulfillment and prevent risk behaviours that lead to occupational deprivation, alienation and dysfunction
	Manage own time, resources and responsibilities appropriately for different levels of service and comprehensive (promotion, prevention, therapeutic and rehabilitation) occupational therapy programmes

One way of achieving this profile is to pay particular attention to the contexts in which practice development occurs, that is, where students gain 'hands-on', practical experience in the field. The practice learning curriculum will differ in developed and developing countries because of access to different resources. The variance, however, deserves closer scrutiny as practice learning opportunities have implications for the evolution of the profession in the long term. The extent to which education addresses new forms of practice in previously uncharted territories and alternative practice paradigms will determine the extent to which future practitioners will be prepared to break the mould of conventional methods of working in response to emerging social needs.

CONCLUSION: ACTING BOLDLY NOW

In essence we have argued for new forms of professional practice education in order to situate health professions at the forefront, not only of comprehensive healthcare, but also of social change. As indicated throughout this chapter, the challenges are varied. On the one hand, there are external or exogenous pressures, relating to challenges in society more broadly, for example, changing mindsets about the nature of professional practice. On the other hand, there are challenges that are endogenous or internal to systems of higher education in many contexts. This includes the political will and commitment to curriculum transformation and to viewing the role of the university in contributing to social justice, development and equity. By acting boldly and by creating a responsive professional development platform through new forms of curricula, critical practice competencies amongst future practitioners will be acquired, thereby enabling them to make a contribution towards the betterment of society.

REFERENCES

Christiansen, C.H. & Baum, C.M. (1997). *Occupational therapy: enabling function and well being*, 2nd edn. Thorofare, NJ: Slack.

Cliff, A., Parsons, P., Sharwood, D., Radloff, A. & Samuelowicz, K. (1996). Underprepared students or underprepared teachers or both? Is there a mismatch between students' and academic teachers' expectations of the processes of learning and teaching in higher education? *Different Approaches: Theory and Practice in Higher Education.* Proceedings HERDSA Conference, Perth, Western Australia, 8–12 July. Available at http://www.herdsa.org.au/confs/1996/cliff2.html

Council for Higher Education (CHE) (2001). *Towards a New Higher Education Landscape: Meeting the Equity, Quality and Social Development Imperatives of South Africa in the 21st Century.* Pretoria: Council for Higher Education.

Dahlgren, M.A., Richardson, B. & Kalman, H. (2004). Redefining the reflective practitioner. In J. Higgs, B. Richardson & M.A. Dahlgren (Eds.), *Developing practice knowledge for health professionals.* Edinburgh: Butterworth Heinemann, pp. 15–34.

Duncan, M., Alperstein, M., Mayers, P., Olckers, L. & Gibbs, T. (2005). Not another multi-professional course: rationale for a transformed curriculum. Part 1. *Medical Teacher 28*(1), 59–63.

Eve, R. & Hodgkin, P. (1997). The restructuring of professional work. In J. Broadbent, M. Dietrich & J. Roberts (Eds.), *Professionalism and medicine-the end of professions?* London: Routledge, pp. 69–85.

Freire, P. (1972). *Pedagogy of the oppressed.* New York: Pelican Books.

Galgeigo, S.M. (2004). Occupational therapy and the social field: clarifying concepts and ideas. In F. Kronenberg, S. Simo Algado & N. Pollard (Eds.), *Occupational therapy without borders: learning from the spirit of survivors.* Edinburgh: Elsevier Churchill Livingstone, pp. 87–98.

Gibbons, M. (1998). Higher education relevance in 21st century. Unpublished paper presented at the UNESCO World Conference on Higher Education. The World Bank, Washington, October.

Goduka, I.N. (1996). Challenges to traditionally white universities: Affirming diversity in curriculum. *South African Journal of Higher Education, 10*(1), 27–38.

Higgs, P. & van Niekerk, M.P. (2002). The program of Indigenous Knowledge Systems (IKS) and higher education discourse in South Africa: a critical reflection. *South African Journal of Higher Education, 16*(3), 38–49.

Higgs, P., Higgs, L.G. & Venter, E. (2003). Indigenous African knowledge systems and innovation in higher education in South Africa. *South African Journal of Higher Education, 17*(2), 40–45.

Higgs, J., Andresen, L. & Fish, D. (2004a). Practice knowledge – its nature, sources and contexts. In J. Higgs, B. Richardson & M.A. Dahlgren (Eds.), *Developing practice knowledge for health professionals.* Edinburgh: Butterworth Heinemann, pp. 51–70.

Higgs, J., Richardson, B. & Dahlgren, M.A. (Eds). (2004b). *Developing practice knowledge for health professionals.* Edinburgh: Butterworth Heinemann.

Hocking, C. & Ness, N.E. (2002). *Revised minimum standards for the education of occupational therapists.* Perth, Western Australia: World Federation of Occupational Therapists. Available at http://www.wfot.org

Hocking, C. & Ness, N.E. (2004). WFOT Minimum standards for the education of occupational therapists: shaping the profession. *WFOT Bulletin, 50,* 9–17.

Hocking, C. & Ness, N.E. (2005). Professional education in context. In G. Whiteford & V. Wright-St Clair (Eds.), *Occupation and practice in context.* Sydney: Elsevier Churchill Livingstone, pp. 72–86.

Kronenberg, F. (2003). *Position paper on community based rehabilitation.* Forrestfield, Western Australia: World Federation of Occupational Therapists. Available at www.wfot.org

Kronenberg, F., Simo-Algado, S. & Pollard, N. (Eds.) (2005). *Occupational therapy without borders: learning from the sprit of survivors.* Edinburgh: Elsevier Churchill Livingstone.

Makgoba, M.W. (1999). *African renaissance.* Cape Town: Mafube Publishing and Tafelberg Publishers.

Marks, D. (1999). *Disability: Controversial debates and psychosocial perspectives.* London: Routledge.

Mayers, P., Alperstein, M., Duncan, M., Olckers, L. & Gibbs, T. (2005). Not another multi-professional course: nuts and bolts of designing a transformed curriculum for multi-professional learning. Part 2. *Medical Teacher (in press)*

Max-Neef, M. (1991). *Human Scale Development.* London: The Apex Press.

Ministry of Education (MoE) (1997). *Education White Paper 3: A Programme for the Transformation of Higher Education. General Notice 1196 of 1997.* Pretoria: Ministry of Education.

Ministry of Education (MoE) (2001). *National Plan for Higher Education in South Africa.* Pretoria: Ministry of Education.

Moore, R. & Lewis, K. (2004). Curriculum responsiveness: The implications for curriculum management. In H. Griesel (Ed.), *Curriculum responsiveness: case studies in higher education*. Pretoria: South African Vice-Chancellors' Association, pp. 39–56.

NCHE (National Commission on Higher Education) (1996). *Discussion Document: A Framework for Transformation*. Pretoria: Human Sciences Research Council.

National Qualifications Framework (NQF) (1997) Education White Paper 3. A programme for the transformation of higher education. *Government Gazette*, *386*(18207), 48–73.

Ntuli, P.P. (1999). The missing link between culture and education: are we still chasing gods that are not our own? In M.W. Makgoba (Ed.), *African Renaissance*. Sandton, Johannesburg: Mafube Publishing and Tafelberg Publishers, pp. 184–199.

Shutte, A. (1993). *Philosophy for Africa*. Cape Town: University of Cape Town Press.

South African Universities Vice-Chancellors' Association (SAUVCA) (1999). *Facilitatory handbook on the interim registration of whole university qualifications by June 2000*. Sunnyside, Pretoria: SAUVCA.

UN (1994). *The standard rules on the equalization of opportunities for persons with disabilities*. New York: United Nations Department of Public Information.

UNESCO (1998). *World declaration on higher education in the twenty-first century: vision and action*. Retrieved 22 August, 2005, from http://www.unesco.org/eduprog/wche/declaration_eng.htm

wa Thionga, N. (1990). *Decolonising the mind*. London: Heinemann.

Watson, R. & Swartz, L. (Eds.) (2004). *Transformation through occupation*. London: Whurr.

Whiteford, G. & Wright-St Clair, V. (Eds.) (2005). *Occupation and practice in context*. Sydney: Churchill Livingstone Elsevier.

Wilcock, A.A. (1998). *An occupational perspective of health*. Thorofare, NJ: Slack.

Wilcock, A. & Hocking, C. (2004). Occupation, population health and policy development. In M. Molineux (Ed.), *Occupation for occupational therapists*. Oxford: Blackwell Publishing, pp. 219–230.

World Health Organization (1978). *Declaration of Alma-Ata*. Geneva: World Health Organization. Available at http://www.who.int/hpr/archive/docs/almaata.html

World Health Organization (1986) *Ottawa Charter*. Geneva: World Health Organization. Available at http://www.who.int/hpr/archives/docs/ottawal

World Health Organization (2001). *International Classification of Functioning, Disability and Health*. Geneva: World Health Organization. Available at http://www.who.int/icidh

Zwarenstein, M., Reeves, S., Barr, H., et al. (2002). *Interprofessional education: effects on professional practice and health care outcomes (Cochrane review)*. Oxford: The Cochrane Library, Issue 3, 2002 Update Software.

3 Reflecting on Contexts of Service Learning

ROBIN JOUBERT, ROSHAN GALVAAN, THERESA LORENZO and ELELWANI RAMUGONDO

OBJECTIVES

This chapter discusses:

- the role that history plays in shaping professional education
- different contexts within which practice learning may occur
- the complexities of practice with individuals, groups and populations.

HISTORICAL ORIGINS

Occupational therapy in South Africa was 'born' about 1945, sandwiched between a strong post-colonial influence and the birth of apartheid, the child of the Nationalist Government that came into power in 1948. Van Staaden (1998) maintains that the philosophy of Western imperialism and the colonial strategies of government depicted 'the dark world other' as the savage opposite of the civilized Western citizen. In this way, it both homogenized the 'other' and simultaneously separated the 'other' into distinct groups, tribes or categories from the colonizer. This system of separation continued into the apartheid era and resulted in a serious disregard for the existing indigenous knowledge of the black ethnic people of South Africa.

It is important to reflect on the possible motives of Western imperialism in depicting 'the other', against the notion of 'the European'. In addition to distinguishing 'other' groups and separating these from Europeans, the Apartheid State expected different racial groups to have unequal status. Racial categorizations of 'white', 'coloured', 'Indian' and 'black' were needed to maintain control, with the term 'white' aimed at depicting a superior social status based only on physical appearance (Biko, 1978). This myth maintained economic gain and preserved white supremacy. To address current inequalities, and

Practice and Service Learning in Occupational Therapy. Edited by Theresa Lorenzo, Madeleine Duncan, Helen Buchanan, Auldeen Alsop
© 2006 John Wiley & Sons Ltd

the continuing disregard of indigenous knowledge systems, we have to challenge past and current myths, assumptions and biases about ourselves and others.

Occupational therapy in South Africa was parented largely by fathers who were European doctors and psychiatrists, and mothers who were mostly British occupational therapists. Control over the content of the curriculum was wielded by the conservative South African Medical and Dental Council, which was, for the most part, administered by white English- and Afrikaans-speaking doctors and psychiatrists (Davy, 2003). Thus, the powerful medical model influenced the development of occupational therapy. Whilst occupational therapy as a profession may have broken away from that control in recent years, it is important to bear in mind that medical science still holds a dominant influence on the profession. Wilcock (1998) maintains that the values of medical sciences are so integral to the post-industrial culture's thinking, it is difficult for those brought up in such a society to perceive health other than from a medical science perspective. This, and dominant Western philosophical world-views, have provided the background to contemporary curriculum discourses.

The South African occupational therapy curriculum was almost entirely based on Western Eurocentric ideological foundations. In addition, therapists selected for training in the early days were mostly white, English-speaking, upper middle-class, Judaeo-Christian females. It is difficult to imagine how such a group, however well-meaning, could have adequately served the majority of this country's people, who were mostly of African origin or belonged to one of the other marginalized groups such as 'coloured' and Asian people. The profile of occupational therapy graduates in South Africa has been changing over the years, with a growing number of the formerly marginalized groups being represented in their numbers. It cannot be assumed, however, that the Western Eurocentric ideological foundations, on which the South African occupational therapy curriculum was initially based, have shifted.

Changes are beginning to occur in the way in which occupational therapy departments approach teaching and learning. Non-traditional students (those formerly excluded from occupational therapy training) have generally had to adjust to the prevailing environment and the culture of departments, meeting expectations based on years of experience with young white middle-class females. Teaching departments are attempting to find ways to integrate appreciation and respect for student diversity into the curriculum and its educational strategies, and to benefit from the insights, perspectives and cultural knowledge that non-traditional student populations can offer.

A transformed curriculum, according to Marchesani and Adams (1995), goes beyond including exceptional individuals at the periphery of an otherwise unaltered curriculum. Instead, it is characterized by efforts to analyse and understand the reasons for and conditions of exclusion for non-mainstream groups. Differences in culture, gender and ability are no longer viewed in relation to the dominant ideas and contributions of those that have traditionally set standards and defined norms of participation.

It is thus necessary to explore and put in place curricula with a philosophy that transcends and may even replace contemporary ones (Slattery, 1995). Extending an occupational therapy service to communities who have been subjected to social ills, such as poverty, discrimination, marginalization and underdevelopment, necessitates 'a reinterpretation of the profession's orientation' (Watson, 2004).

HOW THE PAST INFLUENCES THE PRESENT AND FUTURE

Opportunities are provided throughout the practice education curriculum for students to gain first-hand experience of contexts where occupational therapy has to adapt to and reflect the needs of marginalized people, whilst being appropriately guided, supported and supervised by qualified occupational therapists and others working in the field. Objectives for each year of study ensure the progressive integration of theoretical constructs with exposure to practice in different, and often challenging situations. A variety of challenges and growth experiences are offered, representing the scope of the profession and different service/practice settings. These include exposure to physical and mental healthcare services, education, social and community development, work, vocational rehabilitation and economic empowerment situations.

The acquisition of the necessary competencies to work within communities is contingent on an understanding of, and engagement with, the historical and socio-political circumstances of each context. This requires the development of a political literacy and a strong sense of social justice and responsibility, particularly when students are exposed to socio-political circumstances that impact on the health and wellness of individuals, groups and communities with which they might work (Duncan, Buchanan & Lorenzo, 2005).

A holistic approach to, and an understanding of, all people irrespective of their health status is indicated if occupational therapy is to embrace more fully its potential role as a change agent in society. If occupational therapy curricula transform in a way that reflect an appreciation and respect for student diversity, and the vast indigenous knowledge systems in the country, current students will be the pioneers of new interpretations of practice in the future. The capacity to challenge existing paradigms and to identify potential niche domains for occupational therapy in the 'brave new world' will demand practitioners who can 'think outside the box'. They will be inspired to work together with their clients and colleagues in a partnership relationship of mutual respect, shared responsibility and cooperation. Students will learn to make decisions within the context of historical, social, economic, political, cultural and scientific information.

The principles from a range of current and evolving occupational therapy practice models will guide education and service depending on context and client needs. For example, in some contexts the primary healthcare approach and community-based rehabilitation will direct the practice. Students will acquire the ability to contribute to the health and well-being of individuals and their supporters (such as families, caregivers, employers) as well as groups and communities through occupation as means and as an end. New graduates should be able to provide comprehensive (promotive, preventative, curative and rehabilitative) occupational therapy services, either directly (hands on) or indirectly (through consulting), and to identify the need for referral and consultation.

CONTEXTUAL ISSUES IMPACTING ON SERVICE LEARNING

In an attempt to illustrate the different contexts to which students may be exposed, and within which they may now work during their undergraduate education, three scenarios are described. They offer insights into service learning experiences in different social contexts, first with an individual, then with a group and lastly with a population. The first narrative explores an individual case story about 'Khulu' who lives in a rural area. The second narrative describes a group experience in a peri-urban area known as Lavender Hill.[1] Lastly, the South African Christian Leadership Assembly (SACLA) health project illustrates how students can learn from a population approach to occupational therapy practice in informal settlements.

CONTEXT ONE: AN OCCUPATIONAL THERAPIST'S EXPERIENCE IN A RURAL AREA

Khulu's Story[2]

Every Thursday morning during the term, I join a multi-disciplinary group of students at the Amaroela first-aid centre in the beautiful Acacia Valley. This provides the students with the opportunity to engage in a service learning experience in a semi-rural setting, during which they work in partnership with the mothers or caregivers of children with disabilities, the children themselves and the community health workers. Although it is tarred, the route to the first-aid station is an extremely steep and treacherously winding road of approximately 6 kilometres. I travelled in my own car and the students travelled by taxi mini-bus.

[1] Actual name used with permission.
[2] All names in this story are fictitious.

On several occasions during this trip I passed a most extraordinary sight: a severely disabled man, pulling himself up this steep, winding road by his hands while sitting on a skateboard! The students said they had seen him begging in a shopping mall in the suburb of Industria, some 20 kilometres away. Wanting to investigate further I phoned Sipho, a community rehabilitation facilitator in this area, who set up an interview with the man in question.

One hot and humid, mid-summer morning, when the sun is close to its hottest, Sipho and I parked the vehicle halfway up the steep tarred road and commenced on foot down some 300 meters of very steep, winding and slippery gravel pathway. On the way we passed several homesteads, typical of the area, some traditional mud, wood and thatched rondavels,[3] others a variety of umjondolo[4] type homes. Each had its human residents who waved and greeted us as we passed and the usual contingent of skinny, aggressive dogs, clucking hens and gregarious goats nibbling at the surrounding vegetation.

Finally, we reached the last homestead at the end of this path. On enquiry, a middle-aged lady pointed to a small, corrugated iron-roofed house. Arriving at the open door of this home we were greeted by a middle-aged man with a very friendly smile, his name was Khulu.

There was a single bed with a dilapidated mattress upon which he lay, a ragged blanket covering his legs and a small cupboard next to the bed. The sun beat down relentlessly on the corrugated iron walls and roof and I felt overwhelmed by the heat before even commencing the interview.

Khulu was born in the district approximately 38 years ago. When he was a small boy, his parents sent him to Umkomaas to assist in looking after the cattle of a man who lived there. He was not a relative of the family, but it appears the family was poor and in this way the owner of the cattle provided food for the mouth they could not feed. Khulu never went to school and when he was approximately 9 or 10 years old, his problem started.

He informed us that the cause of his impairments was witchcraft. There was no illness or accident. He tells a story about a fight he had with some young boys and a Ford bantam bakkie.[5] It was after this he became paralysed, implying that the boys had obtained the services of an umthakathi.[6] He was sent to hospital where he appears to have had some physiotherapy. On discharge he never saw his parents again and returned to live with his brother and sister-in-law. She is a friendly and caring lady who joined us during the interview.

---

[3] Rondavel is the term used for the round tribal huts with conical thatched or tin roofs typical of this area.

[4] Umjondolo is the vernacular name given to houses built in informal settlements, which are often very creatively made using whatever materials the builder can obtain. They are usually vulnerable to bad weather and are a sign of extreme poverty.

[5] A 'bakkie' is a small lorry.

[6] Known as umthakathi, this was probably a form of 'day sorcery' that occurs in situations rife with competition and rivalry in which a sorcerer is consulted, who then administers various noxious potions, 'ukudlise', which are added to the victim's food, or harmful substances that are placed along the victim's path (Ngubane, 1977, p. 35). The umthakathi (sorcerer or wizard) is considered an enemy of society because they use their powers for magic and antisocial reasons (Krige, 1965, p. 321).

She feeds him. He has a disability grant and sometimes he pays her. There was a tin plate with a half-eaten sandwich on the cupboard next to his bed.

Apparently, some years ago, a man in Hilly village saw Khulu pulling himself along the road without any form of assistive device and gave him a skateboard. This was the beginning of a much more independent lifestyle. His sister-in-law confirms that he gets himself up the winding path I described earlier completely independently, using his sound right arm and semi-paralysed left arm. He also pulls himself up the rest of the steep, tarred section of the road for about 3 kilometres until he reaches a tavern at the top. There he catches a taxi mini-bus into Hilly village and from there to Industria some 15 kilometres further. Once there, Khulu goes to the shopping mall where he begs. He spends anything from a week to two weeks living there where he has many friends and spends a lot of time socializing and having a good time. He sleeps in covered parking lots or alleys where he is protected from the rain and makes enough money from begging to buy food and drinks, which he shares with his friends. He smiled and laughed constantly when reciting this part of his story. He returns 'home' periodically to rest himself for the next trip.

Finally, we said farewell and so began the walk up the steep, winding and slippery gravel path to our vehicle. As I puffed and sweated up this difficult incline, using both my legs and occasionally, when I slipped, also my arms, I wondered in utter amazement how this intrepid man managed to do the same with the type of impairments I had observed in my visual assessment of his limbs. It revealed the clash between Western cosmology and African cosmology, that is, my immediate seeking for a diagnosis and my hesitancy in accepting his story of umthakathi.

From this account, several questions and issues emerge:

- If Khulu had received occupational therapy in the early 1970s when he became paralysed, assessment and subsequent interventions at the time might have prevented some of his contractures. But it is reasonably predictable that the conventional treatment of the day would have been applied, i.e. provision of a wheelchair, possibly some splints for his hands and provision of an 'acceptable' income-generating activity, such as shoe repairing or leatherwork to do at home had his hand-function been improved. Worse still, he might have been sent to an institution such as a Cheshire Home. This would have robbed him of his current level of independence and control over his life and isolated him from the social opportunities and quality of life that his current existence provides.
- Knowledge of, and respect for, those aspects of the African lifestyle, value systems and cosmology are essential components in assessing needs and bringing about meaningful rehabilitation to the many Khulus we meet in our daily work.

- Could it be that that very African world-view which, unimpeded by the cynicism of our Western views and values, gave Khulu the extra-ordinary 'guts' to achieve what he has achieved today?
- What competencies would we need to assess in a student who would have facilitated Khulu on his journey to where he is today?
- Is begging an occupation?

CONTEXT TWO: AN OCCUPATIONAL THERAPIST'S EXPERIENCE IN A PERI-URBAN COMMUNITY MARKED WITH POVERTY AND VIOLENCE

The Facing Up Project

Facing Up is a development project that was initiated in 1999 by Galvaan (Galvaan, 2004). Facing Up attempts to interpret occupational science, health promotion, social action and social change theories and apply this to occupational therapy practice. It aims to contribute to community develop-ment and social change through comprehensive occupational therapy health promotion services. These services are offered to learners at mainstream primary schools in Lavender Hill, Cape Town. The services were initiated based on interpretations of the experiences of young adolescents in their lived environments, experiences that were perceived as placing their health at risk (Galvaan, 2004).

It is significant to note that despite the ten years of South Africa's libera-tion, Lavender Hill is one of the many communities that continues to reflect the segregated living spaces that were typical of the apartheid government's Group Areas Act. This is significant because much of the present occupational therapy programme is driven by the need to deal with this legacy. The primary schools had not had any occupational therapy services before the first, final (fourth) year, occupational therapy students from the University of Cape Town were placed there for service learning in March 2000. The occupational therapy students are now engaging with the learners at the mainstream primary school for an average of eight weeks. For many occupational therapy students, this is their first experience in a predominantly coloured community and in a role-emerging occupational therapy service setting.

Facing Up runs groups facilitated either by an occupational therapist or by occupational therapy students aimed at enabling agency in learners through creating opportunities to change the learners' occupational repertoires. During the group process learners develop their skills and divert their atten-tion from harmful occupations. Each year a new cohort of learners is selected to participate in these occupational therapy services. The nine boys recruited this year have participated in the programme for about three months. The boys are aged between 10 and 12 years and are in grade six. The group meets twice weekly, when fourth-year occupational therapy students are placed at the school, and once a week at other times, when the group is facilitated by a university practice educator.

Facing Up Boys' Group Story (as Told by the Group Facilitator)

Today is the third time that we meet since the last group of student's left. I describe my experience before and at the beginning of a group session. The sessions are conducted in a classroom allocated to Facing Up by the school. It is upstairs, next to a row of grade six classes.

The school bell has just sounded signalling the end of break. I sit in a circle of chairs, awaiting the boys' arrival. Many children excitedly pop in on their way to their classes, to say hello and enquire what the group will be doing. Slowly, the group participants arrive, ushering non-group members out as they enter. As we sit waiting for everyone, Anthony questions whether the previous students will be returning. I explain that students rotate between blocks (placements) and that a new pair of students will be placed there. Group members describe their dissatisfaction with the change and their wish to have consistent facilitators. Together we decide to flag this as an issue and explore how best to manage the changes. This 'pre-group' discussion allows members to begin to settle down and become conscious of the space that they are entering. Everyone arrives and we lock the room door to ensure that we are not disturbed by curious passers-by.

The group starts by members agreeing to work on their attentiveness and listening skills. I introduce charades as a warm-up activity. We divide into teams, which they name 'Baby Burns' and 'Dare Devils'. They then enact their chosen charade while the competing team attempts to correctly identify the scenario. The Dare Devils pretend to be robbing a drug merchant – the other group guessed that they were robbing a bank. The Baby Burns pretended to have found someone who had been shot in a drive-by shooting and were now helping this person after two people just walked past the man. I note that these scenarios are concerning since they reflect a part of the children's lived experiences or perhaps what is foremost on their minds. We briefly discuss the violent nature of these skits. The boys are attentive and enjoy being in control of the group content. We continue with a quiz/competition that encourages them to become more familiar with one another.

On another occasion, I arrived during an interval for the group and decided to spend some time observing children in the playground. I see Anthony walking around confidently and briskly, with broad shoulders. His shirt collar is up and he has an earphone hanging from his ear. He has a group of about five boys following him. On a few occasions he goes up to a group of three girls to flirt. In between this he is observed to beat up a few boys and swear profusely. The school bell rings and they enter the group room. As the boys enter, they ensure that their pant's zips are up and shirts tucked in. Anthony's shirt collar is down. We begin the group by reflecting on what the change in dress code means. The boys describe who has power on the school playground, with clear reference to Anthony's behaviour. This is the one place where he can be challenged and he expresses his dissatisfaction with this. The group is able to recognize how they idealize the gangsters' way of dressing and relating in their play and how they consciously decide to behave differently in the group. They consider how they would like to change what happens in the playground.

From this account, several questions emerge:

- How do we, as university practice educators, assist occupational therapy students to become familiar with the sociological nuances of a community and interpret these within the service setting?
- How do we instill the social and political commitment in students so that they assume a human rights and social justice approach to this work? This service setting does not have an established occupational prevention and promotion role for occupational therapists. Traditionally, occupational therapists would only see these children (learners) if they found themselves in places of safety (these are, homes for children and youth as a consequence of entering social welfare or juvenile justice system).
- How do we create appropriate opportunities for occupational engagement that are respectful of the communities where people live? Occupational therapy has a history of favouring (prejudicing) European, Western ways of behaving and relating to others. As occupational therapists attempting to create opportunities for change we have to ensure that we work on possible ignorance and the devaluing of different modes of engaging in occupations. Occupational therapy students face the challenge of promoting social change as they learn more about the people.

CONTEXT THREE: AN OCCUPATIONAL THERAPIST'S EXPERIENCE IN INFORMAL SETTLEMENTS

The SACLA Health Project's Community-based Rehabilitation Programme, Khayelitsha

The South African Christian Leadership Assembly (SACLA) Health Project is a non-governmental, primary healthcare organization that works in the disadvantaged communities of Khayelitsha and Nyanga. Parents of disabled children from these communities have been trained as community rehabilitation workers (CRWs) since 1987. The CRWs promote resilience of both disabled children and adults through providing rehabilitation, facilitating access to opportunities and mobilizing groups towards social inclusion.

In 1995, the SACLA Health Project initiated a partnership with the Division of Occupational Therapy of the University of Cape Town as a service, teaching and research affiliate. Given the political changes in the country, higher education institutions were faced with the need to change their curricula to ensure relevance in the education of future practitioners and policymakers. The Division of Occupational Therapy was no exception. Since then, occupational therapy students have been able to work with the CRWs in addressing population needs through various aspects of SACLA's work described briefly here. The centrality of accessible transport is illustrated as a critical factor in addressing poverty and disability in impoverished communities.

People from impoverished communities have struggled to gain daily access to economic and social resources because of long distances, inaccesible transport facilities and an overall poor level of service. Work opportunities are not close to where the majority of poor people live, so travel increases the financial burden. Few people are fortunate enough to own a private vehicle. Those who do, offer a service at a cost higher than public taxis, which are 16-seated mini-buses. In some situations, families have no option but to pay for the convenience and accessibility of private transport, especially in times of illness or emergencies.

The Dial-A-Ride Project was initiated as a pilot project of the Department of Transport in 1999 and 2000 as a result of lobbying from the Disability Rights Movement. It provided a limited accessible mini-bus service for disabled people who have difficulty in using existing public transport. Individuals were assessed for their mobility and ability to use public transport. If they were registered as a user, they had to phone in and book the service each time they needed it. Disabled People South Africa (DPSA) continues to campaign for accessible public transport as a strategy to equalize opportunities for development.

The OT students have been involved in different projects run by SACLA , which are briefly described here.

Community Rehabilitation Worker Education and Training

Students have the opportunity to participate in the continuous education programme of the CRWs as a means of gaining an understanding and appreciation of their role in community-based rehabilitation. The CRWs teach the students about community entry, Xhosa culture and beliefs related to disability. The students gain knowledge about life with a disabled child from home visits with the CRWs. They link with other organizations as part of developing a referral and support system between different levels of healthcare and other sectors. This has extended into an approach that addresses the needs of the wider community, with a particular focus on youth and employment opportunities for women.

Community Disability Entrepreneurship Programme (CoDEP)

The CRWs involved the students in doing participatory action research related to the social economic conditions of disabled adults, with a particular focus on the entrepreneurship development of women. The students ran lifeskills programmes to develop leadership skills in the groups. They were involved in facilitating access to resources and opportunities for skills development, such as organizing business skills training run by other Non-Government Organizations (NGOs). These interactions helped to develop a strong sense of a new identity as the groups participated enthusiastically in different opportunities to increase their productivity. One young woman was excited since she was now able to perm her hair, which made her feel more like her friends:

> I did not know what to expect from the workshops, but I wanted to learn how to make money and start a small business. So I was determined to go to the training workshops on catering organized by SACLA . . . I felt very proud when I received a certificate at the end of the course. I went around showing my neighbours what I had made and let them taste it. They were very surprised. I felt GREAT! I am singing and dancing now. Especially now that I'm cooking. I now offered that the women could work from my house to run a catering business until we found a space from the local council. I changed the front room of my house into an entertainment area where young people can come and play snooker and listen to music from the duke box. This helps keep the young ones off the streets. I also have a vending machine for chocolates and chips. In the afternoon and evening the room becomes a shebeen and I sell beer and cooked meals. We want SACLA to carry on with us so that even at home they can stop feeling sorry for us. They like saying 'don't do much, you are sick'. Other women need to know that there are opportunities for learning skills to run our own businesses.

Day Care Centre Development and Accessing Schooling

The occupational therapy students were involved with the CRWs in the day care centres for disabled children where they trained volunteers as carers. Their role was to assist the CRWs and carers to create opportunities for the disabled children to learn and play. In some situations, they helped the mothers manage situations of abuse that occurred in the family or community. Students were exposed to the tensions experienced by mothers of disabled children because of poor schooling and the struggle to cope. One mother shared how her child was sent home from school as the teachers said he was disrupting the class:

> Another problem that I have is that of my son who is mentally disabled. I cannot explain what I'm going through because of him. Even if I beat him he does not have any feelings for pain and he just laughs. I've taken him out of school because he beats others at school. When the teachers punish him, he laughs.

Masiphatisane Disability Forum: Advocacy and Awareness

An exploratory week-long workshop was facilitated by a change management and organizational development consultant involving the University of Cape Town, the DPSA, service providers and NGOs in the disability field and disabled people living in Khayelitsha, Nyanga and Gugulethu (three of the peri-urban areas of Cape Town in the Province of the Western Cape). Its purpose was to look at addressing disability issues in public health services and poverty initiatives at a community level. The Masiphatisane[7] Disability Forum was constituted to address the need for better coordination of services and strengthen support systems through the participation and self-representation of disabled people in decision-making processes. The Forum meets every second month to look at issues of disability related to service delivery, public awareness and advocacy, skills development and accessing resources and lobbying for accessible transport (Saunders, pers comm). Students were therefore able to participate in these forums as part of service learning. One woman identified the difference that community participation had made:

> Before I never talked about my disability, but now I'm talking. I'm even respected by the taxi drivers. It was difficult for me to get to the monthly workshops because the taxis did not stop for me. I usually arrived late. Now, the taxi will stop and wait until I am settled in because they know I'm their best customer.

Learning about Monitoring and Evaluation

The students gained first-hand experience of the importance of good information management systems and the value of monitoring and evaluation from their involvement in all the different projects. The opportunity for students to learn monitoring is seen in the words of one of the women:

> I know that some of the women in the workshops have not been happy with the progress. They say that we are waiting for the goal of these workshops that we have been doing to see if what they do will make a difference . . . They feel that we need a way forward regarding our needs so that there can be more progress because there are still many women who are not working.

The following questions emerge:

- To what extent do training institutions value and recognize CRWs as learning facilitators and non-traditional clinicians from whom students can learn an enormous amount? Students had to shift their expectations as they learnt to work with the CRWs, mothers and dis-

---

[7] In Xhosa, this means 'holding together', which reveals the spirit of cooperation in a group. The initial workshops were coordinated by the SACLA Health Project to facilitate NGOs working in disability to begin working collaboratively with disabled peoples' organizations. After the first year, the chair for each workshop was rotated to build the capacity of disabled people in leadership and development.

abled people in a flexible and reflective manner. It provided a rich learning experience in how the different sectors need to coordinate their efforts if poverty alleviation and sustainable inclusive development is to be a reality for disabled people.

- How do occupational therapists engage in public health issues without losing their identity, and value the unique contribution that an occupation-focus can bring to poverty alleviation and development initiatives? The service learning experience reflects the need for public health policies and services to integrate disability issues rather than addressing them separately.
- How do occupational therapists address transport as a critical success factor for inclusion and participation?

REFLECTIVE THOUGHTS

These scenarios and emerging questions illustrate the complexity of cultural and contextual circumstances in meeting the needs of communities through individual, group and population approaches that frequently face occupational therapists where there are high levels of poverty. The competencies expected of students in each of these settings are very different to those expected in the traditional clinical and well-equipped confines of a hospital occupational therapy department. In addition, because of the cultural diversity of the South African population, students need to have an understanding and critical awareness of the need for sensitive adaptability and a respectful approach within such transcultural and transcontextual settings. The ability to be flexible and tolerant of differences in values and needs across both socio-economic and cultural groups is integral to being an effective occupational therapist.

Competence is a dynamic and multifaceted quality that is woven into and throughout the student's practice learning. Competence requires more than having an understanding of essential knowledge; it also requires clinical and interpersonal skills, problem solving, clinical reasoning and technical skills (Youngstrom, 1998) and a special type of professionalism embracing culturally-responsive attitudes and values. Practice learning opportunities offer real-life illustrations of classroom learning and provide students with the time for personal reflection; the development of professional practice competencies; and the consolidation of personal values and beliefs about the profession, the service and intersectoral liaison and collaboration.

This chapter has illustrated the importance and richness of service learning. It describes how students are challenged to move beyond their comfort zones to work in environments that build their capacity. Here they can see people in their own environments, speaking with their own voices. Students come to appreciate professional practice where hope is seen more clearly in the eyes and hearts of those served.

REFERENCES

Biko, S. (1978). I write what I like. In A. Stubbs (Ed.), *A selection of his writings*. Oxford: Heinemann.

Davy, J. (2003). *SAAOT: The first thirty years plus 1975 to 1995*. Pretoria: OTASA offices.

Duncan, M., Buchanan, H. & Lorenzo, T. (2005). Politics in occupational therapy education: a South African Perspective. In F. Kronenberg, S. Simo Algado & N. Pollard (Eds.), *Occupational Therapy without Borders – learning from the Spirit of Survivors*. Edinburgh: Elsevier, pp. 390–401.

Galvaan, R. (2004). Engaging with youth at work. In R. Watson & L. Swartz (Eds.), *Transformation through occupation*. London: Whurr, pp. 186–197.

Kinsella, E.A. (2001). Reflections on Reflective Practice. *Canadian Journal of Occupational Therapy*, 68(3), 195–199.

Krige, E.J. (1965). *The social system of the Zulus*. Pietermaritzburg: Shuter and Shooter.

Marchesani, L.S. & Adams, M. (1995). Dynamics of diversity in the teaching – learning process: a faculty development model for analysis and action. In M. Adams (Ed.), *Promoting diversity in college classrooms: innovative responses for the curriculum, faculty, and institutions*. San Francisco, CA: Jossey-Bass pp. 9–20.

Ngubane, H. (1977). *Body and mind in Zulu medicine: an ethnography of health and disease in Nyuswa-Zulu thought and practice*. London: Academic Press.

Slattery, P. (1995). *Curriculum development in the Postmodern Era*. New York: Garland.

Van Staaden, C. (1998). Using culture in African contexts. In P.H. Coetzee & A.P.J. Roux (Eds.), *Philosophy from Africa: A text with readings*. London: Thomson, Chapter 2.

Watson, R. (2004). New horizons in occupational therapy. In R. Watson & L. Swartz (Eds.), *Transformation through occupation*. London: Whurr, pp. 3–18.

Watson, R. & Swartz, L. (Eds.) (2004). *Transformation through occupation*. London: Whurr.

Wilcock, A. (1998). *An occupational perspective of health*. New Jersey: Slack.

Youngstrom, M.J. (1998). Evolving competence in the practitioner role. *American Journal of Occupational Therapy*, 52(9), 716–720.

4 A Quality Framework for Practice Education and Learning

MADELEINE DUNCAN and THERESA LORENZO

OBJECTIVES

This chapter discusses:

- the domains of practice education that need to be monitored and adapted to ensure optimal outcomes for all role-players
- the academic and logistical infrastructures that need to be available to support student learning in different contexts
- how accountability mechanisms promote ethical and evidence-based practice.

INTRODUCTION

Institutions providing education programmes face numerous ethical and logistical challenges in accessing suitable, well-supervised practice learning opportunities for undergraduate health professional students. The logistics of synchronizing academic, organizational, governmental, legal and community expectations; securing access to resources and budgets; aligning timetables and regulating student support structures (for example, transport and supervision) require efficient administration and explicit accountability mechanisms. Practice learning outcomes and expectations are usually negotiated based on the capacity of a particular learning site at a point in time and monitored in ways that comply with professional codes of ethics and service quality assurance indicators. Performance benchmarks need to be put in place in order to protect the persons with whom students work from adverse events resulting from their professional inexperience. The mounting influence of public and consumer demand for accountability by professional groups suggests that higher education institutions must pay particular attention to the ways in which the practice competence and service contributions of students are monitored (Curry,

Practice and Service Learning in Occupational Therapy. Edited by Theresa Lorenzo, Madeleine Duncan, Helen Buchanan, Auldeen Alsop
© 2006 John Wiley & Sons Ltd

1993). While the responsibility for monitoring client or community welfare and for ensuring high-quality services rests primarily with the supervising, registered health practitioner (Allen, Oke, McKinstry & Courtney, 2005), both the student and the person(s) with whom they work are also accountable for monitoring standards, rights and responsibilities.

This chapter considers a quality framework for practice education and practice learning. The interactions between the four key role-players: the university practice educator, the student, the site learning facilitator and the participants (individuals, groups or communities), who receive services in practice and service learning contexts, are addressed. Principles and methods for maintaining educational and professional standards are highlighted. The chapter includes examples of academic guidelines and infrastructures that bring coherence, accountability and structure to student learning, whilst promoting the development of professionalism and ethical behaviour.

A QUALITY FRAMEWORK

The quality framework proposed here represents the essential domains of practice education (see Figure 4.1). It depicts the relationship between various role-players, including their critical functions and roles, and identifies the focal points at which quality assurance needs to occur. The figure is dynamic and three-dimensional with the various dimensions, domains and role-players interacting in varying degrees depending on where, when, with whom, why and how the interaction is occurring.

In this framework a distinction is made between practice education and practice learning. The former refers to the curriculum that guides professional training. It draws on adult education principles and informs how professional concepts and methods are applied in the practice context. The latter refers to the process through which students become professionally competent by collaborating with individuals, groups or communities in assessing, defining and addressing their self-identified needs and aspirations using appropriate professional actions that are guided or monitored by a university practice educator or site learning facilitator.

CONTEXT

The preceding chapters have illustrated how international and national policies of governments and professional bodies influence or create the context in which practice education occurs. There is an interrelationship between these policies; the development of theory and practice that informs learning and promotes competence. Performance and assessment of students are guided by professional and academic standards.

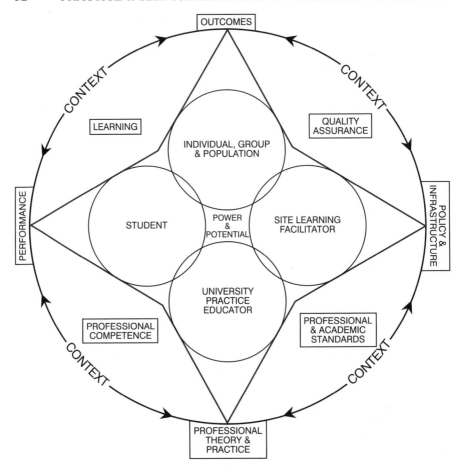

Figure 4.1 Dimensions of practice education in context

POTENTIAL

Situated at the centre of the quality framework (Figure 4.1), potential refers to the essential attribute of human functioning that makes it possible for individuals to develop through learning and, as a result, live more fully and authentically. The equalization of *power* and the development of *potential* is placed at the centre of the interaction between the four role-players to highlight the imperative of mutual accountability to negotiated rights, roles and responsibilities in the practice education context. Potential points to the innate capacity of humans to become more than they are able to conceptualize at a particular stage in their development. In the context of practice education, a focus on potential ensures that professional values, such as dignity, prudence, justice, autonomy and cooperation, guide the actions of students, educators and practitioners. Whilst professional values guide practice, their impact should also be evident in the practice education curriculum. The philosophy of the profession needs to be experienced by the students during professional socialization. Potential unfolds in enabling environments. The quality framework proposed here seeks to create such an environment. Belief in the potential of individuals (including students) and communities to act responsibly and creatively on their environment opens up possibilities for positive change, development and the actualization of capacity through self-directed learning, to occur. Potential and power operate in creative tension during the learning process. People who experience, understand and act on their world in enquiring, critical ways do so because they feel secure, have access to knowledge and are able to exert their power to effect change in their spheres of influence (Aleksiuk, 1996). The quality framework describes the elements of practice education that advance a sense of security, promote the exchange of information, and facilitate the co-construction of knowledge and the negotiation of power in order to achieve desired outcomes for all role-players.

POWER

Power warrants overt consideration in a quality framework for practice education because it is present in the multiple and heterogeneous social relations that occur during professional socialization. Role-players in practice education are subject to the same social dynamics that operate in society. Social stratification and position implicitly assigns certain roles and positions to individuals, groups and communities based on assumptions about their material resources (wealth), power and prestige. Roles and position are not merely convenient classifications; they have intrinsic significance in the interactions between students, educators and the people with whom they work. The amount of influence that people are able to exercise over their experiences of practice and service learning, whether as educators, students or consumers, impacts on the quality of learning and development that occurs. A fundamental premise of practice education is, however, the empowerment of participating role-players to strive towards the actualization of their capacity and potential. Practice education is ultimately concerned with attaining generative power.

According to Nelson and Wright (1995), power is a description of a relation, not a 'thing' that people 'have'. Aleksiuk (1996) describes personal power as the perception by the individual that they have the ability to take effective action, and social power as the ability to take effective action through others. Nelson and Wright (1995) have identified three levels of power related to the process of empowerment. Firstly, 'power to' is 'power [that] grows infinitely if you work at it and [where] the growth of one person does not negatively affect another' (Nelson & Wright, 1995, p. 11). Generative power stimulates activity in all role-players to realize those capacities and knowledge that can be developed collectively or in ways that promote positive outcomes for everyone. The personal level involves developing confidence and abilities including undoing the effects of internalized oppression. The second level of power encompasses 'power over'. This involves gaining access to political decision making, often in public forums. Nelson and Wright caution that what may appear as a 'bottom-up' approach to power may in fact perpetuate and disguise continued top-down attitudes. At this level, power is seen as a 'thing' of which there is a finite amount in a closed system. Power relations in public forums are potentially coercive and centred in institutions of governance. 'Power over' often spills over into other structures of society. At the second level, power is gained at the expense of others. According to Chambers (1995), the professional and institutional authority of researchers and developers characterizes them as 'holding the stick' – a symbol for having knowledge and the right to speak. This can be extended to professionals and service providers and, by implication, health professional students who are working with individuals, groups and communities.

The third level of power is identified as 'decentralized power'. This level refers to power that is not possessed or exercised by a person or institution who may be conceived as a 'powerful' entity (Nelson & Wright, 1995). Decentralized power is subjectless and an apparatus consisting of social discourses, institutional cultures and a complex flow of events that moves power to the lowest denominator. This power interacts invisibly in a way that may only be apparent in hindsight as a system of networks is developed that are based on democratic values.

ROLE-PLAYERS

Irrespective of where practical professional learning occurs, it usually comprises interactions between some or all of the following four role-players. The terms may not be defined universally in the same way. The framework here draws on terminology commonly used in the South African context, although parallels can be drawn for other contexts. The roles are:

- The *university practice educator*, who monitors academic expectations and standards, promotes professional development and acts as performance assessor
- The *student*, placed at the site for the purpose of learning how to practise their chosen profession
- The *learning facilitator*, who may be a *health therapist* or *health worker* (for example, *home-based carer* or *community rehabilitation worker*). The learning facilitator is ultimately responsible for the

welfare of the persons with whom the student works. They ensure a functional on-site infrastructure and monitor ethical, efficient and effective service provision. The learning facilitator may mediate between the student and the individual, group or community by acting as a translator as well as a guide for appropriate cultural behaviour through role modelling and coaching

- The *individual, group or community*, who are either partners in the process of joint learning and development, or those who require specialist professional intervention in identified domains of health or social need.

Figure 4.1 depicts the interaction between these four role-players in a practice learning context as well as the dimensions of practice education that require on-site regulation and support in order to effect positive outcomes.

INDIVIDUALS, GROUPS AND COMMUNITIES

The voice of individuals, groups and communities has often been absent in practice learning in South Africa (Lorenzo & Friedlander, 2005). The communities with whom students work have, however, become increasingly aware of their rights. The social model of disability has brought the rights of disabled people to the fore in the relationship between service providers and users. Whilst mechanisms, such as disability and patient rights charters and public service quality assurance guidelines, promote the interests of the public, they may not necessarily be used to guide practice education. The danger of exploitation therefore exists as communities become integrally involved in teaching students. A number of questions must be addressed in order to promote mutual benefit. Whose agenda drives the relationship between the higher education institution and the community? Who decides what constitutes 'service', 'learning' and 'need'? How may the process of integrating intentions with actions be done so that a just relationship between all role-players can be ensured? Are universities as concerned about the integrity of their actions in dealing with communities as they are about the academic intentions of placing students in the field? These and other questions deserve careful consideration by all role-players at regular intervals to promote transparent, sustainable and progressive partnerships.

UNIVERSITY PRACTICE EDUCATOR

The work pressures of learning facilitators makes the additional function of monitoring a student's practice learning particularly difficult, especially if the amount of time dedicated to assessment is taken into account. University faculty staff members may therefore act as part-time university practice educators for a designated number of students. Due to the low number of faculty staff and the large number of students, the university may also appoint occupational therapists such as private practitioners, post-graduate students or temporarily unemployed clinicians as sessional university practice educators.

University practice educators are responsible for monitoring the professional development (theoretical, methodological and philosophical) of the student and for ensuring that academic standards are achieved and maintained by:

- negotiating entry for students to the organization or learning site
- identifying appropriate learning objectives
- ensuring opportunities and academic expectations within a particular site at a point in time
- assisting the student to formulate personal learning goals against site-specific learning objectives (see Table 4.1)
- performing summative and formative assessment, monitoring learning needs and discerning the progress of students
- assisting the student to translate theory into practice and use critical incidents to identify theory in action
- ensuring that the organization, community and/or clients are satisfied with the liaison with the university and with the output and attitudes of students. This helps to maintain a vigilant, ethical stance to liaison between the university and the learning site.

The widening scope of professional practice suggests that practice learning and service opportunities must be identified within the various contexts where students are placed on an ongoing basis. In the past, universities were able to prescribe the curriculum requirements for practice learning commensurate with students' stage of learning because of relatively stable, well-resourced practice settings. Prescriptive requirements included, for example, the type and number of individual cases and written requirements, such as number of case studies or daily reports and assessment procedures.

A prescriptive approach to learning requirements is considered counter-productive because it limits access to potential learning opportunities and restricts the creativity of students, university practice educators and learning facilitators in response to a constantly changing environment. A responsive, flexible approach ensures that learning expectations and academic requirements can be adapted to the needs of students and their stage of development with due consideration of prevailing conditions and available resources at a particular site. The emergent practice learning and, if indicated, service opportunities at a learning site at a particular point in time may, therefore, be informally negotiated and contracted between the university practice educator and the relevant learning facilitator.

Negotiation tends to occur prior to the start of each placement in order to develop a flexible, practical yet academically well-grounded curriculum pitched at the appropriate level for the student's stage of professional development. Whilst this approach to the practice learning curriculum may appear to be labour intensive, it ensures that:

- all parties gain from the exchange because the expectations and anticipated outcomes of the university and practice learning site are based on mutual agreement
- the practice learning curriculum is responsive to current client and site needs and goals
- a wider range of practice learning opportunities may be developed.

Table 4.1 provides an example of a practice learning contract between an institution of higher education (in this instance the UCT Division of Occupational Therapy) and a practice learning site/organization. It consists of four sections:

1. What the student will do for the site/organization, that is, what the constituency will gain from the student's outputs during a specified period of time.
2. The learning outcomes that may be achieved by the student, that is, what potential shifts in knowledge, skills and attitudes may have occurred by the end of the practice learning experience at the site.
3. The negotiated academic expectations, that is, what the student can reasonably deliver for academic accreditation and formative and summative assessment purposes.
4. What the site/organization will make available to the student, that is, what the constituency will contribute to enhance the outcomes of the practice learning partnership.

THE STUDENT

As an adult learner, the student is responsible for their professional development and learning through goal directed actions aimed at achieving both personal change and positive outcomes for the persons with whom they work. The student provides evidence of progress through performance and competence assessments that are monitored by the university practice educator and learning facilitator. Students are expected to conduct themselves and undertake negotiated tasks in a manner commensurate with their developing professional status, respecting the rights of individuals and cooperating with practice educators, learning facilitators and other role-players for the attainment of mutually agreed learning outcomes.

Health professional students in South Africa must register with the Health Professions Council of South Africa (HPCSA) at the start of their undergraduate education. This may be different from other countries. In the UK, for example, students complete their professional education and then apply to the UK Health Professions Council for Registration. At the University of Cape

Table 4.1 Example of a practice learning contract (based on negotiations between UCT Division of Occupational Therapy and a non-governmental organization offering home-based care to disabled persons in informal settlements)

Services offered by student(s) (What the student(s) will **do** for the organization, i.e. what the organization and its clients will **gain** from accommodating students for professional training.)	Learning outcomes (Potential knowledges, skills and attitudes that the student may **gain** by working at this site.)	Academic expectations (What the student will **do** for academic accreditation during nine weeks full-time placement at this site.)	Infrastructure offered by organization (What the organization will make available to student(s) to promote an optimal partnership.)
Students will: • contribute to the skills development of home-based carers (HBCs) in mutually identified training needs • promote implementation of the National Policy on Home-Based Care (Dept. of Health, 2003) as well as other relevant disability and rehabilitation policies • expand the existing data base of the organization with particular reference to participants' impairment, activity limitations and participation restrictions using appropriate data gathering tools • contribute to health promotion of the clients and caregivers through purposeful and meaningful occupation and other profession-specific techniques and methods	Students will gain: • resilience in coping with the emotional impact of witnessing extreme poverty, the effects of AIDS/HIV and other adverse social conditions • the ability to identify and prioritize occupational therapy contributions in under-resourced contexts • knowledge of indigenous health beliefs and cultural practices • skills in negotiating priorities for action in collaboration with key role-players in a non-governmental organization • community entry skills using primary health care principles • knowledge of the district health system • networking and resource management skills • ability to transfer professional knowledge and skills through adult education methods	Students will: • run **two** workshops with +/− 12 HBCs on mutually agreed topics. • transfer specific skills to individual HBCs based on the emerging needs of individual clients, e.g. transfers, assistive technology, splints, mental health • develop an appropriate functional assessment form to complement the data gathered through the existing HBC Report. • facilitate **one** event that promotes integration, networking and inclusivity amongst clients, their carers, HBCs and the community. • have enabled a positive shift in the autonomy and occupational performance of one individual case-study client in collaboration with the client, their HBC, and other significant role-players • write **one** individual case report • complete **two** group reports of workshops done with HBCs • complete **one** programme report **or** mindmap on the developing OT service • start a resource and network database based on a survey of resources and services	The organization will: • provide a secure, dedicated working space at the NGO head office • negotiate roles and responsibilities with HBCs who students will accompany into the community • transport to and from clients • allow professional staff and HBCs to attend in-service training workshops and/or student performance assessment events • release negotiated financial and other resources to support the work of students

Town Division of Occupational Therapy, each first-year class makes a collective public declaration called a Statement of Intent specifying their commitment to professionalism and good practice prior to entering practice learning. The Statement of Intent is used as an accountability indicator for professionalism in the field throughout the practice education curriculum.

As in many countries, health professional students in South Africa are required to abide by and/or contribute to the implementation of professional rules and regulations, for example, the Rules of Conduct of the HPCSA (n.d.) and a professional code of ethics. Professionalism may be monitored by including professional behaviour and conduct as an explicitly assessed competence. Critical instances of unprofessional behaviour should be factually documented and due process followed in alerting the student to the consequences of unprofessional behaviour. Due process may entail clarifying with the student their perspective on the critical incident(s). Remedial and/or alternative action may be negotiated. Depending on the severity of the critical incident or repeated violations of professional codes of conduct, the student may be given a written warning based on professional regulations and local disciplinary policies and procedures and, as an ultimate measure, be required to withdraw from the professional course with due consideration of legal and other implications.

THE LEARNING FACILITATOR

The ideal practice learning environment includes a qualified health practitioner who ensures that the on-site infrastructure supports student learning. The practitioner should also have enough time to role model professionalism, demonstrate specialist skills and explain the praxis between theory and practice. Learning facilitators, committed to the advancement of their profession by educating future practitioners, do not get paid for the time they spend with students. Additionally, they may not have the academic expertise to assess student competencies so this falls to the university practice educator. Some countries have a more formal system for educating and accrediting learning facilitators so that they can take full responsibility for promoting and evaluating the student's learning.

PROFESSIONAL COMPETENCE

Competence is a dynamic and multifaceted quality that is woven into and throughout the student's practice learning. Competence requires more than having an understanding of essential knowledge; it also requires clinical and interpersonal skills, problem solving, clinical reasoning and technical skills (Youngstrom, 1998) and a special type of professionalism embracing culturally-responsive attitudes and values. Practice learning opportunities offer real-life illustrations of classroom learning and provide students with the time for personal reflection, the development of professional practice competencies and the consolidation of personal values and beliefs about the profession, the service and intersectoral liaison and collaboration.

PROFESSIONAL AND ACADEMIC STANDARDS

Professional and academic standards refer to monitoring student performance against WFOT minimum standards, regulating outcomes of practice education according to stage of training, as well as ensuring that professional values are instilled through appropriate role modelling. An analysis of students' reflective journals and verbal accounts during supervision may reveal instances of apparent professional misconduct amongst learning facilitators. Students themselves may deviate from standards of professional behaviour. University practice educators should encourage both site learning facilitators and students to process what they have witnessed using ethical reasoning, drawing explicitly on known facts. In certain instances the apparent misconduct may need to be reported through the appropriate channels. The following are examples of behaviour that may be deemed as unprofessional, as putting public interests at risk, or as misconduct warranting disciplinary action:

- behaviour that brings the profession into disrepute
- conduct that is prejudicial to the best interests of clients and communities
- theft, deliberate falsification of facts or records as in lying, cheating, fraud or attempting to defame colleagues and/or clients
- breaches of confidentiality, misuse of confidential material relating to clients or service providers
- assault and violent behaviour or serious acts of insubordination
- conduct that demonstrates inappropriate emotional involvement with a co-worker or client
- unprofessional dress that may be culturally offensive (for example, transparent clothing revealing underwear, exposed midriff with belly piercing)
- serious negligence that causes unacceptable loss, damage or that puts others at risk
- misuse of equipment, materials or deliberate damage to property
- incapacity to work due to substance abuse, mental illness, or inappropriate substance use on site such as smoking in non-smoking zones
- absenteeism without permission or failing to follow due process (i.e. notification in writing) in event of unavoidable absenteeism
- persistent lack of motivation such as poor time use, failure to hand reports in on time, arriving late and leaving early; avoiding duties; frequent absenteeism.

Whistleblowing refers to the process of making perceived unethical behaviour of colleagues known to relevant authorities following the due process of either reporting anonymously or by submitting a written complaint. Students should be equipped with the necessary knowledge about whistleblowing procedures within the public service sector and their respective professional boards. The ethical responsibility of maintaining professional and academic standards needs to be a shared effort.

LEARNING

The range of clients and practice domains have broadened significantly since the mid-1990s, firstly, due to necessity because the available education facilities in the public health and education sectors have dwindled; secondly, due to the imperative of intersectoral collaboration within the primary healthcare approach (Watson & Swartz, 2004); and thirdly, due to international trends within the profession itself (Kronenberg, Algado & Pollard, 2005). Students may gain practical experience across five possible practice domains in a wide variety of practice settings. Table 4.2 captures some examples of practice learning sites that are aligned with five domains of occupational therapy practice emanating from a primary healthcare interpretation of the profession's role and scope in a developing country.

Evaluation is a means of understanding the effects of the service learning environment on the students' learning. It implies collecting information about university practice educators and the contexts in which student education takes place, interpreting the information and making judgements about the actions to be taken to improve practice (Ramsden, 1992). Evaluation is an analytical quality assurance process that should be intrinsic to good teaching and practice education. Feedback from students about the performance of university practice educators and site learning facilitators promotes competence development in the specific roles. Likewise, feedback given sensitively on the service being provided at the site is a valuable accountability mechanism for increased efficiency and effectiveness.

The student should be invited to complete the evaluation prior to being given his or her mark for practice education and before performance evaluation is discussed. The student may elect to give the feedback directly to the relevant person on the last day of the practice or by using the form and submitting it to the relevant person via the Head of Division.

QUALITY ASSURANCE

Part of the responsibility of all health professionals is to ensure that clients receive quality care or 'best practice'. It has been suggested that occupational

Table 4.2 Examples of domains, sites and possible outcomes of practice learning

Practice domains	Examples of practice learning settings	Practice education in these domains will enable the student to learn about:
Employment equity and economic empowerment	Insurance and medico-legal industry; income-generating projects run by disabled or socially disadvantaged workers; work assessment and work hardening units; occupational health facilities in factories; mining and agricultural industry; supported employment agencies	Professional philosophy and values Clinical and population reasoning Indigenous human occupation Occupational science Occupational therapy for impairment, activity limitations and participation restrictions related to psychiatric disorders
Child and youth learning and development	Special schools; disabled children in mainstream schools; places of safety; post-acute convalescent children's homes; agencies dealing with children with special needs; organizations dealing with youth at-risk, such as street children; youth on parole from prison	Occupational therapy for impairment, activity limitations and participation restrictions related to medical, surgical and neurological conditions Lifeskills coaching
Mental health and psychosocial rehabilitation	Private clinics; prisons; group homes and day programmes; community-based self-help and advocacy groups	Employment equity Supported employment Poverty alleviation projects
Community-based rehabilitation and social development	Non-governmental organizations and agencies promoting rural, peri-urban or urban support networks for specified populations for example: disabled children and adults, persons living with HIV/Aids; homeless shelters; service centres for the elderly, abused women, refugees and other marginalized groups; home-based care organizations; adult education service centres; Independent Living Centers	Entrepreneurship learnerships and micro-economic skills development Early identification of health and development risk Health promotion policies Disability policy and politics Poverty and occupation Development policies and practices Social action and change
Medical rehabilitation	Specialist/private rehabilitation centres, public sector hospitals, primary healthcare clinics	Management and administration Organizational development

therapy best practice 'occurs within the union of client-centred and family-centred practice, evidence-based practice and practice based upon occupation' (Strong, 2003, p. 197). Dawes et al. (2005) further advocated for evidence-based interventions as an important aspect of quality assurance. Part of the role of the site learning facilitator, therefore, is to ensure that students provide a quality service to their clients through implementing interventions based on sound research wherever possible. Role modelling is seen to be more effective than theoretical teaching in developing attitudes in students, such as those required to foster a commitment to best practice (Reece & Walker, 2002, cited in Dawes et al., 2005). It therefore follows that learning facilitators need to role model the evidence-based practice (EBP) process so that students are able to see how EBP can be applied in real situations. This implies that learning facilitators need to know the principles of EBP, be able to implement EBP and should have a critical attitude to their own practice (Dawes et al., 2005). In addition, learning facilitators should role model the ethical principles stipulated by the Health Professions Council of South Africa, and should adhere to The Standards of Practice for Occupational Therapists (Professional Board for Occupational Therapy and Medical Orthotics/Prosthetics, 2004).

Becoming a professional places various responsibilities on the students. Engaging ethically in providing services of high quality with interventions, wherever possible, based on evidence of effectiveness are some of those responsibilities. A further responsibility is to view their own learning and professional development as an ongoing process of lifelong learning that helps to develop their competence to practise in their chosen profession. Professional education also demands that students view competence as a temporary phenomenon that is constantly called into question (Clarkson, 1994). As a result, they must learn to engage in a process of continuing professional development in order to maintain their competence in the light of changing circumstances and raise professional standards wherever possible.

QUALITY ASSURANCE THROUGH CONTINUING PROFESSIONAL DEVELOPMENT

University practice educators and learning facilitators require additional support and continuing education in managing the professional development of students (Alsop & Ryan, 1996). Continuing professional development is one of the most important mechanisms for overcoming the impact of unstable and under-resourced contexts on student practice learning. In fact, the ethical, practical and effective education of students cannot proceed without regular contact between the university and staff in the field. Structure, based on clear guidelines for action in a climate of collaboration and mutual learning, creates a sense of containment in the midst of instability and constant change.

Professional development programmes for university practice educators and learning facilitators may include a range of topics such as:

- logistics, for example, year plans, dates, timetables, guidelines
- employment contracts, including parameters, benefits, roles and responsibilities
- the university practice educator/student relationship
- adult learning processes
- the supervision process
- clinical and population reasoning
- reflective practice
- formative and summative assessment and evaluation
- uniform occupational therapy terminology
- development of site-specific learning objectives
- professional standards, including ethics and human rights
- contemporary practice theories and models.

Professional development sessions may also be used to evaluate the practice learning curriculum and be a forum for visiting lecturers to run workshops and for communities (for example, representatives from community organizations who are willing to accommodate students) to interact with the university in negotiating appropriate student projects.

QUALITY ASSURANCE THROUGH RISK ASSESSMENT AND MANAGEMENT

Practice learning is enhanced when educational expectations are negotiated, explicit and achievable. Support systems and structures that back-up the actions and experiences of all role-players in order to achieve desired outcomes are also necessary. The onus lies with the education institution to put adequate academic and personal support structures in place to support students who may feel overwhelmed by the apparent lack of onsite guidance and role modelling. Thus, the institution is responsible for developing a risk assessment and management policy.

Whilst not all risks can be identified before students enter practice education, active measures are taken to identify where the risks are so that an infrastructure can be put in place to support the management of those risks identified. The risks often relate to students moving out of the comfort zones into situations that are unfamiliar and culturally different to their own. The university practice educator needs to manage the reluctance and resistance of students to engage in new learning settings, be they hospital or community contexts. Risks also include the emotional costs for individuals, groups and communities, parents, students, university practice educators as well as the site learning facilitators. The growth of transdisciplinary engagement in development work means that there is a blurring of boundaries, which challenges set standards. Higher education institutions have to share responsibility for ensuring the safety of all role-players. Thus, it is essential that sufficient human resources are provided for managing factors that contribute to effective community entry, such as time to negotiate and build trust and to maintain the relationship, deal with conflict management and change.

The benefits of the investment of time and resources include: increased confidence; relevant competence development; service development in areas where there is no service; and contributing to the relevance of the profession in critical local and global issues in a way that demonstrates the values of the profession and the wider role of the profession in meeting community needs. All role-players develop coping strategies and form productive partnerships.

QUALITY ASSURANCE THROUGH ACCOUNTABILITY

Accountability is concerned with proper stewardship of public goods; compliance with standards of best practice, efficient and effective performance of roles and responsibilities, and the exercise of appropriate control in the execution of duties. Numerous tensions exist in a developing society between the privileged who may exercise choice in a private economy and those who are dependent on the State (or public) to meet their health and development needs. Those without a voice are most vulnerable to exploitation because the balance of power is socially constructed around class, education and privilege. The notion of 'service learning' may, for example, be associated with philanthropy and charity aimed at 'uplifting the poor'. It may also be a democratic activity aimed at social change and the promotion of communal well-being. Learning cannot be uni-directional. If it is, the potential for exploitation exists. As a fundamental human right, it should be a reciprocal process meaning that all parties participating in mutually agreed actions should be enabled to change and benefit from citizenship and the practice education process.

Accountability structures should therefore be set in place to monitor the implementation of health professional education. Education institutions operating within a rights-based paradigm should ensure that student practice learning is:

- explicitly negotiated with relevant role-players with due consideration of representation and the affirmation of diversity
- based on universal and culturally relevant ethical principles
- compliant with human rights charters
- compliant with quality assurance principles
- committed to inclusion, the affirmation of diversity and client-centred practice
- responsive to feedback from participants.

CONCLUSION

The work of occupational therapists in South Africa is strongly influenced by an awareness of the need for redress of past shortcomings. The aim is to move progressively towards participation with clients and the communities within which they live, work and play. This shift in focus has necessitated substantial flexibility in the structure and processes of service learning. Captured in this chapter are some of the examples of how adaptations have been made, and some of the systems now in place to help guide students in their work with clients, or educators in the evaluation of student progress. These adaptations accommodate the range of sectors, clients and programmes associated with primary healthcare whilst ensuring congruence with professional standards for education of occupational therapists set by the World Federation of Occupational Therapists and the relevant professional boards in each country.

REFERENCES

Aleksiuk, M. (1996). *Power therapy: maximizing health through self-efficacy.* Cambridge: Hogrefe and Huber.

Allen, R., Oke, L., McKinstry, C. & Courtney, M. (2005). Professionalism and accountability: accreditation examined. In G. Whiteford & V. Wright-St Clair (Eds.), *Occupation and practice in context.* Sydney: Churchill Livingstone Elsevier, pp. 87–103.

Alsop, A. & Ryan, S. (1996). *Making the most of fieldwork education.* Cheltenham: Stanley Thornes.

Chambers, R. (1995). Paradigm shifts and the practice of participatory research and development. In N. Nelson & S. Wright (Eds.), *Power and participatory development: Theory and Practice.* London: Intermediate Technology Publications, pp. 30–42.

Clarkson, P. (1994). *The Achilles syndrome: overcoming the secret fear of failure.* Dorset: Element Books.

Curry, L. (1993). *Educating professionals: responding to new expectations for competence and accountability.* San Fransisco, CA: Jossey Bass.

Dawes, M.G., Summerskill, W., Glasziou, P., Cartabellotta, A., Martin, J., Hopayian, K., Porzsolt, F., Burls, A. & Osborne, J. (2005). Sicily statement on evidence-based practice. BMC *Medical Education* [Electronic], 5(1). Retrieved 27 July, 2005 from http://biomedcentral.com/1472-6920/5/1

HPCSA (n.d.). Rules of conduct. Retrieved 25 January, 2006, from http://www.hpcsa.co.za

Kronenberg, F., Algado, S. & Pollard, N. (Eds.) (2005). *Occupational therapy without borders: learning from the spirit of survivors.* Edinburgh: Elsevier Churchill Livingstone.

Lorenzo, T. & Friendlander, S. (2005). *Hearing the voice of rural communities: the perceptions of occupational therapy students in the Swartland municipal district, Western Cape.* Paper presented at Service Learning Symposium, CHED/JET, University of Cape Town, Cape Town, 1–2 September.

Nelson, N. & Wright, S. (Eds.) (1995). *Power and participatory development: Theory and Practice*. London: Intermediate Technology Publications.

Professional Board for Occupational Therapy and Medical Orthotics/Prosthetics (2004). *Standards of Practice for Occupational Therapists*. Retrieved 27 July, 2005 from http://www.hpcsa.co.za

Ramsden, P. (1992). Evaluating the quality of higher education. In R. Ransden (Ed.), *Learning to teach in higher education*. London: Routledge, pp. 217–247.

Strong, J. (2003). Seeing beyond the clouds: best practice occupational therapy. *Canadian Journal of Occupational Therapy*, *70*(4), 197–200.

Watson, R. & Swartz, L. (Eds.) (2004). *Transformation through occupation*. London: Whurr.

Youngstrom, M.J. (1998) Evolving competence in the practitioner role. *American Journal of Occupational therapy*, *52*(9), 716–721.

II Developing Professional Identity

Introduction to Part II

Part I has provided contextual information about the evolving status of practice and service learning in an occupational therapy curriculum. Part II offers a collection of chapters that each address an issue relating to the preparation, support and experiences of students who undertake practice or service learning in a variety of situations. As will be shown, risk management, the safety of all role-players and the promotion of learning in challenging situations feature prominently in the various chapters.

Part II addresses the development of professional identity, resilience and capacity through practice and service learning. Based on qualitative data analysis of student writing (learning logs) and focus group discussions, various strategies, used by them to negotiate complex practice situations, are highlighted and principles for enhancing learning extrapolated. Chapter 5 suggests practical guidelines for preparing students for practice and service learning in complex, culturally unfamiliar contexts. Based on adult education principles, recommendations are made for ensuring that students feel contained whilst acting professionally, appropriately and ethically in accordance with local cultural norms. In Chapter 6 the authors provide an overview of the professional and personal competencies that may be developed during service learning, including an appreciation of how power operates and how it may be channelled to promote positive outcomes. Chapter 7 deals with social change as learning in role emerging service settings. Detailing the role of occupational therapy in health promoting schools in a historically disadvantaged community, the chapter describes the impetus that social and occupational justice can provide for professional practice education. Chapter 8 discusses group learning experiences and community-based education in rural contexts by highlighting significant principles of community entry, liaison and feedback. Chapter 9 provides novel solutions to staff shortages by describing the practical and educational principles of group supervision in mental health. It expands on the principles of supervision and makes suggestions for promoting learning through peer feedback and evaluation. The service contributions that students make in are described in Chapter 10. It illustrates how their own potential may be enhanced through mobilizing the potential of the people with whom they work. Chapter 11 introduces the perspectives of service users. It describes the principles of a socially responsive practice education curriculum

Practice and Service Learning in Occupational Therapy. Edited by Theresa Lorenzo, Madeleine Duncan, Helen Buchanan, Auldeen Alsop
© 2006 John Wiley & Sons Ltd

that is grounded in community-based rehabilitation philosophy, and discusses how the use of formative service evaluation by community members enhances the quality and relevance of the work that students undertake.

In this part of the book, the unique approaches of the various authors to practice education have been retained. The reader can dip in and out of chapters, according to personal interest, gleaning ideas that may be applied or modified in their own work and context.

5 Preparing Students for the Complexities of Practice Learning

HELEN BUCHANAN and LIZAHN CLOETE

OBJECTIVES

This chapter discusses:

- the contextual complexities that students may encounter during service orientated professional practice learning
- strategies to equip students to remain safe and to be effective at practice learning sites
- the role that practice learning plays in preparing students for the realities of primary healthcare-led practice
- the ethical dilemmas of exposing undergraduate students to the complexities of practice learning.

RESPONDING TO NEW PRACTICE POSSIBILITIES

The scope of occupational therapy practice has expanded globally with services being provided to clients who previously did not receive them (Whiteford & Wright-St Clair, 2002). As a result, new practice possibilities have emerged. This changing scope of practice calls for the re-examination of occupational therapy practice curricula. Educating students for the realities of practice demands the re-alignment of practice learning objectives and the development of suitable models of education that encourage students to 'embrace the unique and uncertain situations that contemporary practice presents' (Ryan, 2001, p. 525). It has been argued in Chapter 1 that service learning is an appropriate model for practice education in resource-constrained, disadvantaged communities. To this end, health professional education programmes have an ethical responsibility to ensure that students are competent to deal with local health and development needs whilst also having an appreciation of international professional trends (Joubert, 2003).

Practice and Service Learning in Occupational Therapy. Edited by Theresa Lorenzo, Madeleine Duncan, Helen Buchanan, Auldeen Alsop

The clinical reasoning process occupational therapists engage in when making decisions about the best course of action for their clients requires that they grapple with the complexities of both occupational therapy practice and the practice learning context. Creek (2003, p. 31) described occupational therapy as 'a profession that focuses on the nature, balance, pattern and context of occupations in individual's lives, and therefore, it is often concerned with multiple and complex long-term needs and problems'. The social context in which intervention occurs has an important influence on occupational therapy practice. Although Creek (2003) described the changing nature of the social context of intervention for the United Kingdom, she did not make reference to pervasive poverty, poorly developed public sector infrastructures, social unrest and structural violence related to the legacy of injustice. When individuals receiving occupational therapy live in adverse social environments that are characterized by, for example, poverty, unemployment and poorly regulated public services, therapists have to reason not only at a clinical, but also at a population, level. The nature, balance and patterns of the individual's occupations may need to be considered against the backdrop of available population-based comprehensive primary healthcare services. Students are more likely to succeed in negotiating the challenges they will encounter in such contexts if they are equipped with some insights into these challenges, and knowledge of available structures to support them in their learning. This requires a carefully planned programme to prepare students for entry into practice learning. Whilst it is impossible to prepare students for every eventuality, practice educators need to provide opportunities for students to engage with them about the risks involved and the most sensible ways of minimizing and managing these. The challenge lies in ensuring that students are sufficiently equipped to manage the realities of practice and to respond appropriately to needs as they emerge.

THE CONTEXTUAL COMPLEXITIES OF OCCUPATIONAL THERAPY PRACTICE

Service learning is a type of experiential learning in which contextual issues play an important role in shaping student learning. An understanding of the context of service learning is crucial for clinical reasoning to take place (Cook & Cusick, 1998). To equip students to understand the demands of the contexts in which they may be placed during practice learning, university practice educators need to familiarize themselves with the particular contextual issues students are likely to face, so that the curriculum is shaped accordingly.

University practice educators should ensure they remain aware of the realities students face in practice learning, for example, when they visit students at learning sites, during individual or group supervision, and when marking written work. Some of the contextual issues that occupational therapy students in South Africa encountered were described in interactive journals kept by the students. Analysis of these journal entries (Buchanan, 2002) identified the following issues:

- poverty
- diverse cultures and languages
- violence, crime and abuse
- uncertainty due to constantly changing institutional and societal structures.

It is argued that these are fast becoming a global reality, making it increasingly important for students in both undeveloped and developed countries to acquire the knowledge, skills and attitudes to be effective in such contexts. Contextual issues that South African occupational therapy students encountered will be described briefly. This will be followed with a discussion about how contextual factors influence the preparation of students.

WORKING WITH PEOPLE LIVING IN POVERTY

'Poverty is a global phenomenon affecting an estimated 2.8 billion people worldwide and 25% of the population of the developing world' (Watson & Fourie, 2004: 44). Disability 'exacerbates poverty by increasing isolation and economic strain, not just for the individual but for the family' (Coleridge, 1993, p. 64). Furthermore, strong correlations between poverty and levels of education, unemployment, access to basic services, and ill-health have been identified (People's Dialogue, 1998). The high prevalence of poverty increases the likelihood that occupational therapy students will work with clients living in extremely poor socio-economic circumstances. Clients in these contexts often experience family difficulties in addition to their own health problems. The complexity involved in making decisions about the best course of action for the client is well illustrated in the following extract from a student's practice learning log. It is about a client who was living in an informal house in a squatter community. The house was overcrowded, being shared with five family members, all of whom were unemployed. The entire household was dependent on the client's old age pension.

> EB had a stroke. She has limited family support. Two children are alcoholics, one grandchild had an abusive boyfriend, she has a son who is HIV positive and it is thought that the son's wife is also positive . . . EB's daughter with whom she is presently living seems to neglect her children and is often rude to and verbally abuses EB.

A student working with EB, would need to understand the importance of enabling EB to deal with all the other issues in her life that may prevent her from reaching her potential, whilst also providing rehabilitation to address the consequences of her stroke. The reasoning skills required in weighing up a number of factors and then deciding on the most appropriate course of action need to be developed and facilitated. Whilst theory about reasoning and strategies to facilitate reasoning can be taught in lectures, the skills required to reason-in-action can only be developed during practice learning when students work with real clients in real contexts. Facilitating the development of reasoning skills is one of the most important tasks of university practice educators and learning facilitators.

It is argued that students need to be exposed to situations of poverty so that 'their work will [not] be contextually impaired or . . . irrelevant' (Fourie, Galvaan & Beeton, 2004, p. 70) when they start work as qualified therapists. However, it is also acknowledged that they may be immobilized when confronted with situations of such overwhelming need. Most occupational therapy students are from middle- or upper middle-class backgrounds and have not been exposed to the harsh realities of living in poverty. In the face of overwhelming need, it is possible (and probably even likely) that students will fail to engage with the context in ways that enable them to maximize the learning opportunities available whilst providing an effective service to their clients. Developing strategies to prepare students to work effectively in such contexts is thus crucial to achieving positive learning and service outcomes. Strategies to support and facilitate learning and to develop awareness of self and others will be explored in more detail later in this chapter.

RELATING WITH PEOPLE FROM DIVERSE CULTURAL BACKGROUNDS

Globally, occupational therapy educators are faced with the challenge and responsibility of preparing students to become competent in working with diverse groups of clients in diverse settings (Lim, 2004; Whiteford & Wright-St Clair, 2002). The complexities of the interaction between culture and health, together with differing opinions about how best to provide services to address health needs, present major challenges to the education of occupational therapists. Becoming competent to work with people from diverse cultures requires an understanding of cultural issues so that practice can be client-centred and culturally sensitive. Whilst students may have knowledge about the centrality of culture in their interactions with clients, they also have to be able to deal with it (Camphina-Bacote, 1995, cited in Whiteford and Wright-St Clair, 2002). Experiential learning is generally agreed to be a suitable method for educating students about socio-cultural diversity (Whiteford and Wright-St Clair, 2002).

Occupational therapists in many countries have to be able to work with clients with whom they may not be able to communicate directly. Language differences are frequently a barrier to realizing client-centredness. Learning to work across the barriers of language is thus a vital skill to the realization of a client-centred approach. Service delivery by therapists who cannot speak the language of the client with whom they are working, can result in communication barriers and mistrust (Brodrick, 2004). Language barriers may limit a therapist's understanding of client needs and could result in misunderstandings, incorrect interpretations and inappropriate (or even incorrect) service provision (Brice & Campbell, 1999, cited in Brodrick, 2004).

Students need to learn to work with interpreters and to appreciate the difficulties and challenges of translating occupational therapy terminology into other languages. They also need to develop awareness of using non-verbal cues to communicate with people from different cultures in a non-offensive way. While some of this may be gained through experience, basic principles of working with interpreters should be included in the preparation for practice learning. Guidelines outlining the principles of working with interpreters, such as the *Guide to working with interpreters in health service settings* (n.d.) should be discussed with students before entering a service learning site. These principles should be revisited during, as well as after, practice learning experiences to enable students to continue learning how to apply them in practice. A survey completed with community service occupational therapists in South Africa, identified the ability to speak an African language as a critical skill (OCP News, 2005). Thus, opportunities should be created in the curriculum for students to learn how to communicate in an indigenous language relevant to the context in which they will practice.

Practice learning plays a central role in developing intercultural competence, but students need to learn skills first so that they can then apply them in practice (Whiteford & Wright-St Clair, 2002). Students may worry about being able to provide appropriate services to people from different backgrounds when they have a limited knowledge of the community (Manderson, 2003). Brodrick (2004, p. 245) suggested that 'only a process of gradual engagement and deepening trust can develop the occupational therapist's confidence, competence, and acceptability by the community'. This is clearly the ideal, but if students are placed in a particular community for a limited period, gradual engagement is not possible. An alternative model could be to structure a learning opportunity within the same community over the three or four years of study. It is argued that if students are equipped with an understanding of the principles of community entry (see Chapter 2) and skills of engaging with people from differing cultural circumstances (often using different languages), they can begin to develop their competence to work effectively.

Equipping students for practice in culturally diverse contexts is complex and is largely determined by the student's receptiveness to critiquing personal biases and assumptions about how people's lived reality is interpreted. Opportunities to explore biases and assumptions can be provided through median groups (Duncan, Buchanan & Lorenzo, 2005) or learners' logs (Buchanan, Moore & Van Niekerk, 1998), and should also be facilitated by university practice educators and learning facilitators at learning sites. Within education programmes, students also need to foster a culture of engaging with each other about cultural diversity issues. They need to be active learners, open to new ways of thinking about practice.

RESPONDING TO VIOLENCE, CRIME AND ABUSE

Although students may be confronted with issues related to violence, crime and abuse at any practice learning site, they may feel safer working within the confines of a hospital rather than in the community where they may feel uncontained and vulnerable. In some communities, students may be seen as strangers or even outsiders. They will have to get to know people, systems and processes that fall outside their personal frame of reference. In addition, the realities of living in some communities become much clearer as students see how violence, crime and abuse impact on the daily lives of their clients. Being placed in an unfamiliar setting often evokes fear in students. Some fears are real, for example, physical safety in communities where violence and unrest may occur, whilst others may result from misperceptions and media reports. Either situation may result in a student being reluctant to enter a service learning site. The learning facilitator and university practice educator need to explore such situations with the student to identify the root of the problem so that the correct action can be taken. For example, the university practice educator may need to explain the safety mechanisms that have been developed to ensure the student's physical safety. Students placed at any practice learning site should be proactive in recognizing risks to their safety, have a thorough knowledge of the correct procedures to follow when faced with unsafe situations, and be able to implement appropriate strategies to manage these effectively. Risk management strategies will be discussed in more detail later in this chapter.

WORKING WITH UNCERTAINTY

The unprecedented changes occurring globally impact on professional practice (Kronenberg, Algado & Pollard, 2005). It is 'within this context that occupational therapists and other health professionals seek to practise and generate knowledge in confusing circumstances and at local and global levels, in addition to having to cope with the uncertainty of dealing with people' (Higgs & Titchen, 2001, p. 526). For example, in South Africa, the Government of National Unity has made it their goal to redress past inequalities in the delivery of health services. Adoption of the primary healthcare approach has triggered the shift of services from tertiary to secondary and primary levels of care. As a consequence, the number of acutely ill people in tertiary hospitals has decreased due to shortened hospital stays. Clients are discharged home in a more physically and emotionally vulnerable state than before, and many clients are discharged before receiving occupational therapy to prepare them for going home. Occupational therapists have had to be proactive and creative in both accommodating and responding to this shift in service, whilst simultaneously being involved in creating posts at primary levels of care. To ensure that students are accommodated within this changing service delivery platform, education must be a central focus in any discussions related to service delivery.

The process of transforming the South African health system has led to an inevitable need for occupational therapy services to change their focus and methods of service delivery, and adopt new models of practice. Students no longer have the luxury of working with clients for undefined periods of time. Instead, they have to make decisions quickly about the assessment and treatment priorities for clients during their short stay in hospital. Sometimes, clients may be able to continue receiving outpatient occupational therapy, but opportunities for longer term rehabilitation are often limited. Even when outpatient occupational therapy services are available, these are often inaccessible to clients as they have no access to transport, or live so far from the hospital that ongoing treatment is impractical. As a result, students are confronted with an environment that is constantly changing and evolving. This in turn has demanded a 'living' curriculum that is responsive to changing service needs (Duncan, 2002). Students need to be able to identify contextual disjunction, be flexible in their expectations and able to adapt their approaches to clients accordingly. The following extract from a student's journal shows how the student was able to identify (and then respond to) disjunction within the context of the practice learning site:

> Community mental health is a developing area in the transformation of health services in South Africa . . . Public policy in line with the model of psychosocial rehabilitation is being drafted . . . but implementation is still in the very early stages.

It is suggested that unless students are adequately prepared and equipped for the realities of working in contexts where cultural diversity, scarce resources, uncertainty, social disintegration and poverty occur in the actual contexts of people's lives, they are at risk of becoming overwhelmed by the needs and thus becoming ineffective. Practical ways in which students may be prepared for effective engagement with the challenges of practice learning now follow.

STRUCTURES TO SUPPORT PRACTICE LEARNING

Practice learning preparation is an on-going, continuously evolving process involving the student, the learning facilitator, the practice educator and the context. Adult learning principles, such as those of Paulo Freire (Hope & Timmel, 1995), guide the process so that students take responsibility for their own learning. However, specific educational structures enable students to explore issues that emerge during practice learning. Structures that are both creative and meaningful tend to be more attractive and useful to students. The next section discusses several structures that may be used in preparing students for the realities of practice. These are grouped into three main categories, namely structures to facilitate learning, structures for emotional support and structures for developing awareness of diversity.

STRUCTURES TO FACILITATE LEARNING

If students are taught how to access information rather than being provided with it, they are able to collaborate in the knowledge construction process. This demands a curriculum that has a strong ethos of self-directed learning, so that from an early stage, students become resourceful in accessing and using information. Students need to learn about the different forms of thinking and reasoning that are used in occupational therapy problem identification and problem solving. Clinical reasoning skills are vital for effective practice in community settings (Lysack, Stadnyk, Paterson, McLeod & Krefting, 1995, cited in Mason, 1998) and should thus be introduced as central to the occupational therapy process. Reflection should be embedded in the curriculum and formats such as interactive journals (Buchanan et al., 1998) and portfolios (Buchanan, Van Niekerk & Moore, 2001) may be introduced as suitable vehicles for developing the skills of reflection. Journals provide a mechanism for facilitating reflection on their own learning and their developing competencies. Students must be able to identify and utilize appropriate writing formats for capturing the occupational therapy process. Through the use of workshops, good instances of writing are modelled and critiqued to facilitate student learning. Written and verbal feedback from university practice educators during practice learning facilitates further development of reasoning and reflective skills. Some strategies to facilitate learning and support students during practice learning will now be briefly discussed.

Providing Pre-placement Information

The anxiety of starting at a new learning site can be substantially reduced by providing students with relevant information beforehand (Duncan et al., 2005; Steele-Smith & Armstrong, 2001). Packages containing essential information, such as maps, physical addresses of learning sites, contact details of people they need to meet at learning sites, transport routes and details of transport arrangements, hours of work, uniform expectations, services provided and suggestions for pre-reading, can be developed for this purpose (Gilbert & Strong, 1997; Steele-Smith & Armstrong, 2001). Students should also be encouraged to do their own preparation, for example, checking the requirements for their next learning site and reflecting on their learning from a previous site to determine the focus of their learning for the next one. They may also be proactive in requesting information from other students who have been to the same learning site (Buchanan, 2002). It is helpful to create a forum for students to voice their expectations, fears and anticipated challenges to contain their anxieties (Lorenzo, 2002). Workshop formats enable students to brainstorm and problem-solve around expected difficulties. Case studies presented to small groups of students facilitate debate around issues such as professionalism, ethics and transformation. Handover between students can be built into a tutorial system, and records and resource files kept thus ensuring sustainability of services (Duncan et al., 2005).

Safety and Risk Management Strategies

Learning about safety and risk management strategies must be a non-negotiable prerequisite for students who are to be placed at any practice learning site where risk is an issue. Experiential problem-orientated learning tasks in small groups may be used to explore appropriate safety and risk management strategies. Students need to be encouraged to identify their fears and the challenges they anticipate when they enter learning sites so that they can begin to address the potential obstacles to their learning.

Students must be familiar with the safety and risk management policies and procedures developed by Departments or Faculties to ensure their safety at learning sites. For example:

- Students should always work in pairs or even small groups
- Students must notify the learning facilitator when they leave the premises and inform him or her about the time they expect to be back
- A community member must always accompany students during home visits (preferably someone who is well-known in the community)
- Students should make use of transport provided by the institution wherever possible to reduce the likelihood of theft from their private vehicles.

Procedures with established actions must be developed for situations where student safety is threatened, and students must be clear about what to do should the need arise. For example, students must report incidents in which their safety is threatened to the learning facilitator, who will inform the practice learning coordinator. In volatile situations, such as incidents of violence, students must be removed from the site as soon as possible until such time that the context is stable. In such circumstances, students need to ensure the safety of their clients before attempting to leave the context themselves. Students should be equipped with the department/faculty handbook outlining risk management strategies and the details of a named person who they can contact should the need arise. Student safety must be monitored carefully on a daily basis by the practice learning coordinator with support from faculty.

During practice learning preparation, students are often concerned about being exposed to communicable diseases, such as tuberculosis and HIV/Aids. It is vital that the facts about the contraction and treatment of all communicable diseases are made known and that students have a clear understanding of the precautions they need to take. Universities must develop policies about exposure to communicable diseases with clear guidelines for action to protect clients, students and staff. Appropriate insurance and medico-legal cover must also be in place.

Learning Contracts and Learning Objectives

Students need to have clear learning objectives before entering practice learning. These should be negotiated and agreed through dialogue between the university practice educator, learning facilitator and practice learning coordinator. Clear objectives inform students about the expectations of the university and the learning site, and enable them to develop their own personal objectives for the learning experience (Christie, Joyce & Moeller, 1985; Duncan et al., 2005). A learning contract allows the student to identify and direct their own learning needs. In a learning contract, students set their own learning goals with appropriate time frames, together with plans of how these will be achieved (Steele-Smith & Armstrong, 2001). Contracts should be specific to the context so that students can learn to evaluate themselves and identify their progress towards their learning goals in their weekly meeting with the university practice educator. The practice educator can then be a resource for facilitating the student's learning towards reaching these goals.

Developing Skills of Learning Facilitators

Learning facilitators require opportunities to discuss issues pertaining to student learning, and prospects for self-development. Continuing professional development programmes provide ongoing training in the skills required for effective facilitation of student learning. These programmes may also provide a forum to discuss practice learning and educational issues (Duncan et al., 2005).

STRUCTURES FOR EMOTIONAL SUPPORT

During practice learning, some students may be exposed to situations they have difficulty handling, or may struggle to engage effectively with their clients and/or colleagues due to difficulties they are experiencing in their personal lives. Mechanisms must be created for students to process such issues in a contained environment so that their learning is not hampered. These may range from peer support to professional counsellors, depending on the severity of the issue.

Peer Support

Peers can be utilized, not only to further learning, but also as a support. This is particularly valuable in situations where human resources are scarce. Opportunities can be created for students to support one another. For example, if students are placed in pairs or larger groups at the same learning site, they learn from one another and do not need to rely solely on the learning facilitator or practice educator (Molineux, 1999). They also find the support they receive from each other indispensable for learning (Duncan et al., 2005; Steele-Smith & Armstrong, 2001). In fact, taking two or more students can be more time efficient than one due to the support and assistance they provide each other (Duncan et al., 2005; Steele-Smith & Armstrong, 2001). Students also feel more confident if they can share work with peers and learn to work as part of a team.

On-site Learning Facilitation

On-site learning facilitation may be provided in small groups or individually with regular written and verbal feedback provided by learning facilitators and/or university practice educators (Duncan et al., 2005). Within a group learning-facilitation structure, students are encouraged to 'discover, articulate, listen and share knowledge and personal meanings' (Mason, 1998, p. 125). Such groups encourage students to discuss their experiences openly as well as to support each other in difficult situations. (Learning facilitation in groups is discussed further in Chapter 9.) Individual facilitation of learning can have similar benefits but has the added advantage of being able to address specific learning needs on a one-to-one basis.

Tutorials

Involvement in weekly tutorials with peers from similar learning sites under the guidance of, and with input from, a university practice educator or expert learning facilitator provides a safe space for students to teach, and learn from, other students and with reference to their clients (Duncan et al., 2005). Student-led tutorials allow students to explore issues and grapple with solutions together, which reinforces learning and reasoning (Steele-Smith & Armstrong, 2001).

Educators and University Counsellors

An open door policy enables students to have easy access to university practice educators. Designated educators can be identified to monitor the progress of individual students where necessary. Mechanisms are required to refer students for counselling and/or academic development where indicated (Duncan et al., 2005). A counsellor may be appointed to see students on a weekly basis for support (Steele-Smith & Armstrong, 2001). This kind of service provides students an opportunity for debriefing with a staff member who is not involved in evaluating their performance.

STRUCTURES FOR DEVELOPING AWARENESS OF SELF AND OTHERS

Mechanisms are required within the curriculum to encourage self-awareness, to enable students to explore their attitudes towards others, and to enable the development of a sense of agency. It has been argued that only when students have developed an awareness of their own values and perceptions about culture and diversity can they be truly sensitive to the cultural issues of clients (Duncan et al., 2005; Fitzgerald, Mullavey-O'Byrne & Clemson, 1997). It thus follows that an essential aspect of the practice learning curriculum is the enhancement of cultural competence. As discussed earlier in this chapter, vehicles such as median groups may be used to provide students with opportunities to explore their beliefs, attitudes and assumptions about others, particularly people from different cultural backgrounds (Duncan et al., 2005). Making transformation an explicit part of the curriculum, for example, by drawing up a class constitution may foster attitudes of inclusiveness.

In a study of final year occupational therapy students at the University of Cape Town, it was found that students used their spirituality to manage their anxieties during practice learning (Buchanan, 2002). Meaning and purpose can be explored in a range of ways, such as through keeping a journal and taking time to reflect or meditate. Students should be encouraged to substitute the urgency of 'doing' with the ability to listen deeply to themselves and their clients (Duncan et al., 2005; Lorenzo, 2002). Through *being,* they become sensitive to the unspoken needs of others, as well as themselves, and are more likely to be able to respond to a particular situation in an appropriate way. Creating a space for reflection enables students to become aware of both their competencies and their limitations.

Agency can be developed by encouraging students to be independent thinkers and to take charge of their own learning rather than having a need to follow 'recipes' or to expect constant guidance from others. Students may find this liberating as well as daunting but, over time, should develop confidence in their solution-generating abilities (Duncan et al., 2005). While students do struggle with many difficult and challenging issues during service learning, in the process of grappling with these issues, they may develop their own personal strategies to manage them more effectively (Buchanan, 2002).

CONCLUSION

Students work in a variety of contexts during practice learning. It is important that every effort is made to ensure that these provide a positive learning experience. Steps must be taken by the education facility to guide, advise, prepare and support students so that their learning is maximized and they develop the competencies to work in similar contexts when they graduate. Some contexts can make students feel powerless because of the often overwhelming real-life issues they are required to face. Is it necessary to expose students to such complex and difficult circumstances to enable them to develop professional competence? Some would argue that students should be protected from difficult issues and that the long-term cost of making occupational therapy education so challenging is not justified. But then how will students learn to deal with these issues?

If we are to respond to Watson's (2002, p. 7) challenge that students need to become 'agents able to address change in their world of work', then surely the best way to do this is through practice in 'real-life' contexts during undergraduate practice learning where they can receive adequate guidance and support. Students are more resilient than they are given credit, but adequate support mechanisms and thorough preparation are crucial to achieving successful outcomes in practice learning. By acknowledging the complexities that students encounter during practice learning, university practice educators and learning facilitators may become better equipped to prepare students in their learning endeavours.

REFERENCES

Brice, A. & Campbell, L. (1999). Cross-cultural communication. In R. Leavitt (Ed.), *Cross-cultural rehabilitation.* London: WB Saunders, pp. 83–98.

Brodrick, K. (2004). Grandmothers affected by HIV/AIDS: new roles and occupations. In R. Watson & L. Swartz (Eds.), *Transformation through occupation.* London: Whurr, pp. 233–253.

Buchanan, H. (2002). *South African contextual factors: impact on occupational therapy student learning, education and practice.* Poster presented at the 13th International Congress of the World Federation of Occupational Therapists, Stockholm, Sweden, June.

Buchanan, H., Moore, R. & Van Niekerk, L. (1998). The fieldwork case study: writing for clinical reasoning. *American Journal of Occupational Therapy, 52*(4), 291–295.

Buchanan, H., Van Niekerk, L. & Moore, R. (2001). Assessing fieldwork journals: developmental portfolios. *British Journal of Occupational Therapy, 64*(8), 398–402.

Camphina-Bacote, L. (1995). The quest for cultural competence in nursing care. *Nursing Forum, 30*(4), 642–648.

Christie, B., Joyce, P. & Moeller, P. (1985). Fieldwork experience, part II: the supervisor's dilemma. *American Journal of Occupational Therapy, 39,* 675–681.

Coleridge, P. (1993). *Disability, liberation and development.* Oxford: Oxfam.

Cook, C. & Cusick, A. (1998). Preparing students for their first fieldwork placement using on-campus practicums. *Australian Occupational Therapy Journal, 45,* 79–90.

Creek, J. (2003). *Occupational therapy defined as a complex intervention.* London: College of Occupational Therapists.

Duncan, M. (2002). *Living curriculum as transformation strategy in occupational therapy education*. Poster presented at the 13th International Congress of the World Federation of Occupational Therapists, Stockholm, Sweden, June.

Duncan, M., Buchanan, H. & Lorenzo, T. (2005). Politics in occupational therapy education: A South African perspective. In F. Kronenberg, S. Algado & N. Pollard (Eds.), *Occupational therapy without borders – learning from the spirit of survivors.* Edinburgh: Elsevier Churchill Livingstone, pp. 390–401.

Fitzgerald, M., Mullavey-O'Byrne, C. & Clemson, L. (1997). Cultural issues from practice. *Australian Occupational Therapy Journal, 44*(1), 1–21.

Fourie, M., Galvaan, R. & Beeton, H. (2004). The impact of poverty: potential lost. In R. Watson & L. Swartz (Eds.), *Transformation through occupation*. London: Whurr, pp. 69–84.

Gilbert, J. & Strong, J. (1997). Coping strategies employed by occupational therapy students anticipating fieldwork placement. *Australian Occupational Therapy Journal, 44*, 30–40.

Guide to working with interpreters in health service settings (n.d.). Retrieved 29 June, 2005 from http://www.health.qld.gov.au/multicultural/pdf/guideto.pdf

Higgs, J. & Titchen, A. (2001). Rethinking the practice-knowledge interface in an uncertain world: a model for practice development. *British Journal of Occupational Therapy, 64*(11), 526–533.

Hope, A. & Timmel, S. (1995). *Training for transformation: a handbook for community workers*, revised edn. Gweru, Zimbabwe: Mambo Press.

Joubert, R. (2003). Are we coming of age or being born again? How does this impact on the education and assessment of competence of occupational therapy students in South Africa? *South African Journal of Occupational Therapy, 33*(3), 2–4.

Kronenberg, F., Algado, S. & Pollard, N. (Eds.) (2005). *Occupational therapy without borders – learning from the spirit of survivors.* Edinburgh: Elsevier Churchill Livingstone.

Lim, K.H. (2004). Letters to the editor: Occupational therapy in multi-cultural contexts. *British Journal of Occupational Therapy, 67*(1), 49–50.

Lorenzo, T. (2002). *Developing competence for partnership: the voice of occupational therapy students in Cape Town*. Poster presented at the 13th World Congress of the World Federation of Occupational Therapists, Stockholm, Sweden, June.

Lysack, C., Stadnyk, R., Paterson, M., McLeod, K. & Krefting, L. (1995). Professional expertise of occupational therapists in community practice: Results of an Ontario study. *Canadian Journal of Occupational Therapy, 62*, 138–147.

Manderson, L. (2003). Cultural diversity – a guide for health professionals. Retrieved 29 June, 2005, from http://www.health.qld.gov.au/multicultural/cultdiv/default.asp

Mason, L. (1998). Fieldwork education: collaborative group learning in community settings. *Australian Occupational Therapy Journal, 45*, 124–130.

Molineux, M. (1999). Making changes: a clinical reasoning journey. In S. Ryan & E. McKay (Eds.), *Thinking and reasoning in therapy*. Cheltenham: Stanley Thornes, pp. 121–132.

OCP News (2005). First feedback from our Community Service Therapists. *Newsletter of the Professional board for Occupational Therapy and Medical Orthotics/Prosthetics, February*, 1–3.

People's Dialogue (1998). *Poverty and inequality in South Africa: summary report.* Cape Town: Information Publication.

Ryan, S. (2001). Breaking moulds – shifting thinking. *British Journal of Occupational Therapy*, *64*(1), 525.

Steele-Smith, S. & Armstrong, M. (2001). 'I would take more students but . . .': student supervision strategies. *British Journal of Occupational Therapy*, *64*(11), 549–551.

Watson, R. (2002). Competence: a transformative approach. *WFOT Bulletin*, *45*, 7–11.

Watson, R. & Fourie, M. (2004). International and African influences on occupational therapy. In R. Watson & L. Swartz (Eds.), *Transformation through occupation*. London: Whurr, pp. 33–50.

Whiteford, G. & Wright-St Clair, V. (2002). Being prepared for diversity in practice: occupational therapy students' perceptions of valuable intercultural learning experiences. *British Journal of Occupational Therapy*, *65*(3), 129–137.

6 Working in the Real World: Unlocking the Potential of Students

THERESA LORENZO and HELEN BUCHANAN

OBJECTIVES

This chapter discusses:

- perceptions of final (fourth) year occupational therapy students of their practice learning experiences[1]
- students' competence and resourcefulness developed through diverse learning experiences
- personal strategies students may use to manage complex contextual and professional challenges
- the nature of power and participation in practice.

SETTING THE SCENE

When you're going into the community it's only 20 km from where you live, except it's so different it's like going to another world. And you think you are going to these shacks [informal houses] that you see on the side of the road, they look grubby and terrible but they are actually homes and they are a community and they are beautiful. They have gardens and it's liveable and it's not what you ever imagined.

The chapter draws on the findings of two separate studies related to students' experiences of clinical practice and service learning in and around Cape Town. In the research, the specific competencies and personal strategies that students developed through 'working in the real world' were identified. In particular, questions were posed about what happened to students when they worked in complex environments: could they manage the challenges they faced, and did these challenges foster or inhibit learning?

Practice and Service Learning in Occupational Therapy. Edited by Theresa Lorenzo, Madeleine Duncan, Helen Buchanan, Auldeen Alsop
© 2006 John Wiley & Sons Ltd

The sense of resilience that students develop as they learn to manage in situations that they initially perceive to be beyond their level of competence emerges. The studies show how much students were able to draw on their inner resources to enhance their learning. Finally, the chapter highlights questions that arose through the investigation for practice educators and students that, for the time being, remain unanswered.

TAKING AN ACTION LEARNING APPROACH

Occupational therapy students at the University of Cape Town are placed at different practice and service learning sites over the four years of study. While the philosophies of these learning sites may differ, the students are generally involved in some aspect of service delivery and programme development in previously disadvantaged communities. To bring about a change in the situation of disadvantaged people, different ways of learning, teaching and evaluation are needed.

Learning may be viewed as a lifelong, cyclical process related to becoming competent in the workplace (Clarkson, 1994; Jarvis, 2001). An action learning approach enhances the relevance of practice learning because it requires reflection in and on practice (Hope & Timmel, 1995; Taylor, Marais & Kaplan, 1997) and helps to prepare students for community development work. Action learning brings about real change because it facilitates a move from viewing disadvantaged people as passive recipients of health care and social services to seeing them as active participants in their own well-being and development. An action learning approach embraces mistakes by encouraging individuals, groups, university practice educators and students to sit, observe, ask, listen and reflect on everyday practice in order to promote real change (Higgs, Richardson & Duhlgren, 2005; Schön, 1991). Such flexibility in partnerships allows for the exploration of diverse needs and ideas, including an appreciation of different experiences and perceptions of power. An inclusive learning process promotes a sharing of power. By transferring initiative to disadvantaged people and allowing them to offer information to the body of centralized knowledge and understanding, an attitude of 'cognitive respect' on the part of the more educated, which is more liberating and empowering, is generated (Chambers, 1993; Taylor & Conradie, 1997).

However, it is here that the problems and pitfalls of participation and action learning are pertinent. Chambers (1995) maintains that the needs of the poorest may go unrecognized and unmet because marginalized people are often missed as potential facilitators. They are hurried though the facilitation process by more educated or 'outside' facilitators intent on either following a development 'agenda' or on achieving measurable outcomes. Unequal power relations may lead to mutual deception. For example, those marginalized may hope to gain an advantage through the relationship, whilst facilitators may fear

being penalized if certain outcomes are not achieved. The practice of participation and action learning may therefore be cosmetic in that, whilst the right
language or terminology is used, little change occurs in the behaviour and attitudes of facilitators or in the lives of the people with whom they work.

These concerns have implications for involving students in community
development initiatives and designing appropriate practice learning curricula.
Students learn how to practise within an action learning and participatory paradigm by joining or initiating such a process with a particular group of persons
(for example, mothers of disabled children or persons living with mental
illness) in a particular context (such as a non-governmental organization
working with people living with HIV/Aids in an informal settlement). In so
doing, they render a service by partnering with the group as 'resource-full'
members committed to seeking mutually identified and feasible solutions
through collaboration and focused actions.

RESEARCHING HOW STUDENTS EXPERIENCE AND
MANAGE PRACTICE LEARNING

An inductive, thematic documentary analysis was undertaken of 12 final year
undergraduate student portfolios (Buchanan, Van Niekerk & Moore, 2001).
The analysis explored the contextual issues that students faced and the competencies they developed as a result of their exposure to unfamiliar environments and impoverished communities (Buchanan, 2002). The students felt
daunted by the overwhelming needs with which they were faced. This was not
surprising as most students were from privileged backgrounds and these learning experiences were likely to be their first exposure to squatter camps and
informal settlements. As one student explained:

> There's a lot of chaos, a lot of underlying things, not on the surface but a lot of
> emotional things underneath. You are working with a physical problem and sud-
> denly something else comes up and [there is] a lot of chaos people tend to hide
> behind.

A second study (Lorenzo, 2002) emerged from an informal initiative that
was originally established to provide students with a structured space to share
their experiences of service learning. It was intended to help contain some of
their anxieties by helping them reflect on and process their personal reactions
to the disjunctions between their world and that of the people with whom they
worked. During focused group discussions, students were asked to create individual collages reflecting their experiences of service learning. The collages
were a trigger to explore the process of building partnerships with clients and
their families, community members, community health workers and community rehabilitation workers. The projective use of creative media for exploring
their concerns raised issues that may not otherwise have become apparent to

them at a conscious level. Inductive thematic qualitative analysis revealed that students developed competence and personal strategies to engage positively with contextual demands.

The next section of the chapter draws on emerging principles to describe aspects of working in unfamiliar social and cultural environments.

EVIDENCE OF DEVELOPING COMPETENCE

According to Bossers, Miller, Polatajko and Hartley (2002, p. 1) 'professional competency is the behavioral definition of knowledge, skills, behaviors, values and personal characteristics that underlie the adequate performance of professional activities'. It is argued that despite working in initially daunting circumstances, students can develop competence essential for practice in diverse and challenging contexts.

BRACKETING POWERLESSNESS

In South Africa, impoverishment has resulted in high incidences of violence, crime and abuse, which impact on the daily lives of the people with whom students work (Watson & Swartz, 2004). The poor social circumstances were an initial shock for many students who had lived 'protected' lives with little reason to go into informal squatter areas. Students sometimes felt uncertain about their safety within learning sites where they came face-to-face with the daily realities of many families. They became aware of the multiple concerns that affected individual clients and the complex issues with which they were also expected to deal. Knowledge of these issues impacted on their decisions about the best course of action for their clients. The students soon discovered that they were not able to significantly change the different contextual circumstances. Nevertheless, they learnt to put their feelings of powerlessness to one side, so that they could act on other issues where they were able to make a difference. As one student commented:

> I realized that, although I had felt helpless at not being able to change the family circumstances, we could work on other stressors in [my client's] life, and independence. This would help lift her out of the depression.

ENTERING THE LIFE WORLD

Students encountered a diversity of relationships and learnt to appreciate difference as they worked with people from many different cultural backgrounds who spoke a variety of languages. They had to understand the phenomenological world of the person and family if they hoped to form a meaningful relationship, and offer contextually relevant intervention.

A young man was not going to tell me that he was suffering. Firstly, because it was not culturally appropriate for him (as pointed out to me by an African colleague working within the unit) and secondly, because the meaning this man gained from the sense of responsibility he felt as a worker far outweighed the alternative of admitting 'weakness' and being asked to stop working and rest.

Students formed relationships with people they would otherwise never meet or learn from. The concept of 'culture shock' impacted on how soon or well they were able to start forming relationships. During home visits, students found that they had more time to establish rapport with individuals and get to know the family situation, which was different from hospital-based learning experiences. This rapport enabled them to give and receive more.

The extent of poverty was clearly evident for many of the people with whom students worked. Many parents were unemployed so there was little money in the homes for basic necessities, such as food and clothing for the children. Some students who worked in schools found they were expected to work with children for two hours before they received their first meal of the day. This was a stark contrast to the students' own childhood experiences.

Many white students had to face the harsh reality of the opportunities and privileges they had obtained under apartheid. Whether students could speak the language of their clients, whose first language was either isiXhosa or Afrikaans, made a difference to the ease with which students formed relationships. Students who had an open approach and an awareness of their differences and biases were able to manage the transition more effectively.

NEGOTIATING TRANSITION

Occupational therapy practice has evolved to encompass a population-based occupation focus and not just an individual or group focus, and this has expanded the occupational therapist's role from using mainly curative and rehabilitative approaches to incorporating prevention and promotion strategies (Duncan, Buchanan & Lorenzo, 2005; Watson & Swartz, 2004).

We found it very difficult to decide what our roles need to be in different programmes. We had to realize that we were not going to have leadership roles, but that we are going to support people. Community is a team. Everyone plays different roles that complement each other. It's a journey that you go together. It's a life. The networks in the community are quite amazing. Everybody knows each other. I realized that I couldn't be up at the top looking down; I had to be on ground level and amongst them. Otherwise I wouldn't see the small, little work inside.

The challenge of working with these new approaches to service delivery were particularly evident at learning sites where mental health practitioners and policymakers had succeeded in gaining more prominence for the incorporation of specific mental health policy and related services in the national health plan for the country.

RECOGNIZING PRAXIS

Students experienced 'aha' moments when they recognized specific theory being applied in practice. Many students commented that they understood their role more clearly once they got out there and started doing. Repeated opportunities for students to learn how to apply theory enabled the development of skill or competence. The process of integrating theory into practice provided opportunities for feedback to ensure that teaching and practice remained relevant.

> For me service learning has been a long journey of learning about me (and occupational therapy and clients) but mainly about me. But my greatest lesson during this [placement] was the translation of theory into visible practice. I was able to observe the group process occurring as we had learnt about it in class.

Students discussed the interplay between being a 'person' and a 'professional', and found that often they were not dealing with a problem, or treating a disease as the person was not ill. The personal–professional boundaries had to be continuously negotiated to address the complexities of 'doing' and 'being'. This will be explored further under personal strategies.

OWNERSHIP OF RECIPROCAL LEARNING

Students recognized that learning was a two-way process between themselves and their clients. They learnt the process of identifying and prioritizing client needs together with the person, family and/or caregiver, which resulted in a sense of reciprocity and shared responsibility. It was liberating for students to realize that they did not have to have all the answers, but that solutions could be found together:

They became excited by the sense of agency and interdependence that had developed through recognizing praxis and reciprocal learning. Development of competence in service learning is challenging for both students and educators alike. It needs to be a dynamic process in which students learn to respond to the needs identified at the learning site. It is suggested that the nature of service learning enables students to become equipped for future practice as they have to adjust and develop competence in response to changing needs (Duncan et al., 2005; Watson, 2002).

UNDERSTANDING PARTICIPATION AND WORKING WITH POWER

The richness of learning to 'work in the real world' becomes evident in the students' voices as they develop competence for professional practice. The areas of competence that emerged provide insights into how students begin to understand participation and learn to work with power. Nelson and Wright (1995) commented that participation involves looking at a shift in power and working in partnerships. The students' accounts illustrate how people stand in relation to each other in the different systems (political, economic, family) that are described as power (Nelson & Wright, 1995). Two aspects that merit further exploration are: 'the power to act' and the 'power to take risks'.

THE POWER TO ACT

The power to act reflects students' ability either to engage people in activities, or to develop programmes of action to address identified needs. Students realize they are able to influence service delivery by changing expectations and adjusting goals. In the process, students develop their self-confidence, communication and organizational skills, ability to cooperate and participate in decision making and to self-evaluate. The context also provides the opportunity for them to learn the value of teamwork, collaboration and networking.

Nelson and Wright (1995) found that in everyday encounters, individuals are both reproducing and challenging or changing systematic relations. Students' expectations of the focus of practice change as they find themselves having to shift from providing traditional occupational therapy intervention to addressing basic needs. However, students' experiences also confirmed their power to act and so enable people to gain spaces of control through building their confidence.

Working collectively has greater impact than working alone. The social model of disability calls for a shift in paradigm from seeing disability as a tragedy and individual issue, to viewing it as a social and political issue (Barnes & Mercer, 2004; Oliver, 1996). The disability rights movement has prioritized the development of community-based support systems to provide an organized power base for disabled people from which to build a partnership with professionals (Coleridge, 1993; Finkelstein, 1993). For example, students can learn how to engage disabled peoples' organizations as partners.

Structures, such as parents' support groups, playgroups or day care centres, small business and entrepreneurship projects, provide an organized power base from which disabled people can establish a partnership with professionals. These structures also provide models for other disabled people and the community at large. The partnerships help to break down attitudinal, institutional and physical barriers. They also provide a training ground for developing knowledge and skills of disability and rehabilitation issues for disabled people, caregivers and community members. These participants learn how organizations work and how services are set up. Students learn how professionals can act as allies and resource people.

THE POWER TO TAKE RISKS

Participation is always risky because it challenges local power structures (Nelson & Wright, 1995). Marginalized groups need to access resources so that they can be involved in decision making on a long-term basis. They need to be treated as equal partners in the process of development by people in positions of power. However, any notion of empowerment given by one group to another can hide an attempt to keep control (Nelson & Wright, 1995).

Townsend (1995, p. 12) commented that marginalized people 'show great faith in the power of the written word, the power of experts. They set a great value on our level of education, making them very vulnerable to exploitation.' Students have to continually reflect on personal and professional boundaries. Initially, some students may experience 'power over' the people with whom they work because of a perception of being needed. As friendships are established, they find they have to juggle personal and professional boundaries. Students find themselves in unfamiliar situations where they are compelled to take risks, or to think outside of the occupational therapy box, in order to learn the best way of approaching problems and perceived obstacles. Chambers (1995, p. 42) noted that:

> The new challenges for the 21st-century face the rich and powerful more than the poor and weak, for they concern reversals, giving up things . . . for uppers to give up dominance at the personal level, putting respect in place of superiority, becoming a convenor and provider of occasions, a facilitator and catalyst, a consultant and supporter, is less difficult . . . perhaps one of the biggest opportunities now is to enable more and more uppers to experience those satisfactions personally, and then themselves to spread them upwards, downwards and laterally to their peers.

Students learn to provide structure for themselves, in what are sometimes fairly unstructured work environments, to prevent them from being overwhelmed. As they are often on their own (without a qualified therapist), they learn organizational skills. They become aware of the need to develop essential skills for effective management of community-based rehabilitation projects, such as planning, time management and programme development, problem solving and trust building (Thomas & Thomas, 2002). Students' experiences echo the writings of Gronow (1995), who claimed that before shifting power in a system, the basis of existing and future institutional arrangements need to be well understood. As students become more aware of the complexity of contextual issues and feel more confident in managing them, they are able to identify and value the personal strategies that have helped them make meaningful changes.

PERSONAL STRATEGIES

Students developed competence as they used personal strategies to manage the complex contextual and professional issues of practice.

USING EXISTING RESOURCES CREATIVELY

Students differed in their approach to new tasks and their willingness to take risks and show initiative. In so doing, they learnt about themselves and realized their desire to make a significant contribution in the lives of people with whom they worked. They experienced the ongoing demands of community projects as emotionally draining.

Some students appeared to thrive on accessing resources when they worked in resource-constrained environments, while others found this difficult. Learning to identify potential resources in such contexts requires creative solutions, and is an essential strategy for facilitating the occupational potential in individuals, families and communities.

USING OPPORTUNITIES TO TEACH AND LEARN

The students created structures in what were sometimes fairly unstructured work environments to contain a sense of being overwhelmed. Some students found reflection helped them make sense of their experiences (Buchanan, 2002). Other accounts revealed how they struggled with feelings of inexperience and incompetence in situations where they were given the status of professionals (Lorenzo, 2002). Many students realized that while there was a tendency to hide behind professionalism in institutional settings, this strategy could not be used in the community. Listening was a valuable strategy for learning and developing a growing self-awareness.

> Being left on my own I have learnt in other ways. I realized my potential and limitations. I enjoyed the elderly as they have thought about life, about where they are going, about their families. By listening to them I learnt a lot.

CREATING DIVERSE SUPPORT SYSTEMS

A major consensus amongst all students was feeling valued by community members and not just by project staff. Students found that respect from others increased their confidence in their ability to achieve set goals. This suggests that a 'belief in self' needs to be engendered, whilst simultaneously creating an awareness of personal limitations.

> While I was building a professional image, I felt very fragile. Support from someone who valued me gave me such a boost to hold onto. We all have mental health concerns. I felt like running away – sometimes it got too much being empathetic, being a professional, being an OT.

Varied life experiences help students to develop coping strategies on which they can draw for support. Students were able to support each other, particularly those working at the same learning site. Sharing enabled them to learn to appreciate different interpretations and perceptions of a situation, and helped them realize the need to remain open to different views.

DRAWING ON THEIR SPIRITUALITY

Spirituality was identified as both a strength and a strategy, as students drew on or developed inner resources to manage in contexts that were unfamiliar and often characterized by suffering and unpredictability (Lavin, 2005). Students became aware of existing support systems, such as their family and belief systems (faith, culture and traditions). Feeling hopeful helped them to persevere despite their struggles.

> It's much easier working with people who appreciated me and whom I appreciated. I realized that each one of us is our own person, but we have a lot to give each other. I have learnt that it is all about nurturing myself and people, bodies and souls. It's about trusting yourself.

Some students entered different learning sites with a sense of freedom to explore and discover new things. They realized that having a positive attitude made a difference in managing the challenges. The spiritual qualities of hope, courage, trust, humour and creativity often unlocked hidden potential. Their spirituality offered a sense of agency and a vision of how things actively contributed to achieving the identified goals in collaboration with different role-players.

NEGOTIATING BOUNDARIES TO NURTURE SELF

Students grappled with the issue of boundaries between their personal and professional lives. There was an early realization of the need to protect themselves against burn-out in response to the seemingly never-ending needs of clients. This meant having the confidence to take responsibility for themselves and learning to develop boundaries to ensure emotional well-being. It involved recognizing their own needs, and finding ways to meet these needs. Students realized that as they learnt to develop boundaries to protect emotional well-being despite working with complex issues, they experienced the freedom to discover more about oneself. These life experiences contributed to resilience as seen in their comment 'When you're out there you learn to cope'. They realized that they could only help others if they also cared for themselves.

PROMOTING EMOTIONAL RESOURCEFULNESS

Students seem to have the capacity to develop their sense of agency when 'thrown' into situations they find challenging. These experiences encourage

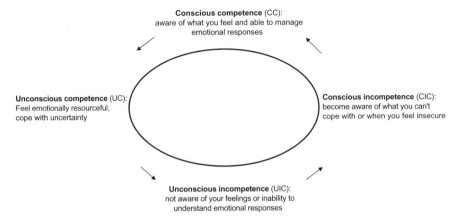

Figure 6.1 The cycle of competence in emotional resourcefulness (adapted from Clarkson, 1994. *The Achilles Syndrome: overcoming the secret fear of failure*, Element Books)

students to develop strategies to help their learning thereby enabling them to become competent for practice. Adapting Clarkson's (1994). four-staged cyclical process of achieving competence (Figure 6.1) is helpful in describing the process students may go through to become emotionally resourceful as part of their professional development. Students are initially unaware of the range of emotions they may experience in different contexts. Once they become aware, they fear not being able to provide adequate intervention, especially in communities different to their own. Through developing personal strategies to manage the changing circumstances in which they work, students gain a degree of emotional resourcefulness. However, in moving to a new learning site, they invariably encounter feelings of emotional and professional incompetence again and so repeat the cycle.

Aspects of power related to becoming emotionally resourceful involve finding a balance between the 'power to interact' and the 'power to protect'.

THE POWER TO INTERACT

Students may experience service learning as a period of emotional volatility. They may fluctuate between feeling at home and welcome to experiencing chaos and uncertainty. This may sometimes spark conflict internally, between peers, with university practice educators, learning facilitators and sometimes with clients and their families. As students become confident in building trust and creating friendships with the people with whom they work, the process of relating becomes a mutual experience of hope and courage in which skills are learnt and outcomes achieved. They begin to realize the power and potential that is unleashed through various interactions. The context of poverty, together with the subsequent marginalization and disablement, enables students to engage in their own vulnerability and the need for resilience and flexibility. Peck's (1987) process of community building may help students make sense of their experiences. Nurturance may be fostered through reciprocity and interdependence, placing value on self-care and support systems. Students may initially appear to be too dependent on other professionals, usually the university practice educator or learning facilitator, but they soon realize the risk of working in a manner that creates dependency. To move through this phase, the students need to identify and remove the barriers to communication, which Peck (1987) categorized as: expectations; stereotypes and biases; differences in theories and ideologies; the need to fix, heal and solve; and, lastly, the need to control.

In African culture, the collective is more important than the individual, as expressed in the African philosophy and spirituality of Ubuntu, which means a person is a person through other people (Tutu, 2004). Relationships and belonging to a group are valued above individual achievement. The struggle against racial apartheid in South Africa was won because of collective mobilization and action, often at the cost of personal sacrifice and individual ambition. Students need to recognize the value of support and respite from their emotional struggles in order to deepen their understanding of professional practice and development.

THE POWER TO PROTECT

The power to protect recognizes the importance of taking care of oneself as much as protecting the rights of the people with whom we work. The nature of connectedness to self and others has been identified as the essence of spirituality (Burgman & King, 2005; Ramugondo, 2005). University practice educators need to guide students in developing the skills and knowledge to cope with their own vulnerability as well as the vulnerability of others. At an unconscious level, students may engage with issues of loss that have not been dealt with previously. Resolving these unconscious issues may necessitate referral to appropriate support structures, such as counselling or spiritual guidance.

Potential is enhanced through the strategies that students use to create harmony and balance in contexts that are unfamiliar and unpredictable. Ramugondo (2005, p. 321) argues that 'through resilience ... we can find our spirituality and the spirituality in turn, strengthens our ability to be resilient'. She found that people who experienced marginalization and oppression developed resilience from resistance and were able to instill this resilience in students. Students who learn to manage feelings of hopelessness and helplessness and are able to reconcile themselves to accepting that it is acceptable not to cope, develop the power to protect themselves against future burn-out (Lorenzo & Cloete, 2004).

Suffering is inevitably associated with spirituality, as people are called to respond to circumstance, adapt or find creative power to bring about change. Iwama's (2005) Kawa model reflects the need to find culturally relevant ways of creating harmony and balance, which may be totally unique in different communities and contexts. Spirituality involves a process of meaning-making and finding purpose in daily activities and rituals (Lavin, 2005). It provides a connection to and expression of emotions. Students need to appreciate the flexibility required to respond to needs that are not directly medical or rehabilitative in nature.

CONCLUSION

This chapter has explored the emerging competence students develop as they grapple with contextual issues in practice learning. Students who are given the opportunity to learn in demanding situations seem well equipped to work within a variety of contexts. This observation raises a question about the extent to which educators are able to prepare students adequately for working in complex contexts. Alternatively, as students process their struggles in these contexts, is it possible that they develop strategies that help them practise effectively in these contexts? Do we, as university practice educators or learning facilitators, create spaces where students are able to speak about the inner issues or conflicts that professionals are called to manage?

To ensure that students are well prepared for working in a variety of contexts, they need to become catalysts for change in their world of work where issues of marginalization, discrimination and subsequent inequity are addressed at the same time as professional and emotional competence is achieved and maintained (Duncan et al., 2005). Students seem to be able to learn to be effective no matter what the circumstances of the learning site. They come to appreciate the difference they can make and the relevance of occupational therapy in complex contexts.

REFERENCES

Barnes, C. & Mercer, G. (Eds.) (2004). *Implementing the social model of disability: Theory and research.* Leeds: The Disability Press.

Bossers, A., Miller, L., Polatajko, H. & Hartley, M. (2002). *Competency based fieldwork evaluation for occupational therapists.* Albany, New York: Delmar Thomson Learning.

Buchanan, H. (2002). *South African contextual factors: impact on occupational therapy student learning, education and practice.* Poster presented at the 13th World Congress of the World Federation of Occupational Therapists, Stockholm, Sweden, June.

Buchanan, H., Van Niekerk, L. & Moore, R. (2001). Assessing fieldwork journals: developmental portfolios. *British Journal of Occupational Therapy,* 64(8), 398–402.

Burgman, I. & King, A. (2005). The presence of child spirituality: surviving in a marginalized world. In F. Kronenberg, S. Algado & N. Pollard (Eds.), *Occupational therapy without borders – learning from the spirit of survivors.* Edinburgh: Elsevier Churchill Livingstone, pp. 152–165.

Chambers, R. (1993). *Challenging the professions: frontiers for rural development.* London: Intermediate Technology Publications.

Chambers, R. (1995). Paradigm shifts and the practice of participatory research and development. In N. Nelson & S. Wright (Eds.), *Power and participatory development: theory and practice.* London: Intermediate Technology Publications, pp. 30–42.

Clarkson, P. (1994). *The Achilles Syndrome: overcoming the secret fear of failure.* Dorset: Element Books.

Coleridge, P. (1993). *Disability, liberation and development.* Oxford: Oxfam.

Duncan, M., Buchanan, H. & Lorenzo, T. (2005). Politics in occupational therapy education: a South African perspective. In F. Kronenberg, S. Algado & N. Pollard (Eds.), *Occupational therapy without borders – learning from the spirit of survivors.* Edinburgh: Elsevier Churchill Livingstone, pp. 390–401.

Finkelstein, V. (1993). Disability: a social challenge or an administrative responsibility. In J. Swain, V. Finkelstein, S. French & M. Oliver (Eds.), *Disabling barriers, enabling environments.* London: Sage, pp. 34–43.

Gronow, H. (1995). Shifting power, sharing power: issues for user-group forestry in Nepal. In N. Nelson & S. Wright (Eds.), *Power and participatory development: theory and practice.* London: Intermediate Technology Publications, pp. 125–132.

Higgs, J., Richardson, B. & Duhlgren, M.A. (Eds.) (2005). *Developing practice knowledge for health professionals.* Oxford: Butterworth-Heinemann.

Hope, A. & Timmel, S. (1995). *Training for transformation: a handbook for community workers (Books 1–3).* Gweru, Zimbabwe: Mambo Press.

Iwama, M. (2005). The Kawa (river) model: nature, life flow and the power of culturally relevant occupational therapy. In F. Kronenberg, S. Algado & N. Pollard (Eds.), *Occupational therapy without borders – learning from the spirit of survivors.* Edinburgh: Elsevier Churchill Livingstone, pp. 213–227.

Jarvis, P. (2001). Questioning the learning society. In P. Jarvis (Ed.), *The age of learning, education and the knowledge society.* London: Kogan Press, pp. 195–204.

Lavin, B. (2005). Occupation under occupation: days of conflict and curfew in Bethlehem. In F. Kronenberg, S. Algado & N. Pollard (Eds.), *Occupational therapy without borders – learning from the spirit of survivors.* Edinburgh: Elsevier Churchill Livingstone, pp. 40–45.

Lorenzo, T. (2002). *Developing competence for partnership: the voice of occupational therapy students in Cape Town.* Poster presented at the 13th World Congress of the World Federation of Occupational Therapists, Stockholm, Sweden, June.

Lorenzo, T. & Cloete, L. (2004). Promoting occupations in rural communities. In R. Watson & L. Swartz (Eds.), *Transformation through occupation.* London: Whurr, pp. 268–286.

Nelson, N. & Wright, S. (Eds.), (1995). *Power and participatory development: theory and practice.* London: Intermediate Technology Publications.

Oliver, M. (1996). *Understanding disability: from theory to practice.* London: Macmillan.

Peck, M.S. (1987). *The different drum. The creation of true community - the first step to world peace.* London: Arrow Books.

Ramugondo, E. (2005). Unlocking spirituality: play as a health-promoting occupation in the context of HIV/AIDS. In F. Kronenberg, S. Algado & N. Pollard (Eds.), *Occupational therapy without borders – learning from the spirit of survivors.* Edinburgh: Elsevier Churchill Livingstone, pp. 313–325.

Schön, D.A. (1991). *The reflective turn: case studies in and on educational practice.* New York: Teachers College Press.

Taylor, J., Marais, D. & Kaplan, A. (1997). *Action learning for development: use you experience to improve your effectiveness.* Cape Town: Juta and CDRA.

Taylor, V. & Conradie, I. (1997). *'We have been taught by life itself' Empowering women as leaders: the role of development education.* University of Western Cape: SADEP.

Thomas, M. & Thomas, M.J. (2002). Some controversies in community based rehabilitation. In S. Hartley (Ed.), *CBR: a participatory strategy in Africa.* London: University College London, pp. 13–25.

Townsend, J. (1995). Who speaks for whom? Outsiders re-present women pioneers of the forests of Mexico. In N. Nelson & S. Wright (Eds.), *Power and participatory development: theory and practice.* London: Intermediate Technology Publications, pp. 83–94.

Tutu, D. (2004). *God has a dream: a vision of hope for our time.* Johannesburg: Rider.

Watson, R.M. (2002). Competence: a transformative approach. *WFOT Bulletin, 45,* 7–11.

Watson, R. & Swartz, L. (Eds.) (2004). *Transformation through occupation.* London: Whurr.

7 Role-Emerging Settings, Service Learning and Social Change

ROSHAN GALVAAN

OBJECTIVES

This chapter discusses:

- the professional values that guide practice education in role-emerging settings
- service learning as a contributor to social change
- an approach for optimizing reciprocal learning and development within the community context.

INTRODUCTION

Many of the insights introduced in this chapter arose from my reflections as an occupational therapy practice educator on students' learning processes at a role-emerging occupational therapy service site at a number of health promoting schools on the Cape flats, Cape Town. (The details and background information about the *Facing Up* project can be found in Chapter 3.) I started the service in 2000 and, together with an off-site, voluntary occupational therapist, have been involved since then in discerning what the profession may offer in this context (Galvaan, 2004). Bossers, Cook, Polatajko and Laine (1997, p. 71) describe role-emerging occupational therapy services as occurring at 'sites that do not have an occupational therapy programme, nor an established occupational therapy role. Here, the health student establishes and implements an occupational therapy role'. The student is assigned a university lecturer (in this instance myself as practice educator) as a contact person for site-related issues, and is supervised by an off-site occupational therapist (in this instance the voluntary occupational therapist).

In this chapter, critical issues arising from the impact of role-emerging services on student learning are discussed. The demands placed on students and practice educators when working developmentally in a new service area such

Practice and Service Learning in Occupational Therapy. Edited by Theresa Lorenzo, Madeleine Duncan, Helen Buchanan, Auldeen Alsop

as *Facing Up* are described and principles for managing the many challenges are suggested. The process of change that occurs at many levels for various role-players frames the discussion and raises questions about the potential of service learning as a humble contributor to social change.

LEARNING AND SOCIAL CHANGE IN ROLE-EMERGING SERVICE SETTINGS

Role-emerging occupational therapy services developed at *Facing Up* in response to an interpretation of the contextual needs of local youth. *Facing Up* was initiated within a 'development mindset of possibility', which according to Pieterse and Meintjies (2004), is based on the belief that personal development is possible and that people have the potential to become agents of positive social change. Giddens (2001, p. 698) suggests that social change is ever present and defines it as 'alteration in the basic structures of a social group or society'. The Black Consciousness Movement, based on liberation philosophies and ideologies, made a major contribution to social change in South Africa. The country's journey into post-apartheid South Africa continues to be marked by significant social change. This is evident in the continued efforts towards addressing social divides through social transformation initiatives in historically marginalized communities, such as the one in which *Facing Up* is located. *Facing Up* is based on values that affirm Black Consciousness and aims to conscientise individuals so that they become active agents of change in their local sphere of influence by assuming a positive identity (Biko, 2004).

Occupational therapy literature indicates that the profession does not yet have an established protocol for practice aimed at promoting social change. Although a number of authors have alluded to this emerging domain of practice, very little has been documented about the actual principles, processes and epistemological foundations on which the profession may build in this new and challenging field (Townsend,1993). While occupational therapy's contribution to redressing societal influences, such as poverty or violence, on occupational performance is still unclear, the growing body of occupational science literature about the value of occupation as a catalyst for change provides helpful indicators to guide the actions of therapists (Townsend & Wilcock, 2004). However, learning in an environment that has rudimentary principles rather than established professional procedures is challenging because it requires practitioners, educators and students to 'think outside the box' and to grapple with their personal-political ideologies. Some people become enthused by such challenges, others feel frustrated by the demands placed on their emotional 'comfort zones', whilst others are paralysed by the apparent lack of clear direction. Students' experiences in role-emerging occupational therapy settings, where they have to deal with the unfamiliar, with ambiguities in their experiences and personal disjunction, appear to be similar to those the literature suggests they experience during problem-based learning

(Savin-Baden, 2000). This points to the possibility that the kind of learning that occurs in role-emerging settings may contribute to social change. The following section describes the learning experiences that are facilitated for all participants when an occupational therapy programme explicitly holds ideals of contributing to social change through the actions and attitudes of students, educators and learning facilitators. It details the demands that are placed on students, illustrates how they are likely to respond and makes suggestions about how to enhance learning for social change.

LEARNING AS A CONTRIBUTOR TO SOCIAL CHANGE

Learning can be facilitated in ways that produce change for students by enabling them to reimagine their identities. The primary school learners with whom students work, can also, through consciously exploring and creating a changed occupational self, experience positive shifts in their identity. Learning that leads to expanded understanding and insight involves: deliberate consideration of facts and perspectives; seeking alternative ways of looking at the world; discussing possible outcomes of various choices; and (sometimes) experiencing the consequences of ill-considered choices. Social change is manifested through the process and outcome of learning for the students and through social engagement in a development space for the learners. The learners experience a shift in their occupational selves as a result of responding to invitations by occupational therapists and students to explore alternative ways of interpreting, engaging with, and acting in their world. Students, in reflecting on ways to bring about social change within a liberating ideology and through witnessing the outcomes of their work with learners, begin to experience their own emancipation as agents of change. They come to appreciate subtle nuances of change in learners' sense of identity, seldom expecting or trying to manipulate major behavioural shifts but celebrating those moments when learners take a stand against the oppression of their social context. Students also begin to adopt this stance towards their own learning. The goal of occupational therapy becomes the multiplication of moments or instances of liberation in individual learners and students; adding up over time to a more positive self-identity, which, in turn, influences the social sphere within which they live. Students who adopt an alternative stance to learning come to appreciate the significance of this goal and the personal-professional values that support its attainment.

LEARNING THROUGH NEGOTIATING THE
LEARNER'S STANCE

Stance refers to 'one's attitude, belief or disposition towards a particular context, person or experience' (Savin-Baden, 2000, p. 56). The primary task of the practice educator at *Facing Up* is to facilitate the student's ability for critical enquiry into their personal stance through reflection on and in action. The emphasis of reflection is on exploring multiple interpretations of reality, for example world-views, values and fundamental beliefs about society, difference and power. Documented literature on reflection addresses its role in clinical reasoning (Buchanan, van Niekerk & Moore, 2001). Reflection for and on social change is less concerned with 'clinical' reasoning and more concerned with social critique and transitional learning (Savin-Baden, 2000). Transitional learning refers to shifts in the learner orchestrated by shifts in their life-world. Shifts, such as deeper appreciation of human poverties (Max-Neef, 1991) and the consequences of social injustice, are triggered through critical reflection on the unfolding changes in learners' personal, pedagogical and interactional stance as they engage with the dynamics of the context. Building relationships with learners and other significant role-players in historically disadvantaged communities, and being willing to interrogate their own learning stance, mirrors or complements, for the students, the same process that is facilitated within the learners. They move towards 'becoming' the social change themselves that is desired in the context and ultimately in the learners.

The ensuing discussion describes each of the stances in the student's experience of learning. Difficulties are identified and principles for negotiating these and for enhancing perspective transformation are suggested.

FACILITATING THE PERSONAL STANCE

The personal stance (Savin-Baden, 2000) describes the way that educators, learning facilitators and students see themselves in relation to the learning context. This 'way of seeing' is shaped, for example, by personal history and enculturation into a particular set of beliefs about the world. It gives meaning to the way in which they make sense of and engage with the context. Shifts in the personal stance may be precipitated by a sense of fragmentation, which in turn leads to a willingness to discover the 'self' in and through the 'other'.

Fragmentation

Fragmentation refers to situations in the domain of personal stance where 'students experience challenges to their values and beliefs, which appear to be at risk or are threatened through this challenge and resultant uncertainty' (Savin-Baden, 2000, p. 59). The example presented here is particular to post-apartheid South Africa, but may apply to any social or practice education situation where disparity exists between the life-world of students and the people with whom they work as a result of historical, socio-economic, religious, political, class or other forms of priviledge and/or disadvantage. By 2004, ten years after South Africa's liberation, most occupational therapy students at the University of Cape Town (UCT) had not had the opportunity to form relationships with black and coloured people. The majority of the students studying occupational therapy at the University are white females from the middle and upper socio-economic classes. This contrasts sharply with the predominantly black racial profile of the community within which *Facing Up* is located.

Facing Up presents students with the opportunity to learn about and form relationships with a part of the South African population that they may not have been concerned about or intimately interacted with before. The Cape Coloured culture is conveyed through a colloquial English and Afrikaans dialect (commonly called 'kombuis', or 'kitchen', Afrikaans) (Erasmus, 2001). Unfamiliar with kombuis Afrikaans and the way of life on the Cape Flats, students arrive at *Facing Up* with preconceptions that need to be modified in order to engage fully with the learning opportunities at hand. Their different experiences of social class, race and culture places the responsibility on them to learn about, and from, local residents in order to recognize capacity and opportunities for agentic action. Learning becomes more than just 'getting to know' and 'treating' an individual client. It becomes an opportunity for appreciating the rich diversity of people and cultures in South Africa and for exploring ways in which locally relevant forms of professional action can contribute to social development. Personal stances shift when parts of 'the self' are discovered in relationship with 'the other' (Savin-Baden, 2000).

Discovering the Self in Order to Discover the Other

It takes emotional, physical and spiritual effort and maturity to understand the community and the culture that is valued by its members. The ability to recognize the strengths and areas that need to change within a community is directly related to the students' ability to reflect on their belief in their own capacity and potential. They therefore need to become aware of the following:

- how they manage the unknown
- their ability to find and generate affirmation by looking for cues that indicate the positive influences of occupational therapy
- their ability to challenge existing stereotypes and prejudice they may hold

The learning expectation here is both academic and personal. The personal learning, although often implicit, creates a resilient, resourceful occupational therapist. However, it has to be recognized as an academic exercise so that students can make professional sense of the attitudinal change that occurs within them.

Students usually enter the geographical location of *Facing Up* anxious about their physical safety, possibly because of their lack of familiarity with the group of people and stereotypes about poverty and violence in the surrounding community. This anxiety exacerbates the disjunction they experience when challenged by psychological, social and spiritual questions, arising from the context, for which they have no answers. Disjunction refers to a sense of fragmentation of part of the self and is characterized by frustration and anger and a need for the right answers (Savin-Baden, 2000, p. 56). One student wrote the following in her reflective journal:

> I saw the opportunity as an obstacle. I felt as though I was under extra pressure to create a good impression and set a high standard. It was difficult not having an example of previous work done.

Whilst *Facing Up* presented her with a learning challenge that needed to be negotiated, she would still have preferred an established framework for action. Disjunction may cause students to experience a range of negative emotions that have to be contained through appropriate educational and support structures. The student had also internalized expectations associated with the development of the *Facing Up* occupational therapy programme believing that it would, through students' (like her) involvement, make a difference. She expected ready-made answers and information on how to deliver this.

There is often an assumption that if the learning facilitator and/or practice educator has the expertise (which they do not, given the fact that it is a role-emerging service site), they should be able to provide the necessary information in the form of clear answers. Processing the disjunction through explicit learning activities paves the way for students to recognize what may be entailed in promoting social change in and through the learners. Their personal, internal journey of 'self-discovery' becomes the framework for external action that leads to the discovery of 'the other'.

Facilitating Discovery of the 'Other' and Perceiving the 'Future Self'

Initially the approach to practice education was to meet with the students before they went to *Facing Up* in order to discuss their concerns and expectations. It was hoped that this would contain them, as they would be made aware of possible disjunction and start working on this. The university practice educator assisted the students to familiarize themselves with the service learning setting by having open discussions about what they already knew about the community and how they felt about working there. This led to honest acknowledgment of students' fears and the stereotypes and myths surrounding the community. The supervisor then offered another perspective through providing information on the school and community in the form of newspaper clippings and photographs of people engaging in occupations. This was supplemented by providing documented narratives of the lives of the children and adults.

It soon became evident, however, that, despite preparing students and their subsequent positive intentions, the reality of the disjunction was only felt once they were actually in the service learning setting. This led to the use of transitional learning, that is, rather than specifically preparing students to enter the setting, the emergent opportunities to explore personal psychological, spiritual and social questions would be used to deal with disjunction as it arose. This educational approach calls, on the one hand, on the students' patience and perseverance, and, on the other hand, on the university practice educator's or learning facilitator's ability to recognize instances of disjunction and to coach students through the reflective learning process.

A tacit service learning expectation is that students have the emotional capacity and strength to suspend and contain their own emotional experience and to use themselves as a change agent to benefit the learners. Successful engagement in this process will contribute to the growth of the profession in South Africa so that it is more relevant to the needs of the country. At times, this demand is in conflict with personal events in a student's life. The necessary mechanisms then need to be identified and put in place to enable the students to fulfill the learning expectation.

Assisting students to geographically orientate themselves to the context helps them to feel more secure. They realize that the community where *Facing Up* is based is en route to a beach area with which most of them are familiar. Further orientation within the physical environment of the schools and surrounding community assists students to appreciate how context may shape a learner's life story. This orientation presents the opportunity for students to dispute their political view and personal prejudices. Learning occurs through discussions with the university practice educator and literature is used to orientate students to the socio-political history of the area and its people and how, for example, the legacy of apartheid continues to influence the dynamics within the community. This transitional approach to learning and to dealing with disjunction acknowledges and values who the students are, while gaining an appreciation for learners as the 'other'. They are expected to be sufficiently resourceful to create the necessary support and learning infrastructures for themselves. This requires the student to feel comfortable enough to engage with the fragmentation that they experience. This experience is grounded in a threat to the student's value and belief system.

Students are challenged to find the connection between their roles at *Facing Up* and themselves as future professionals. This demands that they have a vision of where they see themselves practising as a graduate and, in understanding what they need to contribute at *Facing Up*, how this may influence their personal professional vision. This reflection on the values of *Facing Up* could also result in fragmentation of their future vision, for example, possibly only serving an elite segment of the South African population. Achieving success at *Facing Up* sometimes means changing one's values. This is influenced by the way one learns.

FACILITATING THE PEDAGOGICAL STANCE

This stance refers to the way in which one's identity as a learner is viewed. It is constructed through a combination of prior learning experiences and the extent to which learning experiences have been successful (Savin-Baden, 2000).

Moving from 'Not Knowing' to 'Knowing How' to Apply Own Knowledge

The students' approach to learning influences how they engage with the knowledge generation and application process at *Facing Up*. Some students respond to the learning demands at *Facing Up* with enthusiasm and others with despair and anger. Some manage to excel. Others struggle to discover and to develop occupational therapy theory to substantiate and guide practice in this role-emerging setting. Frustration and despair cannot be equated with learning; in fact these emotions are counterproductive. Pedagogical strategies that point students to potential sources of knowledge and ways of generating evidence for appropriate actions therefore need to be made available in a timely way.

Strategies of Knowing

Students are given guidance on the philosophy and basic theoretical framework of the *Facing Up* occupational therapy programme that has evolved to date. They are required to access and interpret a range of related literature and apply it as evidence for how they practise in the context. This approach leaves them feeling 'unclear' about what is expected as if a prescribed format for action exists. Students often express antagonism towards the University and the service learning facilitator for placing, what they perceive to be 'high demands', on them in this setting. They intimate that they have been insufficiently prepared and that what they are being required to do is unreasonable. Their pedagogical stance begins to shift as they learn to use their previous knowledge and build on their emerging experience within the context. They come to appreciate that, by tolerating their mixed emotions and 'not knowing', and by being open to the learning experience, they discover what they need to know when they need to know it.

Sladyk (2002) stressed that to develop positive learning attributes, students should not expect always to equate learning with liking. Since students expect to 'like' the learning, they experience tension upon entering service learning settings and struggle to hold on to their positive attitude(s) to learning. At *Facing Up* students are required to be open to knowledge from all sources to enable them to learn whilst laying the foundation for practice. An autonomous style of learning leads them to previously untapped sources of information, thereby contributing to novel forms of practice.

The academic expectation is that students have, or gain insight into, regional political agendas and social development principles so that they act on this within the occupational therapy programme. For example, the programme aims to confront the risk behaviour that children engage in and to address the negative impact of health-compromising occupational choices on their development and their community whilst also respecting the principle of self-determination. Biko (1978) claimed that the concept of self-determination is essential for ensuring that one group of people is not thwarted by another. This means that students learn to work with the learners and teachers at the school on their self-identified problems, rather than trying to 'fix' problems that appear to be of significance according to their professional insights.

For example, one fourth-year student had difficulty evaluating the progress being made by group members. She questioned: 'If some children can be positive, then why can't others be?' She struggled to shift from labelling and potentially blaming some learners for being negative, to perceiving her role as an occupational therapist as valuing the learner's potential to create more positive ways of being and doing for his- or herself. Initially she thought that she had to fix the identified problem(s) rather than contribute towards social change. Had this student recognized that she had to learn or draw on experience of how to use oneself as an agent, holding on to the potential for change, she may have viewed the outcome of her actions, and the progress of the group, differently.

Negotiating Access to Knowing

The learning facilitator and university practice educator, and the students' personal stances each influence the learning experiences of the other. The facilitator's perspective on what has to be learnt may be in contrast to what the student feels they need or is required to learn. That is, students may not believe that becoming an occupational therapist means valuing 'the other' in ways that spark their potential to become all that they are able to be, and through this approach contribute to social change. A forum where this approach to learning and practice can honestly and openly be addressed on an ongoing basis is necessary. Remaining aware that the students, like the learning facilitator and university practice educator, are 'small' in comparison to the community's contextual dilemmas is the first step towards a liberating personal stance. The learning facilitator, practice educator and students have to contain their, sometimes overwhelming, sense of responsibility and ensuing anxiety. An ongoing process of addressing assumptions helps students and their learning facilitators and university practice educators to find their purpose and contribution to the service learning setting by reconstructing an alternative reality of occupational engagement amongst learners.

Whether the service is effective or most appropriate at its present stage of development is debatable (Galvaan, 2004). The tension of not knowing needs to be held lightly because the 'How do I know if what I am doing is the right thing if no one has done this before?' question will only be answered once the service has been fully developed and evaluated. This requires time and perseverance in interacting with a range of people in the learning context.

FACILITATING THE INTERACTIONAL STANCE

This stance encapsulates the manner in which the learner interacts with others in the learning context (Savin-Baden, 2000). The way in which the student builds and maintains relationships is influenced by their pedagogical and personal stance.

Individualism

Final-year students are placed in pairs at *Facing Up*. They are expected to interact with the volunteer learning facilitator (occupational therapist), the university practice educator, the teachers, learners and the learners' parents. The quality of these interactions shapes the learning and development of all participants in the change process.

For example, let us consider the interactional stance of a group of second-year occupational therapy students who were placed at *Facing Up* for one week. Their task was to conduct a context-related assessment and to identify a health promotion product that would educate the identified recipients appropriately. The students identified the high illiteracy rate as limiting the young adolescents' occupational choices. They recognized that learners were only reading academically and not for fun. Having interviewed the relevant role-players, the students, with the university practice educator's guidance, recognized that two main factors were at the root of this problem. The first was that many parents were illiterate and thus did not read to children when they were young, and secondly that no leisure reading books were available to the children either in their homes or at school.

The students then accessed resources and within a short space of time were able to attract a large donation of suitable books. They also facilitated a meeting between interested parents and a teacher to investigate the possibility of group storytelling sessions. These students were able to respond to the identified need by taking the risk of interacting proactively with others and depending on them to make their project a success. Through the students taking this risk, they modelled a way of doing within the school system that indicated that small steps could be taken as a start to approaching widespread problems.

At a second-year level this interactional stance was considered appropriate. At a fourth-year level, when students interact within the context for between six and ten weeks, a more developmental approach would be expected. Rather than the students themselves accessing resources and attracting a large donation of suitable books, they would be expected to coach senior learners in owning the reading project so that learners would become equipped with skills for accessing resources (for example, writing letters, making phone calls), managing the distribution of books (for example, setting up and running an informal loan library) and acting as a buddy reader to a younger child. Through taking a developmental interactional stance, students unlock the potential within learners to become agents of change themselves rather than relying on the students to do the work for them.

A Binary Perspective

The necessary creativity is blocked when students do not shift their polarized view of 'us' and 'them'. A fourth-year student experienced real difficulty empathizing with the young adolescents. She doubted that she could valuably contribute to the programme and resisted engaging with the children's sub-jective experience beyond acknowledging their social discomfort and emo-tional pain. She formed superficial relationships with learners and avoided interaction with teachers. Her apparent contempt towards the university prac-tice educator and the context was clear during supervision sessions when she opposed attempts to engage her in dialogue about her interactional stance. Her goal was to survive the service-learning placement without having to get too involved, and her approach to the programme became mediocre and pro-cedural. The practice educator could not facilitate a shift in the student's inter-actional stance and had to acknowledge that she was learning by enduring her time at *Facing Up*.

Occupational therapists have different functions. The student's interactional stance indicated that she was not at a stage of her personal–professional development to engage with the function of becoming an agent of social change. The disjunction between the university practice educator and the student's personal stances was difficult to resolve perhaps because of the high value and priority that the educator places on developing occupational therapy services that contribute towards social change. The university practice educator has to be aware of, and deal with, her own attitudes and introjec-tions, as well as the potential projections from students that arise as a result of different interactional stances. Whilst facilitating student learning at *Facing Up*, it became apparent that whoever does the teaching also influences stu-dents' receptiveness to learning. The knowledge source needs to be valued so that meaning can be interpreted in relation to its credibility. Learning is com-promised when a binary perspective is adopted, for example, if the source is undervalued as a result of markedly different world-views, values and belief systems, then the resultant resistance may stifle creativity and an exploratory attitude.

Synchronizing Information

Supervision in pairs, rather than individual sessions is used as a strategy for helping students synchronize information and make sense of their learning as a collective. The students' interactional stance is further facilitated through group tutorial sessions. Students are also encouraged to synchronize information through proactive data gathering from multiple sources.

Another fourth-year student used a reflective approach to learning that allowed her to openly express her feeling of being overwhelmed, but she still wanted to learn as much as she could. This student's learning was also strategic in that she acknowledged the value to the profession of being innovative at *Facing Up*. She openly respected the political stand that was being taken and appreciated the opportunity to work with the unknown. She obtained information from the existing community, teachers, learning facilitator and learners in order to build a knowledge base to inform her service learning. She used this base to deepen her awareness of how familiar occupations were performed differently by the learners. She felt validated by her agentic[1] knowledge generation and realized that she had skills that could be used at *Facing Up*. As a result, she felt able to plan successful group sessions, having a clearer appreciation of the philosophy, values and purposes guiding the decisions of social change agents.

INTEGRATING LEARNING STANCES TO ENHANCE CAPACITY TO BE AGENTS OF SOCIAL CHANGE

Knowing how to learn and facilitate learning in a role-emerging setting is like carving the role and developing the occupational therapy service. That is, the answers are learnt through doing and reflecting and occur through the process of contributing to community development. The fact that the doing has to happen before the student feels confident about their knowledge or competent in their skills is a possible source of tension. This final section attempts to describe some of the mechanisms that facilitate negotiation during and for learning. These mechanisms are intended to assist the students to progress through the various stances so that they are able to effectively contribute to social change.

Terre Blanche and Durrheim (1999) recognized that the way in which we provide accounts of situations is based on our background knowledge. This background knowledge tells us what exists, how to understand it and how to engage with it. The students, in collaboration with the university practice educator and the community, have to reconstruct this background knowledge and find a way of changing what they see. The student, as a social scientist, is encouraged to adopt an interpretive and constructionist approach.

---

[1] 'Agentic' refers to self-directed agency in applying personal power to author choices. According to Polkinghorne (1995, p. 301), agentic individuals are 'clear on what they want to accomplish, understand how intended actions will contribute to their accomplishments and are confident that they can complete the intended actions and attain their goals'.

INTERPRETIVE APPROACH TO INTEGRATING LEARNING STANCES

Within the interpretive approach (Terre Blanche & Durrheim, 1999) the student is compelled to explore the subjective meanings behind the learners' occupational engagement. Open discussions about what is known about the community and how students feel about working there are facilitated. Naming and admitting to the fears, stereotypes and myths surrounding *Facing Up* as a service learning setting is vital to the process of gaining insight and changing personal and interactional stances. Another strategy is to provide information on the schools and community through newspaper clippings, narratives and photographs of people engaging in occupations. Students are invited to use their existing competencies in dealing with diversity in order to make sense of the disjunction that they may experience in the face of working cross-culturally.

CONSTRUCTIONIST APPROACH TO INTEGRATING LEARNING STANCES

Within the constructionist approach (Giddens, 2001), the practice educator aids the student in defining what and how occupational therapy discourse is constructed and how it may be interpreted. The discourse in occupational therapy literature is deconstructed in order to uncover what possible meanings and applications could be of relevance within *Facing Up*. Furthermore, the language that the teachers, children and community members use and the symbolic meanings of kombuis Afrikaans and dialectic English are analysed. This deepens the student's understanding of the social setting and serves as a cue for what issues need to be pursued.

The last and possibly the most fundamental mechanism is that of attributing value to the work being done at *Facing Up*. The need for the service is unquestionable. Students have to be convinced through literature and through facilitating commitment to social change that the problems identified are serious enough to require the redefinition of traditional perspectives of occupational therapy. This shift is possible through observing the impact of incremental changes and valuing the long-term collective contribution of a programme such as *Facing Up*. This involves seeing that, although one therapist may be limited as a person, working with a community on the same goals, much could be achieved over time. The student who only works at *Facing Up* for eight or nine weeks has to appreciate the invaluable contribution they make, no matter how small the shifts may appear on the surface. If this is achieved, then the potential to contribute to social change is ignited. Students begin to act on a political orientation that puts commonly held positive notions about social and occupational justice into occupational therapy programmes of action (Townsend & Wilcock, 2004).

CONCLUSION

This chapter has argued that developing occupational therapy services to address local South African needs, requires that occupational therapists consider how they influence groups and communities. It has presented examples of how students may be prepared to do this by addressing their personal, pedagogical and interactive stances. Most people who decide to become occupational therapists do so because they want to help individuals. Students experience substantial disjunction when their motivation to 'help' individuals has to be replaced with a substantially different professional stance that adopts a socio-political position to practice. This stance means redefining occupational therapy's outcomes and interpreting theory and practice in a distinctly different way. The subsequent conflict that an individual student may experience has to be worked with to enable transitional learning to occur. Transitional learning enables students and practice educators to embrace their roles as agents of social change at an individual and community level, whilst simultaneously shaping new forms of occupational therapy practice.

ACKNOWLEDGEMENT

The author wishes to acknowledge the contributions made by all students who have had service learning experiences at *Facing Up,* and in particular Loren Rubenstein.

REFERENCES

Biko, S. (1978). Black souls in white skins? In S. Biko (Ed.), *I write what I like.* Johannesburg: Picador Africa, Craighall, pp. 20–29.

Biko, N. (2004). Introduction. In S. Biko (Ed.), *I write what I like.* Johannesburg: Picador Africa, Craighall, p. xv.

Bossers, A., Cook, J., Polatajko, H. & Laine, C. (1997). Understanding the role-emerging placement. *Canadian Journal of Occupational therapy, 64*(1), 70–81.

Buchanan, H., Van Niekerk, L. & Moore, R. (2001). Assessing fieldwork journals: developmental portfolios. *British Journal of Occupational Therapy, 64*(8), 398–402.

Erasmus, Z. (2001). Introduction: Re-imagining coloured identities in post-apartheid South Africa. In Z. Erasmus (Ed.), *Coloured by history, shaped by place. New perspectives on coloured identities in Cape Town.* Cape Town: Kwela Books and South African History Online, pp. 13–28.

Galvaan, R. (2004). Engaging with youth at risk. In R. Watson & L. Swartz (Eds.), *Transformation through occupation.* London: Whurr, pp. 186–197.

Giddens, A. (2001). *Sociology,* 4th edn. Cambridge: Polity.

Max-Neef, M. (1991). *Human scale development: conception, application and further replections.* London: Apex Press.

Pieterse, E. & Meintjies, F. (2004). Introduction: framing the politics, poetics and practices of social change in the new South Africa. In E. Pieterse & F. Meintjies (Eds.), *Voices of the transition: the politics, poetics and practices of social change in South Africa.* Sandown: Heinemann, pp 2–12.

Polkinghorne, D.E. (1995). Transformative narratives: from victimic to agentic life plots. *American Journal of Occupational Therapy, 50*(4), 299–305.

Savin-Baden, M. (2000). *Problem based learning in higher education: Untold stories.* Buckingham: Society for Research into Higher Education and Open University Press.

Sladyk, K. (Ed.) (2002). *The successful occupational therapy fieldwork student.* Thorofare, NJ: Slack.

Terre Blanche, M. & Durrheim, K. (1999). Social constructionist methods. In M. Terre Blache & K. Durrheim (Eds.), *Research in Practice.* Cape Town: University of Cape Town Press, pp. 147–188.

Townsend, E. (1993). The Muriel Driver Lecture: Occupational therapy's social vision. *Canadian Journal of Occupational Therapy, 67*(1), 61–69.

Townsend, E. & Wilcock, A. (2004). Occupational justice. In C. Christiansen & E. Townsend (Eds.), *Introduction to occupation: the art and science of doing.* New Jersey: Prentice Hall, pp. 243–273.

8 Group Learning Experiences in Rural Communities

FASLOEN ADAMS and HEATHER WONNACOTT

OBJECTIVES

This chapter discusses:

- the learning that students can acquire through a rural service learning experience
- the rationale for this experience within the evolution of the profession and of South Africa's health system
- how students address personal issues relating to diversity
- the outcomes, drawing on students' journalled experiences.

BACKGROUND

As South Africa enters its second decade of democracy, the health sector is in a process of transformation. Influenced by the constitution, our national health policies are attempting to incorporate principles of democracy, social justice, human rights and equity to redress past inequalities (Duncan, Buchanan & Lorenzo, 2005), thus ensuring health for all. To this end, a Primary Health Care (PHC) Approach (World Health Organization, 1978), has been adopted by the Department of Health (1997) in the planning of comprehensive health services.

The main focus of the PHC approach is to ensure: equitable distribution and redistribution of resources; community involvement; a focus on prevention of health-related problems; the promotion of health; the use of appropriate technology; and a multi-sectoral approach (Department of Health, 1997). This approach advocates a shift from traditional health practices, which only focused on curative and rehabilitative intervention, to a more comprehensive approach that also incorporates primary and secondary prevention as well as health promotion (Department of Health, 1997). Consequently, the context in which health services are being offered shifts (Duncan et al., 2005), with the bulk of services being moved from tertiary to primary levels of care.

Practice and Service Learning in Occupational Therapy. Edited by Theresa Lorenzo, Madeleine Duncan, Helen Buchanan, Auldeen Alsop
© 2006 John Wiley & Sons Ltd

In many places, occupational therapy as a profession has been aligning itself with the PHC approach for decades. Since the 1960s, the focus of practice has expanded to include the social context (Watson, 2004), and the role of occupational therapy within the public health sector has moved beyond traditional medical model approaches (Lorenzo & Cloete, 2004; Townsend, 1999; Wilcock, 1998). Consequently, increasing numbers of occupational therapists have already made a transition from hospital/institution-based practice to the community (Kronenberg, Simo-Algado & Pollard, 2005). According to the Canadian Occupational Therapy Association, by 1996, 37% of Canadian occupational therapists in the health sector were working in the community (Canadian Association of Occupational Therapy, 1996). The trend to shift from institutional to community practice has been similar in the UK. In 1989, Blom-Cooper recommended that occupational therapists in the UK should align themselves with practice in the community. He envisaged that only 20% of occupational therapy practice would eventually take place in institutional settings. Although he advocated that 80% of occupational therapists' work should be in the community, the proportions to date (2005) are not yet as he predicted. However, the trend in favour of community practice is ongoing and strengthening.

This shift in the service delivery domain places pressure on education institutions to ensure that students are well prepared to work within such an environment. This creates a need for students to have opportunities to grapple with the underlying philosophies and principles of these approaches in practice. The need to recognize the changing context of practice applies to students wherever they gain their experience. South African students in particular, need to understand the realities of South Africa's past and present as they relate to poverty and discrimination, the impact such factors have on human and occupational development, and how this should inform occupational therapy programmes guided by PHC principles. Undergraduate programmes in South Africa must therefore change from using traditional practice learning settings, such as tertiary hospitals and rehabilitation centres to using other, less traditional settings such as community empowerment projects and non-profit organizations. As preparation for practice, it is now essential that students gain experience in settings where they are exposed to the various socio-political realities that influence the health not only of individuals and groups, but also of communities (Duncan et al., 2005). One such learning opportunity is the rural service learning experience offered to third-year occupational therapy students at the University of Cape Town (UCT).

LEARNING IN THE SWARTLAND MUNICIPAL REGION

This service-learning opportunity, spanning two weeks, takes place in the Swartland Municipal Region, a rural district, about 60 kilometres north of

Cape Town. This learning opportunity is compulsory for all third-year students and the hours contribute towards their practice learning hours as specified by the World Federation of Occupational Therapy minimum standards (Hocking & Ness, 2002). The aim of the placement is for students to develop their understanding of the role of occupational therapy within a rural area, whilst gaining insight into the realities of working within such an environment. During these two weeks, students are expected to live in the community whilst they complete a specific task relevant to, and identified by, community stakeholders. Examples of such tasks include: individual client and contextual assessments; the evaluation, planning and implementation of identified health projects; and the design and implementation of health promotion and prevention programmes. The class, normally comprising between 40 and 50 students, is divided into five smaller groups to facilitate mobility, learning and practical efficiency. The students work in five different communities within this rural district. Two of these communities are suburbs of one of the largest towns in this district, while the other three are small neighbouring towns.

The three small towns, Kalksteendal,[1] Rygerskraal[1] and Chandel Town,[1] are home to a community whose members are predominantly coloured (people of mixed race, as classified by the South African government during the apartheid regime) from low socioeconomic backgrounds, and who speak Afrikaans as their home language. The population size ranges from 1500 to 2000 people per town, and the average income is about R417 (US$60) per month per household (sometimes up to 12 people or more). The main sources of income are seasonal work on farms, and governmental grants and pensions. These impoverished communities have little infrastructure, high unemployment figures, low literacy figures and a housing shortage. Houses consist of a mixture of formal brick structures as well as informal houses, and not all houses have access to electricity and running water. Only the main road within each town is tarred. Education centres are limited to primary level, and each community has a primary healthcare clinic, usually only open one day a week.

The main town, about 60 km north of Cape Town, lies within a rural district. It is a farming community known for its wheat and wine cultivation, as well as sheep and poultry farming. The town itself has been developing steadily, but the same cannot be said for some of the other surrounding towns. Two suburbs on the outskirts of the town, Dahliahof and Dublamazi,[2] are the other two communities in which students are placed.

Dahliahof consists of about 752 one-room brick houses, with water and electricity. The community members are predominantly coloured and speak Afrikaans. This area has no schools, clinics, police stations, recreational spaces or churches. Unemployment and lack of education are the two major problems identified by students.

---

[1] Pseudonyms.
[2] Also pseudonyms.

Dublamazi is a predominantly isiXhosa speaking, black community. It possesses a slightly better infrastructure than its neighbour, with crèches, small informal shops and churches, but it is still classified as an impoverished community. Primary healthcare and safety services are limited.

This rural district is under-resourced in terms of rehabilitation/health professionals. There is only one community occupational therapist who works across the whole region, which includes this rural district. The occupational therapist focuses more on rehabilitation services than on prevention and health promotion.

THE STUDENTS WITHIN THE COMMUNITIES

The third-year occupational therapy student population contrasts starkly with the demographics of the communities described above. It consists predominantly of white, female students between the ages of 20 and 25 years, from middle to upper socioeconomic backgrounds. The majority come from urban areas, with English as their home language. These differences in demographics create a great learning opportunity for the students, but can also create barriers to learning and make acceptance of the students by the communities difficult in some situations. This will be explored in more detail later in this chapter.

The class must live together on one site. The university organizes and pays for accommodation and transportation for the students and supervisors. Students have to be self-sufficient with regards to subsistence and each student is provided with a daily subsistence allowance of R30.00 (about $4.80 [with exchange rate at R6.25/$] or €3.75 [with exchange rate at R8.01/€]). Groups of students tend to combine their money to buy food and prepare and eat it within these groups. As a group, they also have to negotiate religious and cultural differences, especially where cooking is concerned. Shopping and other leisure activities, such as going to the movies, to restaurants or jogging, take place in the main town. This gives students the opportunity to interact further with the local people. Staying together on one site, not only makes supervision easier, it also has various other benefits, as will be discussed later. Students are supervised either by two occupational therapists, or by one qualified therapist and three final- (fourth-) year undergraduate students. Supervisors are expected to spend these two weeks on site with the students. During their two weeks, students also have lectures focusing on community-based rehabilitation and they meet with the district community occupational therapist to find out about the role of occupational therapy within the district. This further enhances their learning.

Prior to the practice experience, entry to the community is negotiated by the university practice educator. Permission first needs to be obtained from the director of health for that health district. Meetings then follow with the district community sister, community health workers, the community occupational therapist, community developers and other relevant community role-players to plan the placement and to identify a task or an area of focus for the students. It is important that the task is identified by the role-players, is of relevance to the community and fits into national and regional policies. It should either be a task that the students are able to complete within the 10 days or a task that relevant role-players have the means to sustain once the initial programme is implemented. Lastly, the task should be within the scope of occupational therapy. The tasks usually have a health promotion and/or prevention focus. Completing these tasks in the Swartland district provides students with an opportunity to understand and implement PHC principles. It also makes it possible for students to work within and understand the reality of poverty, whilst providing insight into the impact this has on the health and development of community members.

AN EXAMPLE OF A TASK

Proposed Task

Poverty is a big problem in some of the communities. Many community residents do not have access to hot nutritional meals on a daily basis. This can impact negatively on the residents, especially on the children's ability to take part in daily occupations. Feeding schemes are being used as a strategy to assist members of these impoverished communities. The current feeding schemes consist of one or more governmental, or non-governmental, organizations within the community, preparing meals once or twice per week for the needy within the community (e.g. a soup kitchen).

A need to evaluate and coordinate these feeding schemes, within each town, was expressed. There was also a hope that the feeding schemes would develop into health-promoting centres. Together with all relevant role-players, the students had to consider what needed to be planned and implemented in order to make the coordinated programme effective and sustainable.

Students also needed to consider the occupational implications of poverty. They were expected to include strategies to promote occupational health in their plan, e.g. developing a vegetable garden to be run by those receiving meals.

Groups were expected to work within a health promotion framework. Skill development and capacity building were to be considered together with other emerging needs that may need to be addressed. The district does have resources to offer funding, provided students are able to provide a realistic budget.

On their first day in the district, each student group meets with at least one role-player who has agreed to act as a gatekeeper to facilitate students' access into the community. The gatekeeper is usually a volunteer from the community or a health promotion practitioner. The students are verbally and, time allowing, physically oriented to the community. From day two, they are required to set their own schedules and agendas. Students usually spend the first 2–3 days entering the community and conducting a context analysis of the area. During this process they introduce themselves to all the relevant role-players within the community and ensure their role in the community is understood.

The students are transported to their respective communities on a daily basis and spend about 4–6 hours there at a time. Staying in the main town allows them to visit the community at night, to attend workshops and town meetings. It also gives the students the opportunity to live within a rural environment, to face the reality of having to take an hour's drive on a gravel road just to get to work in the morning and to implement a programme with very limited resources. At the end of the two weeks, the students give verbal presentations to community members, to provide feedback on their projects. They leave a written report detailing the progress made.

FACTORS TO CONSIDER

PREPARATION AND PLANNING

There are a number of factors that must be considered in planning a project of this nature. Logistically, it is a big task to plan, especially when there are 40 or more students to accommodate and account for. Finding accommodation has proven to be challenging at times and has even resulted in the students having to stay in tents at a campsite during one of these experiences. Living in such close proximity with each other, whilst also having to work together, can produce tensions between students, which will be discussed later.

The student group is generally a diverse group. Students come from a range of religious backgrounds: Muslim, Christian, Judaism and Hindi, amongst others. Sensitivity is needed and students must accommodate differences. For example, the Jewish and Muslim students cook together with their own cooking utensils and use Kosher or Halaal foods. There are generally few male students, but their needs must also be considered and appropriate accommodation found.

The timing of the service learning experience is another factor that has to be considered. The service learning has to fit into the natural time frames of both the communities and the students. Community projects tend to wind down at the end of the year and start up again in the New Year, with students taking exams in November. By organizing the placement at the beginning of the year rather than at the end, community programmes are starting up and students are more refreshed and willing to contribute to their learning.

TIME FRAME AND SUSTAINABILITY

A further factor to be considered is that of the time frame of the placement. Students only have a short time to gain an understanding of the community, their group and their task. Students often feel that 12 days is not enough time to work effectively with the communities and to ensure projects are sustainable. Sustainability is partially addressed through collaboration with key role-players prior to and following on from the project. Students also need to implement strategies that will facilitate sustainability.

Recent research to explore the communities' perspective of this intervention showed that some communities experienced sustainability of student projects, whilst others did not (Abdullah, Barry, Buddhu & Mienie, Personal communication). A number of factors seemed to impact on this, namely:

- existing structures within the community
- community dynamics and how the students worked as a group
- how students interpreted their task
- level of experience.

Further research is needed to identify the factors that facilitate sustainability of programmes and the intervention that is initiated through the students.

A learning scheme such as this has proven to be an invaluable opportunity for students to experience working within communities where they can not only integrate their theory into practice but also develop competencies and skills in becoming occupational therapists. During the years that this project has been running, insights have been gained, some of which are described here.

LEARNING PROCESS AND OUTCOMES

During the service learning opportunities, a variety of adult-learning approaches are drawn on. Three of the key approaches are: experiential learning, problem-based learning and action learning. *Experiential learning* acknowledges that experience is a critical aspect of adult learning and is said to form an adult learner's living textbook (Lindeman, 1926, cited in Brookfield, 1995). The value of *problem-based learning* is that, within this process, the learner is often faced with different forms of disjunction, which are critical to learning. These disjunctures are made manageable and enabled through facilitation and support (Savin-Baden & Major, 2004). *Action learning* comprises four stages, i.e. action, reflection, learning and planning. These should ideally form part of an upward spiral where the cycle is repeated and builds on the previous cycle, thus improving the effectiveness of future action (Taylor, Marias & Kaplan, 1997).

These three modes of learning form and inform the process, and thus the outcomes that students experience during this rural placement. Through this process, students begin to consolidate and apply much of their theoretical knowledge gained through formal lectures. The insights, reflections and realizations from this learning opportunity are often invaluable in their journey to becoming occupational therapists. These experiences are illustrated in the following section in light of community entry processes and students' development as professionals. Quotes from student journals highlight these experiences.

SUPERVISOR AND STUDENT ROLES

University practice educators and learning facilitators (final-year students) are available for supervision and guidance throughout the service learning. They provide information to help direct the students' learning processes and to guide them through challenging aspects of the experience, including challenges the students face as a group (Gravett, 2001). However, as adult learners, it is up to the students to know how and when to access this resource (Brookfield, 1995). For students, the transition from formal academic lectures to the application in practice can be challenging at times as they grapple with realizing that lectures alone have not taught them how to be occupational therapists. The following quote captured the students' experience of this:

> Sometimes its hard to find a balance in our own minds between wanting to do the job perfectly because we know that these are real people we are dealing with, not textbook case studies, but also then realising that this is all a learning experience and that chances are, our lack of experience will mean we often won't do things as we should. This has been quite difficult for us to come to terms with.
>
> (Chandel Town group journal)

This quote reflects a tension that students often have to face: being students who are in the process of learning versus having the perfect solutions to meet the needs of the people. Learning facilitators guide them through this process during supervision sessions in order to balance independent learning with the inherent demands of the experience.

COMMUNITY ENTRY

Communities have their own dynamics, infrastructures, cultures and ways of interacting. South Africa is a country rich in cultural diversity, which means that working within communities requires a sensitivity, openness and non-judgemental attitude and approach. But in order to be accepted within a community to do any work, it is necessary to gain community entry. This is a sensitive process that requires an awareness and understanding of communities, interpersonal relationships and group processes.

> Another thing this morning, to stretch and challenge our thinking and our professional behaviour, we had been trying to get in touch with the town counsellor for Chandel since we arrived there, but to no avail. Eventually when we did reach her on the phone, she told us in no uncertain terms that she was very busy and would not be able to see us until tonight. Nonetheless she phoned, clearly extremely angry (and perhaps feeling quite threatened) about the workshop we were intending to run. We realised that often as health professionals (and students) it is so easy to step on people's toes when working in their space – even when it is totally unintentional. This can so easily undermine the good that one has

achieved. . . . It also made us aware of principles to remember when entering communities, like getting to know all the members and key role players.

(Chandel Town group journal)

Community entry takes place on a number of different levels in order for learning to take place: between university staff and community; between university staff and students; and between students and the community. The students constitute a community of their own, having been together for over two years prior to this service learning experience. Resistance to this placement from students (discussed below) is common and, for this reason, the first level of negotiation takes place when staff need to negotiate entry into the 'student community' and they involve this community in the planning process.

Paulo Freire's (1974) adult education principles are drawn on throughout this process to facilitate collaboration and to limit resistance from students. Students need to be included in the planning from the beginning, particularly with regards to the logistics of such an experience. Many of the students are resistant to 'being shipped off' to a rural community for two weeks and feel they do not need to bond with their student colleagues anymore or to live in the community for the duration of the project. By including students in the planning process, not only do they contribute to the manner in which things happen, but they also take more responsibility for their own experience, whilst seeing all that is needed in order to make such an experience a reality. In addition, they come to understand the processes and rationale for making decisions regarding their service learning and working in communities.

The next level of negotiation occurs before students arrive in the rural community when staff discuss entry into the community with the community authorities. This part of the process is vitally important in order to ensure key role-players are identified, access is obtained, appropriate tasks are established and sustainability is possible. It has been found to be quite a sensitive process at times with gatekeepers preventing contact with some role-players, making community entry principles even more pertinent. Once the students arrive in the community, they initiate the third level of entry. Students have to negotiate entry into the community at large, that is the district, and then to the individual communities to which each group of students is assigned. The health promotion practitioners (HPPs) play a valuable role in assisting in this process. HPPs are community members who are trained to meet the basic health needs of their community. They screen and make appropriate referrals to community health services and also address issues pertaining to health promotion and disease prevention.

Part of the process of community entry that the students undertake involves defining occupational therapy and negotiating the occupational therapy role within this context amongst themselves and with the people with whom they work. The relationship between occupation, meaning, purpose and health is something the students have to make explicit from the outset as most of the community members, as well as the HPPs, define health intervention within a biomedical framework. This often results in the community placing unrealistic or inaccurate expectations on the students, something that students need to negotiate from the beginning.

> This [focusing on the task] is hard sometimes especially because so many people in the community think that we've come to take all their problems away. It is a very humbling experience to realise that we do not have the answers even though we come across as educated because the answers and solutions are within the people already.
>
> (Chandel Town group journal)

LIVING IN A COMMUNITY

Given that the students live within their own community, whilst working in other communities, a number of parallels emerge. Group dynamics are often influenced by political (power) factors where individuals or small groups come into conflict with others with opposing views, values and beliefs. This process of experiential learning raises the students' awareness and sensitivity to the influences that such dynamics have on communities, including the ones in which they are working. Through reflection, they are able to apply some of these insights and experiences in their intervention process.

> I guess as OTs, the clients we encounter are in essence just people, with similar feelings to myself. If I can understand and empathise through my own experiences what others are going through it will be that much easier to appreciate that every group is made up of individuals and every individual is made up of a unique set of experiences and characteristics. Ultimately it is these that contribute to the big picture. Perhaps this is what working in groups, like communities, etc. is all about.
>
> (Chandel Town group journal)

Students learn simultaneously to negotiate their professional and personal roles. This is a dual process and is often something students struggle to develop. They need to develop the ability to differentiate between being a peer and friend, compared with being a therapist, especially when living and working together. This is a useful tool for future service-learning opportunities, as well as for their future as qualified therapists. The difficulty comes when they all need to develop this within their own community as students. In addition, students develop personal, academic and professional relationships with fellow students, forming a strong basis for interactions during third and fourth years, where service learning and research projects are conducted with class peers. This becomes more than an academic exercise and students learn to draw on each other for support, learning and guidance.

At a logistical level, the reality of living and working in rural communities in South Africa becomes all the more apparent when students have to commute daily to the different communities for their work. The drive in the bus on dirt roads that are usually in a poor condition takes considerable time and has to be accounted for in daily time management. In addition, groups usually need to negotiate between themselves in order to coordinate their time in the communities as more than one group has to utilize one of the two buses. This experience helps students appreciate the struggles these communities are faced with on a daily basis and how this impacts on occupations, especially employment and livelihood.

> Today was the first day that we were able to spend time amongst the community. Our aim was to gather as much info about the context from as many sources as possible. The first thing we realised was how far Chandel Town is from [the main town] and we immediately began thinking about the effect that this distance would have on occupation. It certainly explained why many people are unemployed and those who do work, choose to do so on the surrounding farms.
>
> (Chandel Town group journal)

PROFESSIONAL DEVELOPMENT

> Although we know that our task involves soup kitchens, the needs of these people are overwhelming. We definitely feel quite small in the face of a task, which at the moment seems enormous.
>
> (Chandel Town group journal)

Students need to engage with their understanding of the occupational therapy role within such a context, and explore how their role as students fits with this. Students are familiar with working with disability, ill health and performance components, but through this experience, they gain insight into the role of occupational therapy within a health promotion framework. In addition, they develop their understanding of occupation as the essence of the profession. Preconceptions and assumptions are challenged as they encounter the occupational engagement of a community often very different, culturally and socially, from their own. An example of this was illustrated by one group of students who reported that people living in Rygerskraal experienced occupational deprivation. They described how, when they (the students) walked around the community, no one was doing anything and most people where sitting on their veranda, 'watching the world go by'. When this was explored with students, they came to see the meaning and the experience of being (Wilcock, 1998) in this occupation for these people. Such experiences transform their understanding of what they have been taught, and encourage deeper reflection on the issues and nature of occupation in future settings.

Students also gain insights into their own competencies and abilities, developing their sense of professional identity. They begin to realize the degree to which they have internalized skills and knowledge thus far. Initially, there were high levels of anxiety with regards to their competence and ability to be effective. As they undertake their tasks, however, they discovered they had a range of skills and capacities they were able to offer to the communities. In addition, students' initial resistance to learning was broken down, as they came to realize the extent to which their actions were meaningfully informed by what they had learnt.

> As individuals, we are starting to notice an increase in confidence levels in our interviewing and group skills, compared to that of first and second year. We started to notice how we don't sit and panic about what question to ask next when chatting to a community member or other relevant people, and can tolerate a period of silence much more than before.
>
> (Dahliahof group journal)

> We were talking about how the process we are engaging in is known as reflection-on-action and how we need to reflect-in-action on Monday. We found that a lot more theory than we suspected has become (secretly ☺!) part of our thinking . . . something went right after all that studying.
>
> (Dahliahof group journal)

The realities of this learning experience force students to understand and integrate information on a deeper level, resulting in the development of a more comprehensive and integrated clinical reasoning for future practice.

REFLECTION AS A TOOL

> Also, our supervisor is reflecting on how huge this project is, the fact that this is not some school project, not a little paper project. This is the biggest, most important thing we've ever done.
>
> (Dahliahof group journal)

Students are required to write in their journal each day in order to optimize their learning experience, thus drawing on principles in action learning. The action learning approach recognizes that actions, understandings and feelings, together with thinking, are all important sources of learning. Action learning is a cyclical process of action, reflection, learning and planning that is repeated (Taylor et al., 1997). Through journalling, students become more aware of their experiences on a range of levels, including the dynamics involved through the process, and they are able to identify and explore critical learning experiences (Buchanan, Moore & Van Niekerk, 1998). The journals are handed in at the end of the service-learning experience and are used to gain insight into the experience of students and to inform future planning.

ACCESSING LIMITED RESOURCES

Poverty and limited resources impact on every aspect of the communities' lives. As students develop their understanding of this, the importance of appropriate and realistic intervention becomes clear. They learn from the community how to creatively utilize available resources, including 'waste material' (e.g. using old juice bottles, boxes used for packaging and storage) and assist the community to access resources of which they may not be aware. Through this process, students begin to develop appropriate budgets for intervention and learn about managing available funds in an optimal way. A small intervention budget was at their disposal for the purposes of their projects. These funds tended to be used for running workshops, developing health promotion resources and starting appropriate programmes.

CONCLUSION

This rural service-learning experience provides students with the opportunity to understand the dynamics of working within a community. They are able to gain experience of community entry principles and strategies needed to inform all interactions, not only in the beginning but also throughout the process. As professionals coming from outside the communities, they realize that they are guests in the community and must respect that. It is important that they become familiar with structures and systems through which to work so as not to undermine, offend or incapacitate anyone. Everyone in the community is a valuable resource and they should be treated as such. In addition, it has proven to be very valuable for students to stay together as a class whilst working in the communities in order for them to become aware of community dynamics. Great benefit is drawn on these experiences within their own class community to inform the work they do during this rural service-learning experience.

REFERENCES

Blom-Cooper, L. (1989). *Occupational therapy an emerging profession in health care.* Report of a Commission of Inquiry. London: Duckworth.

Brookfield, S. (1995). Adult learning: an overview. In A. Tuinjman (Ed.), *International Encyclopedia of Education.* Oxford: Pergamon Press. Available at http://nlu.nl.edu/ace/Resources/Documents/AdultLearning.html

Buchanan, H., Moore, R. & Van Niekerk, L. (1998). The Fieldwork Case Study: writing for clinical reasoning. *American Journal of Occupational Therapy, 52*(4), 291–295.

Canadian Association of Occupational Therapists (1996). Annual labour force survey. *The National.* Ottawa, Ontario: CAOT Publications.

Department of Health (1997). *White Paper for the transformation of health systems in South Africa.* Pretoria: Government Printer.

Duncan, M., Buchanan, H. & Lorenzo, T. (2005). Politics in occupational therapy education: a South African perspective. In F. Kronenberg, S. Simo Algado & N. Pollard (Eds.), *Occupational therapy without boarders. Learning from the spirits of survivors.* Edinburgh: Elsevier Churchill Livingstone, pp. 390–401.

Freire, P. (1974). *Pedagogy of the oppressed.* Harmondsworth: Penguin.

Gravett, S. (2001). *Adult learning.* Pretoria: Van Schaik.

Hocking, C. & Ness, N.E. (2002). *Revised minimum standards for the education of occupational therapists.* Perth, Western Australia: World Federation of Occupational Therapists.

Kronenberg, F., Simo-Algado, S. & Pollard, N. (Eds.) (2005). *Occupational therapy without borders: learning from the spirit of survivors.* Edinburgh: Elsevier Churchill Livingstone.

Lindeman, E.C. (1926). *The meaning of adult education.* New York: New Republic.

Lorenzo, T. & Cloete, L. (2004). Promoting occupations in rural communities. In R. Watson & L. Swartz (Eds.), *Transformation through occupation.* London: Whurr, pp. 268–286.

Savin-Baden, M. & Major, C.H. (2004). *Foundations of problem based learning.* Buckingham: Society for Research into Higher Education and Open University Press.

Taylor, J., Marias, D. & Kaplan, A. (1997). *Action learning for development: Use your experience to improve your effectiveness.* Cape Town: Juta & Co.

Townsend, E. (1999). Enabling occupation in the 21st century. *Australian Occupational Therapy Journal, 46,* 147–159.

Watson, R. (2004). New horizons in occupational therapy. In R. Watson & L. Swartz (Eds.), *Transformation through occupation.* London: Whurr, pp. 3–18.

Wilcock, A. (1998). *An occupational perspective on health.* USA: Slack.

World Health Organization (1978). *Primary Health Care. Report of the International Conference on Primary Health Care, Alma Ata.* Geneva: WHO.

9 Group Supervision: Making the Most of Limited Educational Infrastructures

ELKE HAGEDORN and FASLOEN ADAMS

OBJECTIVES

This chapter discusses:

- the role of group supervision in under-serviced contexts
- principles, procedures and outcomes of group supervision
- advantages and disadvantages of group supervision
- a possible structure for group supervision.

BRIEF OVERVIEW OF SUPERVISION

Frum and Opacich (1987), and later Alsop and Ryan (1996), acknowledged that supervision is an intensely focused, one-to-one relationship in which one person is designated to facilitate the development of professional competence in another. The supervisor is said to be one who, by reason of their greater knowledge and skill, establishes a relationship that leads, teaches, supports and provides a barometer of performance for another person (Yerxa, 1994). Despite the age of the references, the described characteristics of supervision and of the supervisor seem to have stood the test of time.

A commonly understood aim of supervision is to allow the student to develop professionally by making good use of evaluation, reflection, effective communication and planning. The student not only has to gain an understanding of how to apply knowledge to practice, they must also learn to reflect on the skills used in the process, and to evaluate the outcomes of various actions and processes. Scheerer (2003) mentioned that students described their practice learning experiences as 'therapy' for themselves. This is an important comment as students are challenged to learn constantly in different situations and sites, but at the same time have to learn to acknowledge and reflect on

Practice and Service Learning in Occupational Therapy. Edited by Theresa Lorenzo, Madeleine Duncan, Helen Buchanan, Auldeen Alsop
© 2006 John Wiley & Sons Ltd

their personal growth. Thus, finding the balance between learning in terms of personal growth and learning through service provision is vital. During supervision, the supervisor needs to guide the student to integrate theory into practice and draw on clinical reasoning to substantiate practice.

A further aim of supervision is to guide the student in their emotional development. In a supervisory relationship, a student is given space to reflect on their own development and to challenge and review personal interpretations or assumptions; for example, regarding cultural differences. More specifically, the student is given the space to identify the occupational therapy role and to reflect on the interdisciplinary teamwork in a given context.

OCCUPATIONAL THERAPY IN A DEVELOPING CONTEXT

Occupational therapy is increasingly recognizing the importance of occupations in social, cultural and physical environments, including broader political, economic, institutional and societal structures. Occupational therapists are thus challenged to think more broadly in terms of population issues and health environments, rather than focusing only on the individual (Letts, Rigby & Stewart, 2003). This is particularly relevant in a developing context such as South Africa where transformation is occurring at many different levels. However, engaging with new ideas and opportunities can be difficult. Factors such as insufficient resources, increased student numbers, unreliable public transport, shortage of supervisors, lack of professional role models and budget cuts continue to have an adverse effect on the quality of learning opportunities for prospective health professionals.

The shortage of learning opportunities raises questions about how best techniques and models of supervision can be made to work in a developing country. For all of the above reasons, universities in under-serviced contexts are being challenged to think of creative ways of facilitating student learning and professional development within available resources. Effective supervision is crucial to the learning process in well-resourced, as well as under-resourced, contexts of work.

METHODS OF SUPERVISION

Supervision is central to student education, professional education and continuing professional development. At most times it is a satisfying, career-confirming, yet exhausting and challenging experience for both the supervisee and supervisor. No matter what method of supervision is used, however, the process of supervision appears to be key to professional and personal growth. For the purposes of this chapter, the focus will be on student supervision. The terms used will be university practice educator (supervisor) and student (supervisee).

The methods currently used in student supervision appear to be dominated by the one-to-one format. On the one hand, this provides a great opportunity for students to reflect on, evaluate and develop or enhance their overall skills and abilities within their field of work. On the other hand, it can be very time-consuming and limiting, as the student is mainly dependent on the views and skills of the university practice educator. Questions can thus be raised about whether:

- individual supervision is always the most effective method for guiding student practice learning?
- other forms of supervision could adequately guide students in under-serviced practice learning contexts?

In addressing these issues, this chapter records the experiences of the second author, as university practice educator, of initiating group supervision in a tertiary psychiatric hospital in Cape Town, South Africa. The case story that follows provides an example for planning future alternatives to combat the challenges related to student practice education in under-resourced contexts. The first author witnessed the adoption of group-based supervision in the UK to meet the growing demand for the supervision of less experienced health professionals. The benefits and limitations drawn from reflections on both experiences are then presented. A study by Milne and Oliver (2000) also examined flexible formats of supervision. Where these had been implemented, supervisors appeared to appreciate the potential benefits. First, however, it is necessary to consider the relative merits of group supervision.

GROUP SUPERVISION AS A STRATEGY

To optimize learning opportunities for students in practice, suitable supervision formats must be developed. Supervision is an integral feature of practice education promoting learning, professional development, maintenance of academic standards and quality assurance during practice learning. Bernhard and Goodyear (1992, p. 72) defined group supervision as 'the regular meeting of a group of students with a designated university practice educator for the purpose of furthering their understanding of themselves as practitioners, or their clients, or of the service delivery in general and who are aided in this endeavour by their interactions with each other and with their supervisor in the context of group process'. This definition indicates the significance of supervision in providing opportunity for peer review, peer feedback and for developing personal insight into interpersonal behaviours relevant to the profession, with due consideration of issues of power between service providers and consumers.

Even though group supervision is practised widely and effectively within various professions, the research to substantiate this practice is minimal. Over the past few years, various disciplines have documented the benefits of group supervision and compared its effectiveness to the more traditional individual supervision structure (Bogo, Globerman & Sussman, 2004; Farrow, Gaiptman & Rudman, 2000; Milne & Oliver, 2000; Ray & Altekruse, 2004). The literature confirms that training remains essential to enable supervisors to feel confident in facilitating the group supervision process.

The following case story describes a group supervision approach to practice learning that has been used for several years at a psychiatric hospital in Cape Town, South Africa. This case story may be seen as a pilot study to assess the effectiveness of group supervision within occupational therapy as an alternative to individual supervision.

CASE STORY

THE CONTEXT AND RATIONALE FOR GROUP SUPERVISION

The practice learning site used for piloting group supervision was one of the larger mental health hospitals in Cape Town. It is a tertiary and secondary level facility as it provides specialized psychiatric treatment and rehabilitation. The hospital consists of 14 units. The occupational therapy department provides input into some of the units, and patients are also referred to the department for treatment. There are six occupational therapists working in the hospital, of which one is responsible for fourth-(final) year students, whilst the other five take responsibility for third-year students.

Due to the challenges faced by the university in locating suitable practice learning opportunities for rising numbers of students, alternative ways of providing the optimum amount of guidance and support to students needed to be found. Budgets for student supervision were reduced and staff downsizing at tertiary and secondary levels of care meant that there were fewer practitioners available on site. Some students were working with the complexities of 'real-life' patients and providing 'real-life' treatment without the direct supervision of learning facilitators and other practitioners. Rather than opting out of providing practice learning opportunities, the head occupational therapist at the hospital requested assistance from the university. Discussions centred around how best to deal with the practical issues of the few available occupational therapists taking on students whilst simultaneously dealing with their own caseloads and their clinical and managerial roles. Staff felt that supervising students was extra work for which they had no time. Additionally, staff felt that time with students was not being used efficiently; for example, there was often duplication of effort completing tasks such as inducting students, teaching group facilitation skills and discussing the impact of mental illness on the person as an occupational being.

In an attempt to solve these problems, a university practice educator was appointed to supervise all the students placed at the learning site. She had previously worked at the hospital and therefore had a good understanding of the organizational structure and the dynamics of the site. Having knowledge of both the university requirements and the given environment was considered important in determining realistic expectations for the students. It was also anticipated that time and costs would be managed more effectively through this strategy. The site learning facilitator thus focused on the practical learning of students with their chosen clients, whilst the university practice educator focused on the professional development of students and making sure they were guided in achieving the outcomes of the curriculum.

GROUP SUPERVISION IN PRACTICE

The student group met weekly throughout a seven-week practice period. The university practice educator acted as both group supervisor and learning facilitator. The first task of the university practice educator was to develop a flexible group supervision programme. In respect of weeks one and two, the university practice educator designed the induction schedule and general programme for all the students, listed each student's duties and responsibilities, and scheduled dates for practical examinations. Students were orientated to the service and were given an opportunity to identify their own learning objectives. Learning objectives were based on site-specific objectives and anticipated learning outcomes, which the university practice educator had developed in collaboration with the practitioners. For the first group supervision session, the university practice educator took the lead, initiating discussion about health conditions that the students had seen, the handling of clients and general principles for working within the given environment.

In weeks three and four, students were increasingly encouraged to initiate and take more responsibility for their supervision session by bringing topics or questions to the group for consideration and reflection. By the final weeks, the focus had shifted to sharing learning opportunities with each other. Students brought case stories to the group and discussed the planned occupational therapy intervention with their peers. The university practice educator facilitated student learning by encouraging active reflection amongst all group members. Group supervision thus provided an opportunity for education to take place in a way that suited the context. Alsop and Ryan (1996) described this as an educational process where the focus is not only on developing therapeutic competence, but also on developing an understanding of self and how theory is applied in practice.

BENEFITS OF GROUP SUPERVISION

From interviews conducted with learning facilitators and university practice educators at the psychiatric hospital, and from written and verbal feedback from the students at the learning site, the various benefits of group supervision were identified and are discussed here.

The Educational Philosophy of Self-directed Learning is Carried Through to the Actual Learning Site

Towards the end of the learning opportunity, the students were encouraged to learn from each other as well as from the university practice educator. Students gained the self-confidence to debate and reflect on situations and occupational therapy interventions with each other rather than focusing purely on feedback from the university practice educator. Supervision was still goal-directed, focusing on aspects such as written work, intervention modalities and application of principles. Whilst the group supervisor provided structure in the early sessions, facilitation eventually promoted self-directed learning. Bernhard and Goodyear (1992) confirmed that group supervision helps diminish student dependence on the university practice educator and decreases hierarchical issues between them.

Shared and Individual Learning Takes Place

Within the group format, students were able to share information, problem solve, reflect together on their practice learning experiences and support each other. In the group, the spectrum of scenarios and experiences with which students engaged was more diverse, and students appeared to benefit from reflecting on each other's performance. Furthermore, by hearing about interventions in other mental health practice areas on a weekly basis, students were given the opportunity to 'fill the gaps' in their knowledge. For example, a student based in an acute ward might gain experience in assessment but little experience of intervention. This gap in knowledge could be addressed in group supervision. 'You experience eight interventions instead of one or two. You also hear about everyone's experiences' (student comment).

A study conducted in the field of social work reported that since mistakes and failures are experienced in relation to others' struggles, students might understand them more as part of professional development than as an indicator of personal inadequacy (Bogo et al., 2004).

Shared Learning Allows Students to Acknowledge the Complexity of Mental Illness and Impact on the Individual

Through sharing experiences from different units, students gained a clearer overall picture of the different stages of recovery a person experiencing a mental illness might go through, for example, the differences in handling a person during a psychotic episode compared to when they are mentally stable. Generalization of knowledge takes place automatically through sharing of experiences. Hayes (1989) suggested that group supervision allows participants to develop more accurate perceptions of self and others through consistent feedback from others. Participants have an opportunity to develop or enhance empathy and social interest and to gain a stronger sense of self by reality testing within the group and letting go of negative perceptions of self.

> Truthfully, I can't imagine being there [psychiatric hospital] alone or with one other person; I really found it valuable to see the other areas.
>
> (Student comment)

> It can be frightening to see people in the ward suffering a mental illness that could be my brother, mother or a friend! For me it was good to have the space to deal with this in the group supervision sessions. I realised that I was not the only one who felt this way – and that it is ok to feel like that!
>
> (Student comment)

Students are More Open to Being Challenged in a Group than Individually

The university practice educator was able to gauge a student's level of competence through the supervision process and could use the group format to challenge individuals. 'It feels less threatening having supervision in a group than individually' (student comment).

The university practice educator was also able to initiate discussion and challenge students in a group format and thus facilitate optimal and effective student learning by also being aware of the occupational therapy curriculum's anticipated outcomes, learning methods and evaluation strategies. 'Eight brains are better than one – everyone can contribute to your learning' (student comment).

Students Acknowledge the Importance of Peer Support within Supervision

Students mentioned that the support from peers gained during the group supervision sessions was as important as the support received from the learning facilitator. This sheds some light on the importance of support from people who are 'in the same boat'. Students come to appreciate the issues that clients deal with and the impact of their illness on their lives. Through support and reflection the student is able to deal with the issues better within the group than alone.

> The group learning process was a very effective and meaningful process, especially at [name of site] where it is emotionally draining. The support from my classmates was vital for me.
>
> (Student comment)

Students are Able to Develop Clinical Reasoning Skills more Adeptly

Learning to verbalize clinical reasoning in a group also enhanced the development of professional identity in that the student was more able to practise being 'part of a team' and express their views in a team. A structured format for prompting discussion and the development of reasoning abilities could be useful during group supervision. A framework for giving formative written feedback according to a student's level of professional development is already in use to guide and prompt professional reasoning and something similar could be used in group supervision. The group supervisor could initiate discussion by asking questions that elicit reasoning according to the various levels described in Chapter 15.

Students are known to question their marks and achievements during their practice learning experiences, in trying to understand why they are where they are. Questions within group supervision drawn from the various levels of feedback that elicit reasoning skills could help students understand their varying levels of competence. Students could be given the opportunity to develop these skills by listening actively to, and reflecting on, questions posed to other students. This opportunity would be unavailable to them in one-to-one supervision.

Students are More Actively Able to Reflect on Cultural Differences and the Impact of Diversity on the Person and Their Occupations

Within the South African context, especially after ten years of political democratic change, citizens are now learning about and developing an understanding of other cultures. The affirmation of diversity is now encouraged compared with the suppression of cultural identity during the previous apartheid era. This attitude towards political change is unique to South Africa at this time and is having an impact on student learning in the sense that students are not only learning to work with clients and students from cultures different to their own, but they are also learning about differences in their own culture. They are, therefore, challenged by their preconceived ideas about what is 'right and wrong', as well as by what is 'culturally different'. For example, how a client conveys their life-story and how they carry out their occupations could be 'culturally different' and not necessarily a sign of mental illness. Through sharing, students are exposed to these concepts more quickly and learn to reflect on them openly. Students find that they have to reflect more on their own perceptions and misconceptions in a group setting than as a lone student.

It Allows Students Time to Reflect on Their Own Perceptions about Mental Illness

Students appeared to use their supervision to grapple with their understanding of mental illness. At some stage during practice learning, students raise questions in supervision about normality. By encouraging these questions in group supervision, the group can explore issues about stigma, prejudice and psychiatric disability in more depth.

It Encourages the Shift in Models

In order to discuss topics relevant for all students, the focus in group supervision tended to be more on occupation and the impact of occupational deprivation, alienation and/or imbalance on the client. It allowed students the space to expand their understanding of the role and scope of occupational therapy at the site. The focus thus shifted to understanding the emerging identity of occupational therapy and the need to transform practice.

LIMITATIONS OF GROUP SUPERVISION

There were also limitations to this type of supervision that need to be taken into account:

- The success of the sessions is greatly dependent on the university practice educator's ability to plan and facilitate the session. The university practice educator has to spend time planning the sessions and making practical arrangements for the group to meet. The university practice educator's group handling and adult education skills are as important as their knowledge of the profession. Effective group supervision requires substantial in-service training, which may be difficult to implement given the resource constraints experienced by some universities.
- In order to use the time effectively the onus lies with the students to take initiative in voicing personal concerns, problems or bringing forth ideas for discussion. This tends to create problems for the quieter or weaker students. Group supervision should aim to draw out the individual student's potential. It is quite difficult to balance the amount of attention given to weaker students with the need to avoid embarrassment. This requires experience in group facilitation skills.
- It is more difficult to identify individual problems within a group setting. Thus, individual supervision might be needed in addition to the group supervision. The university practice educator, as group facilitator plays an important role in addressing this problem. One-to-one supervision is still likely to be favoured by students requiring more individual attention.

GROUP SUPERVISION: A STRATEGY FOR THE FUTURE

One of the aims of practice learning is for the student to gain confidence and ultimately be able to work independently in a variety of work areas. Supervision is the tool used to achieve this. The question arises as to whether group supervision could not enhance this process further as students learn to listen, reflect, evaluate and reason together with other students rather than only with the university practice educator? Further questions that require consideration in this model of supervision include: Should group supervision replace individual supervision or complement it? Would it be viable to apply group supervision to all areas of practice learning? If so, how should such sessions be structured?

An example of the structure of group supervision has been described. From this experience, it is suggested university practice educators consider the following principles when planning group supervision:

- The students' level of experience needs to be taken into account. More guidance is needed for students at early stages of learning.
- Regular times should be planned with all students, for example, once per week for one hour. This ensures that the sessions remain time-effective.
- Consider whether any other participants should be involved, such as other staff or students from other facilities.
- Group norms need to be decided within the first session to ensure the development of group cohesiveness and structure. Alvarez (2002) stated that explaining norms and the approach to be used helps group members 'buy into' the process. Students are more often than not 'involuntary members' and, by explaining the approaches used and why, they are likely to be more involved in the group process.
- The importance of confidentiality needs to be emphasized especially when personal or client issues are discussed.
- An agenda provides structure to the sessions and ensures that goals are met either during the session or are addressed later if time runs out.
- Dynamic interaction is vital within the group in order for students to experience the benefits of group supervision. This needs to be facilitated by the university practice educator, and is thus a key role and skill that they should have.
- The aim should be to promote student independence so that the amount of input from the university practice educator is tapered throughout the learning experience. As the group progresses, students should be encouraged to become more active, initiating learning opportunities for themselves.

- Ensure inclusion of all students. This skill can either 'make or break' the sessions.

For this model of supervision to work, university practice educator training and support is vital (Milne & Oliver, 2000). The principles outlined above should be included in a training programme, and regular support sessions for university practice educators should also be introduced.

CONCLUSION

Questions have been raised about the potential of group supervision to facilitate student learning in resource-constrained environments. The case story used in this chapter focused on supervision of students placed in a mental health setting using the group format. It appears that group supervision is worth pursuing in certain contexts of practice in order to assist students to develop their professional knowledge and skills. Students, however, also proposed that group supervision be introduced into other domains of practice learning despite the practical difficulties that might arise. Conclusions drawn suggest that it is an innovative strategy that may assist universities to respond to the challenges of practice learning in under-serviced contexts.

Occupational therapists have the ability and training to facilitate groups but it may be possible for students to also develop these skills. By facilitating student groups, students are challenged to think for themselves and thus take ownership of their learning. Further research is needed but it appears from the literature that a variety of professions are using group supervision and are also questioning whether individual supervision is in fact the ideal way forward. Milne and Oliver (2000) believed that group supervision might have more benefits than individual supervision and that these benefits needed to be explored. Reflecting on what is done in other countries helps to inform the debate, but the challenge is to assess and understand the process in a given context, working together with all role-players in order to develop the 'custom-fit' idea further.

REFERENCES

Alsop, A. & Ryan, S. (1996). *Making the most of fieldwork education: a practical approach.* London: Chapman and Hall.

Alvarez, A.R. (2002). Pitfalls, pratfalls, shortfalls and windfalls: reflections on forming and being formed by groups. In R. Kurland & A. Malekoff (Eds.), *Stories celebrating group work: it's not always easy to sit on your mouth.* Haworth Press, pp. 93–105.

Bernhard, J.M. & Goodyear, R.K. (1992). *Fundamentals of clinical supervision.* Needham Heights, MA: Allyn and Bacon.

Bogo, M., Globerman, J. & Sussman, T. (2004). The field instructor as group manager: managing trust and competition in group supervision. *Journal of Social Work Education*, *40*(1), 13–26.

Farrow, S., Gaiptman, B. & Rudman, D. (2000). Exploration of a group model in fieldwork education. *Canadian Journal of Occupational Therapy*, *67*(4), 239–249.

Frum, D. & Opacich, K. (1987). *Supervision: the development of therapeutic competence*. Rockville, MD: The American Occupational Therapy Association.

Hayes, R. (1989). Group supervision. In L. Bradley (Eds.), *Counselor supervision: principles, processes and practice*. Muncie, In: Accelerated Development, pp. 399–422.

Letts, L., Rigby, P. & Stewart, D. (2003). *Using environments to enable occupational performance*. Thorofare, NJ: Slack.

Milne, D. & Oliver, V. (2000). Flexible formats of clinical supervision: description, evaluation and implementation. *Journal of Mental Health*, *9*(3), 291–314.

Ray, D. & Altekruse, M. (2004). Effectiveness of group supervision versus combined group and individual supervision counselor. *Education and Supervision*, *40*(1), 19–31.

Scheerer, C.R. (2003). Perceptions of effective professional behaviour feedback: occupational therapy student voices. *American Journal of Occupational Therapy*, *57*(2), 205–213.

Yerxa, E. (1994). Techniques of supervision. In *Guide to fieldwork education*. Bethesda, MD: American Occupational Therapy Association, pp. 184–192.

FURTHER READING

Avi-Itzhak, T.E. & Kellner, H. (1995). Preliminary assessment of a fieldwork education alternative: the fieldwork centers approach. *American Journal of Occupational Therapy*, *49*(2), 133–137.

Jung, B., Martin, A., Graden, L. & Awrey, J. (1994). Fieldwork education: a shared supervision model. *Canadian Journal of Occupational Therapy*, *61*(1), 12–19.

Loyd, C. & Maas, F. (1997). Occupational therapy in group work in psychiatric settings. *British Journal of Occupational Therapy*, *60*(5), 226–229.

10 Engaging Students as Partners in Service Development

THERESA LORENZO and AULDEEN ALSOP

OBJECTIVES

This chapter discusses:

- the misconception that taking students for practice education leads to a drain in resources
- the potential benefits of supporting a student in practice education
- the ways of using student expertise to review and develop practice collaboratively with service personnel.

INTRODUCTION

In resource-constrained environments, practitioners are hard-pressed to provide quality service for their clients whilst simultaneously attending to student learning needs. Practitioners may view the additional responsibility of students as a distraction in the face of significant service demands. Thinking more creatively about what students could offer would enable practitioners to facilitate student learning whilst engaging with them as an additional resource. Students often feel vulnerable and dependent on practitioners for the acquisition of skills to be able to gain their professional qualification. Not only should students have the opportunity to engage in new learning experiences, their assets could be made available and used to maximum effect for the benefit of everyone. Practitioners therefore need to be assisted to find ways of shaping projects for students so that learning and development in the practice environment is reciprocal. Assumptions are often made that students undertaking practice or service learning in any domain of practice have a negative effect on the service delivery and that they tend to make a drain on resources within the organization. Students' contribution to the service is sometimes perceived as being minimal, and more adversely

Practice and Service Learning in Occupational Therapy. Edited by Theresa Lorenzo, Madeleine Duncan, Helen Buchanan, Auldeen Alsop
© 2006 John Wiley & Sons Ltd

affecting the work of an organization than benefiting it. These assumptions can be far from the reality of the situation.

Higgs and Titchen (2001, p. 527) claim that the primary goal of practice development is to move increasingly closer to a 'model of client-centred, clinically and socially effective care', focusing on a greater sharing of power and responsibility between clients and health professionals. This model reflects the profession's humanist origins and acknowledges the increasing drive towards a more social and community-based approach to practice in which partnerships are developed. These authors further advocate that a goal of practice development is to promote and develop professional artistry, whereby students and practitioners find ways of making intelligent professional judgements within complex and unpredictable environments. Both practitioners and students are likely to face unique and challenging scenarios that require the use of problem-solving skills in ways not previously seen. Considering these challenges, learning to practise and develop skills for professional work afterwards is therefore not unique to students. It is a phenomenon also experienced by practitioners: 'Practitioners, like artists, must learn to see, interpret and make new meanings' (Whiteford, Klomp & Wright-St Clair, 2005, p. 13). Given the complex learning environments that now provide opportunities for practice education, both students and practitioners face dilemmas from which they learn. In some cases students as well as practitioners may present novel ideas that enable practice dilemmas to be addressed and resolved. Problem solving in novel situations, therefore, is not just the prerogative of qualified practitioners. The expectation that either or both could be involved redresses the power relationship between novice and expert in some way.

The purpose of this chapter is to define and describe the positive contributions that occupational therapy students, particularly final-year students, can make to service development. The concept of students as a potential resource in terms of ideas, time and energy within a service will be explored.

STUDENTS AS PARTNERS

Through purposeful interactions with practitioners and service users, students can assist both service provision and service development. If practitioners can view students as a resource, this will help to change the perception that students are a burden. It will help address practitioners' anxieties related to taking students and the misconception that students increase their workload with little reward. With these thoughts in mind, the first author completed an analysis of reflective comments and feedback from practitioners and students regarding the contribution students make to service development. The findings were analysed using the reflective stance approach (Meulenberg Buskens, 1999). Five themes on maximizing students as a resource emerged. These were:

a knowledge resource; a marketing resource; a service resource; a team-building resource; and a professional development resource.

STUDENTS AS A KNOWLEDGE RESOURCE

Students bring with them new ideas and products from previous life or educational experiences that may have relevance for practice. Some of these earlier experiences may have provided them with opportunities to develop tools, products and activities that can be tested out in the practice environment. Most students are unlikely to have been exposed to organizational politics or to the customs and practices of service organization that might otherwise inhibit them from voicing their opinions. However, some students may have been involved with civic organizations or student political bodies and would be familiar with those aspects of organizational politics. They should, thus, be able to think creatively and bring forward fresh ideas and possibilities that, with thought and guidance, could be tested out in practice. Some of the new ideas and possibilities might ultimately be integrated into the practice situation or further developed as appropriate. Newly devised assessment tools, models of practice and educational products are then left with the service.

Students are particularly keen to see theory in action and often try to engage practitioners in thinking about, and making explicit, their use of theory in practice. As Mattingly and Fleming (1994) advocated, explaining practice decisions and theoretical underpinnings of their work enables therapists to develop further insights into the reasoning process, a reasonable attribute for students also to acquire. Practitioners may sometimes feel threatened by a perceived challenge from students to 'walk on new ground', but given an open mind, and with a commitment to learning in partnership, both student and practitioner can benefit mutually from the experience. Students are more likely to engage in risk-taking if they are in an environment where practitioners are willing to take steps to advance practice in different ways and to evaluate outcomes with the student. Not every new scheme will go well, but reflecting on the process and outcome will inevitably offer fresh insights into problems and possible alternatives for their resolution. Incentives in the grading scheme may encourage students to be creative in the practice environment but, whatever the situation, their enthusiasm for learning and for the profession itself, should be used to advantage.

A student's presence can also promote the concept of 'individual (or group) as expert'. People with disabilities who contribute to aspects of teaching in order to enhance the student's knowledge and understanding of disadvantage and the consequences of disability will be 'experts by experience'. Similarly, if encouraged to do so, the 'student as expert' might also be revealed. The student could engage in discussion with practitioners about new theory or the evidence base for practice. This exposure to current theories might help the practitioners keep up to date or review their work in light of evidence discussed. Students have the capacity to promote learning between a range of stakeholders if given the chance.

STUDENTS AS A MARKETING RESOURCE

Students' enthusiasm for their profession can have spin-offs in different ways. Students can bring youthful energy and enthusiasm to a service, which help to create a positive image of occupational therapy and of what the profession can do. As an example, students are now increasingly being placed in communities where no occupational therapists are employed. They work instead with other members of the team, such as community health workers, community rehabilitation workers, nurses or social workers. Despite little being known about the role and potential of occupational therapy in the setting, students are still able to identify and meet the needs of service users that would otherwise not be addressed. They demonstrate the unique role and interventions of the profession and educate other team members and their managers about occupational therapy and what it can offer. In some instances, community members have raised questions about the absence of occupational therapy resulting in new posts being created. Examples in South Africa include posts in a children's home, within a unit for children with HIV/Aids (Ramugondo, 2004), with community elderly projects (Broderick, 2004) and an old age home, and in the UK, posts with homeless people (Totten & Pratt, 2001).

Some students who have been placed in a community where there was no occupational therapy service have commented on the poor quality of life for members and how the programme they developed brought small changes that made a significant difference (Lorenzo & Friendlander, 2005). One such example was the provision of appropriate paper technology seating for a child, positioning her so that she could participate in playing and interactions with others in her environment (Beeton, personal communication). Others, such as Totten and Pratt (2001), have commented on the need to work hard to adapt and present occupational therapy in a positive light in a non-traditional setting. Gaining credibility and creating an interest in a project amongst members can be hard to do, yet, in this example, a collaborative project such as producing a newsletter offered group participation, engagement in decision making, a tangible product and sense of achievement at the end. The project needs to be self-sustaining after the departure of the student.

When students develop and provide occupational therapy in areas where there are no existing services, they may challenge how things are done. This is not necessarily negative as it can help facilitate change where change is needed. Fresh ideas can be offered as an alternative to those that currently exist. Students need to be advised, however, to act with sensitivity, respect and discretion if feeling the need to be critical about existing services. They need to learn how to build on existing foundations rather than try to change the world.

Awareness raising and advocacy may be relatively new to occupational therapists but without these activities the potential of occupational therapy may go unrecognized. They are necessary in order to expose others to occupational therapy who would otherwise remain ignorant of the profession. They also promote the benefits of using occupational models for developing the potential of individuals and their families within their environment. They market the profession to sceptics who have never really given the profession a chance to show its potential in environments in which disabled or disadvantaged people exist. Students often demonstrate transitions in occupational therapy practice to ensure that it becomes more relevant in meeting the needs of different individuals, groups and populations.

STUDENTS AS A SERVICE RESOURCE

Students can readily contribute to service needs in areas that would not otherwise benefit from occupational therapy. These include services where no occupational therapists are employed as well as services in which the occupational therapy resource is stretched to capacity. Role overload of practitioners may lead, for example, to long waiting lists or referrals for clients who would not otherwise be seen. Some practitioners no longer have the time to see individual patients and are pressurized into offering only group therapy. Students could address needs on a more individual basis. Students tend to be able to spend more time building interpersonal relationships with individuals with whom they are working and to develop a more comprehensive picture of personal needs and strengths so that an appropriate, individually tailored occupational therapy programme can be offered.

Students can also assist the practitioner with their workload, freeing them up to develop new areas of service. The student and practitioner could even engage in new projects together, developing new ideas collaboratively. Where there are long-term projects on the go, one or more components may be suitable for students to complete alone within a time-limited period. These components would help contribute to the bigger scheme.

STUDENTS AS A TEAM-BUILDING RESOURCE

Whilst operating in the practice learning environment, students should be acknowledged as peers and fully integrated into staff teams. However, students often connect with staff who are at a different level in the 'hierarchy', such as support workers, cleaners and auxiliary staff. They are often able to facilitate teamwork by enhancing the skills and knowledge of auxiliary staff and promoting mutual learning. Students also come to appreciate the role of these members of the team and to develop important management skills for the future. Students have indicated that they tend to feel less intimidated by auxiliary staff, recognizing that it is these staff who often provide students with important knowledge about how different systems operate. Through communication with these staff, who often come from local communities, students also develop an understanding of the dynamics of the communities themselves.

Students share knowledge and skills with people at all levels of the organization, thereby increasing their awareness of occupational therapy and facilitating effective collaboration. In so doing, students gain insights into the power dynamics of organizational systems and the relationships that determine the nature of hierarchies. As team members take an active interest in organizational functioning, it has been known for students to contribute to the development of services. As a newcomer to the service, a student can offer insights from observations that alert the team to new ways of thinking. Discussion, dialogue and the sharing of ideas between team members that include students can result in mutual learning and lead to the development of skills and new approaches to service delivery.

STUDENTS AS A PROFESSIONAL DEVELOPMENT RESOURCE

Students ask questions about various aspects of practice and it is often through deliberating on the more challenging questions collectively that learning and professional development takes place. Critical thinking skills and reflective skills are enhanced through dialogue with students and these may prompt new ideas about the service that can be tried and tested out with the student (Higgs, Richardson & Dahlgren, 2004). Practitioners, however, must be open to being interrogated about their practice and for some practitioners this can be a daunting prospect. In this position, it is easy to forget that no practitioner knows everything and that it is acceptable to admit to not knowing the answer. Debating and discovering new perspectives on practice together can lead to professional development on both sides.

Practitioners are sometimes challenged by the constant questioning of their practice and this can lead to reticence about taking students for practice learning, as practitioners can easily feel that their practice and their decision making are being undermined or criticized. Reasons commonly put forward by practitioners for not taking students often shield the underlying fear that their level of competence to teach, guide and assess students is inadequate, and that they lack confidence in their own ability. In order to overcome this fear, practitioners need to address their attitude to learning. Whiteford et al. (2005, p. 8) contend that ongoing learning is essential. Practitioners today can only be 'temporary experts', so practitioners must know both how to learn and how to think. Thus, if practitioners are willing to engage with ongoing learning then they must accept that learning may be prompted by anyone, including students. Learning together can produce results that are of benefit both to the individuals and families concerned, and to the wider service, including its users.

Questions posed by students can create opportunities for developing evidence-based practice. Issues brought to the attention of practitioners may lead to an audit, or evaluation of service delivery, to determine strengths and limitations, and opportunities for seeking new ways of practising and of advancing practice. A focus on evidence-based practice may lead to a literature search and a review of a service in the light of what is found. Where there is no clear guide, research may be indicated to determine 'best practice' in that environment. Both practitioners and students could contribute to the research process, offering professional development opportunities to all.

SUSTAINABILITY

The essence of sustainability is effective planning and resource management, and the richest resource is often perceived to be the people who do the work. Students are one such resource and, if managed creatively, they can make significant and meaningful contributions to sustainable service development in resource-constrained contexts. But because of the nature of the academic year and other curricular issues, students are not able to provide a continuous service. Strategies thus have to be developed to enable students to contribute effectively to sustainable projects within organizations and in the community. In order to do this, it is imperative that there is a system whereby organizations or community members can sustain a development, but at the same time enable students to contribute meaningfully to the project during the time that they are available.

This means that students must be effective in handing over their achievements and recommendations, both to staff in the organization and to the next group of students, so that interruptions caused by curricular constraints do not impact negatively on the programmes that have been implemented in the various communities. Such challenges provide opportunities for students to develop skills in communication, coordination and collaboration. The contributions of experienced staff, and of those offered by students who have the theory and enthusiasm, create enormous potential for service development, given that teamwork is effective.

Students bring time and energy to service organizations. They not only provide an extra pair of hands but also the capacity to complete small-scale projects in line with the ultimate goal of the service. Action learning and reflective practice are processes that contribute positively to sustainability. Support, encouragement and mentoring are also essential for the development of practitioners and future leaders of the occupational therapy profession.

In the second year, students from the University of Cape Town spend a one-week period as fieldwork assessing the environment in different communities. In the process, they network with diverse stakeholders. The students consult to identify a specific need related to health promotion and occupation in order to develop a community education project for the identified organization or stakeholder group. The project should aim to make a contribution to the community. The students then have allocated time to develop the community education project over a two-month period. They do a class presentation and invite different stakeholders to the presentation.

Projects and programmes developed by final- (fourth-) year students are usually driven by service needs. Students develop the product during their practice experience and are assessed on it in their final examination. The product is often used by either the university or organization long after the students leave. The key to the challenge of continuity of programmes started by students is that they are time-bound and identified in conjunction with the practitioners or community members. Such reciprocity provides a way to explore the nature of power in purposeful interactions that contribute to sustainability of new projects within services.

EMERGING THEMES

From the above comments it is easy to see that two clear themes emerge. Firstly, practitioners learn from students as students bring new ideas into the service, ask questions, challenge current practice and enter into debate with the therapists about possible solutions to practice dilemmas or ways of advancing practice. Students and practitioners reflect together, learn together and grow professionally together. Secondly, students contribute to the achievement of organizational goals. The organization becomes a community of learning to which the student contributes and service enhancement and development can result.

Students represent the profession. Their positive contribution and enthusiasm can go a long way towards providing a positive image of what the profession can do. A student, as a new team member, can challenge stereotypes and preconceived ideas, and can often suggest new ways of thinking about problems and dilemmas in practice. A student can bring new energy as well as extra manpower into the service and may even suggest alternative ways of meeting service goals to open-minded practitioners. The fresh approach, which might entail asking seemingly innocent questions, can draw out new perspectives on practice. If acted on, these might ultimately improve the quality of the service. Students often leave a legacy that makes an impact on the service and its users and to which others can relate.

Any innovation of note, due either to new ideas, service audit or research activity, should be considered as a potential topic for publication. Disseminating new ideas that make quality improvements to service provision and impact positively on service users has to be a responsibility of the different stakeholders. A joint paper, either published or presented at a conference, will acknowledge the work of the practitioner and student in partnership.

SATURATION

Given the number of students in training who require high-quality practice experiences, it is not surprising that a common cry from practitioners is that they are at saturation point with students and no longer able to offer practice opportunities. If a service arrives at this point, then measures need to be taken urgently to explore alternatives that make fewer demands on service personnel. The education of occupational therapy students is a relentless process with new educational programmes emerging regularly to swell the numbers of students who require practice opportunities. Services that are well supported by university staff and have mutual benefits are less likely to arrive at saturation point.

The benefits of taking students into services for practice experience must be advocated, but if placements are offered that only match the custom-and-practice experience of 'yester-year' then both students and services will be disadvantaged. Expectations of student education must shift to reflect the changing nature of practice and allow students to develop and consolidate their skills in new ways. If services ignore the potential benefits of having students, or fail to put themselves in a position where they can learn from them and use their skills to advantage, then students and services collectively will suffer. Different kinds of learning experiences are not necessarily synonymous with poorer learning experiences. Provided that a sound infrastructure for student and practitioner support is available then learning opportunities can be made available in many different services and communities. Mechanisms that can support students before, during and after their practice experience and that can promote their learning are explained elsewhere in this book.

AVOIDING EXPLOITATION

This chapter so far has advocated that students have the energy, ideas and capacity to contribute significantly to service delivery and that practice learning is not a 'one-way-street' that advantages only the student. The benefits of mutual learning, of collaboration and of collective professional development have been promoted here so that practitioners and students together can work on creative ventures that offer mutual learning and opportunities for service development and quality enhancement. Unscrupulous services may, however, focus more on using the student as merely another pair of hands to help them deal with waiting lists, backlogs, service overloads or staff shortages. It is easy to forget that students enter the service in order to learn and to develop their competence so that ultimately they can operate confidently alongside their peers once qualified.

Students should not be exploited and merely offered repetitive work that will neither stretch their thinking and reasoning nor promote their learning. Students need opportunities for learning either through carefully thought-out project work or through caseload management. Projects that practitioners themselves would not tackle are inappropriate for students. It is all too easy to have high expectations of students, but the expectations should be realistic and achievable. Students need guidance, support, and opportunities for: reflection; dialogue; and receiving constructive feedback, reinforcing comments and praise in relation to their work. Students should not be directed, but should be allowed to undertake the project in their own way. Risks need to be both taken and managed. Learning will inevitably take place this way.

DOUBLING UP

Various models of student supervision have been proposed but the one-to-one practice educator/student relationship still appears to dominate. Practitioners do take some convincing that supervising two students at a time is less demanding than only supervising one student, but in many circumstances there are benefits to be gained from working with more than one student at once. These benefits are clear. Primarily, students support each other in the learning process. Their first point of contact will be their peer, and not their practice educator, to check their understanding of situations. They will problem solve together, making project work a favoured learning tool for students. Projects can address service goals, with each student addressing a different aspect. Through trial and error and reflection on experiences, students will learn more as a twosome than if they were in a single supervisory relationship.

Practitioners tend to think that they are being exploited if asked to double up and take two students for practice learning, but those who have tried it are clear that there are benefits for all. The students learn together and therefore seek less guidance and support from the supervisor. They can work collaboratively on projects and individually on a caseload, which they can then share with their colleague, so extending their learning. It would seem sensible to suggest that two students to one practitioner should become the norm and one-to-one relationships the exception to the rule.

THE REAL WORLD OF PRACTICE

Hocking and Ness (2005, p. 73) suggested that, commonly, practice education was about 'placing students in health-care settings for periods of time in order to promote the application of academic knowledge to the real world of health-care'. However, Whiteford et al. (2005, pp. 13,14) argued that the real world of healthcare was immensely complex and that practice within it occurred 'at the very edge of chaos', often involving 'a journey into the unknown'. But, through encounters in practice, new understandings could emerge. Students engaging in practice learning are thrust into this environment and are expected not only to make sense of it, but they must also demonstrate that they can operate effectively within it. Their preparation for practice, their initiation into practice and the experiences they have in practice learning thus becomes critical features of their educational programme. Students can thrive if offered suitable experiences. Jensen and Thomas (2005) reported that students who had engaged in projects in resource-constrained environments had felt confident as they graduated and began to practise as occupational therapists. But not all students feel confident about entering and coping in a work environment once qualified. Stress and the feeling of being unsupported can be common (McInstry, 2005). If practice learning has not provided opportunities for students to take control, to deal with risks and complexities and to learn from being exposed to a variety of challenging experiences then arguably the means to grow in confidence may have been restricted. Where students have been given project work and allowed to take risks, where they have shared and used their ideas in practice, their confidence in their own ability to shape practice should have grown.

THE WAY FORWARD

Practitioners have expressed concern that they feel burnt out and bored from struggling to work in resource-constrained contexts, which leads to frustration, disillusionment and a negative attitude towards student practice learning. This chapter has attempted to address the ambivalence and resistance that practitioners sometimes experience at the thought of taking students for practice learning. By shifting the perception of students as a burden and drain on energy and time to seeing students as a resource for service development and continuing professional growth, practitioners should be able to view student education as an opportunity for mutual learning and for professional growth. It is a responsibility of the practitioner, however, to devise a learning programme for the students through which these benefits can emerge.

There appear to be five broad areas in which students might be seen as a resource for the service, namely, a knowledge resource, a marketing resource, a service resource, a team-building resource, and a professional development resource. In their relationship with the service, students can offer a fresh, positive attitude towards occupational therapy and towards what the profession can achieve.

Students can suggest and initiate change, or contribute through project work to service development. Sustainability of project work appears to depend on good planning and resource management. It is important, however, for students to be viewed as integral to the team and a valuable resource rather than a burden. In their capacity as learners, however, students do become a resource for services to use discerningly in ways that contribute effectively to the life-long learning of practitioners. Dialogue, theoretical debate and reflections on practice are thus of mutual benefit to the university practice educator, practitioner and student. The concept of mutual learning should be introduced to students as they prepare for practice learning. A learning network established between academics, service providers and practitioners in different contexts could serve to develop positive approaches to practice learning that can be seen to benefit to all. It is then the responsibility of the practitioner to engage the student in clinical or service initiatives that are achievable and bring about such results.

REFERENCES

Broderick, K. (2004). Grandmothers affected by HIV/AIDS: new roles and occupations. In R. Watson & L. Swartz (Eds.), *Transformation through occupation*. London: Whurr, pp. 233–253.

Higgs, J. & Titchen, A. (2001). Rethinking the practice-knowledge interface in an uncertain world: a model for practice development. *British Journal of Occupational Therapy, 64*(11), 526–533.

Higgs, J., Richardson, B. & Dahlgren, M.A. (2004). *Developing practice knowledge for health professionals*. London: Butterworth-Heinemann.

Hocking, C. & Ness, N.E. (2005). Professional education in context. In G. Whiteford & V. Wright-St Clair (Eds.), *Occupation and practice in context*. Marrickville, NSW: Elsevier, pp. 72–86.

Jensen, H. & Thomas, Y. (2005). Sustainable practice in resource-poor environments. In G. Whiteford & V. Wright-St Clair (Eds.), *Occupation and practice in context*. Marrickville, NSW: Elsevier, pp. 254–272.

Lorenzo, T. & Friendlander, S. (2005). *Hearing the voice of rural communities: the perceptions of occupational therapy students in the Swartland municipal district, Western Cape*. Paper presented at service learning symposium, CHED/JET, University of Cape Town, Cape Town, 1–2 September.

Mattingly, C. & Fleming, M.H. (1994). *Clinical reasoning. Forms of inquiry in a therapeutic practice*. Philadelphia, PA: FA Davis.

McInstry, C. (2005). From graduate to practitioner: rethinking organisational support and professional development. In G. Whiteford & V. Wright-St Clair (Eds.), *Occupation and practice in context*. Marrickville, NSW: Elsevier, pp. 129–142.

Ramugondo, E. (2004). Play and playfulness: children living with HIV/AIDS. In R. Watson & L. Swartz (Eds.), *Transformation through occupation*. London: Whurr, pp. 171–185.

Totten, C. & Pratt, J. (2001). Innovation in fieldwork education: working with members of the homeless population in Glasgow. *British Journal of Occupational Therapy, 64*(11), 559–563.

Whiteford, G., Klomp, N. & Wright-St Clair, V. (2005). Complexity theory: understanding occupation, practice and context. In G. Whiteford & V. Wright-St Clair (Eds.), *Occupation and practice in context*. Marrickville, NSW: Elsevier, pp. 3–15.

11 Partnerships in Service Learning Evaluation

LUCIA HESS-APRIL

OBJECTIVES

The chapter discusses:

- an example of socially responsive practice learning
- service evaluation as a quality assurance mechanism in practice and service learning
- the principles of qualitative service evaluation
- using the findings of service evaluation to inform and enhance practice and service learning.

INTRODUCTION

The University of the Western Cape (UWC) Occupational Therapy Department has, since the 1980s, embarked on providing students with service learning opportunities to help equip them to deal with the challenges of societal needs. Successful partnerships with service providers and key community representatives from the surrounding communities of Mitchell's Plain and Nyanga have been established. These communities are served by the UWC Community-Based Rehabilitation (CBR) Project, which was launched by the occupational therapy department in 1986. The department has endeavoured to equip graduates to address the needs of these communities innovatively through the promotion of social justice.

This chapter provides a brief description the UWC Rehabilitation Project in order to draw out lessons on a partnership with the community of disabled people in evaluation of students' engagement in service learning. Occupational therapy students at UWC are introduced to CBR in the first year of their four-year undergraduate programme. Students explore concepts of health, development and primary healthcare (PHC) through an interdisciplinary faculty foundation course. Foundation courses are generic to all departments in the

Practice and Service Learning in Occupational Therapy. Edited by Theresa Lorenzo, Madeleine Duncan, Helen Buchanan, Auldeen Alsop
© 2006 John Wiley & Sons Ltd

faculty including physiotherapy, psychology, nursing, social work, natural medicine and dietetics. Another first-year faculty foundation course provides an introduction to philosophies of care. In this course, culture and diversity issues and the concept of service provision are addressed. In year two, students engage with the principles and philosophy of health promotion (WHO, 1986). They also undertake practice learning activities where they apply learned principles of health promotion in the surrounding communities. All these courses are integrated into the profession-specific curriculum (Hocking & Ness, 2002). Principles for student engagement are identified. The findings and principles of a service evaluation process undertaken to ascertain the value and outcome of services rendered through the UWC Rehabilitation Project are explained. The principles for the service evaluation process are derived from qualitative research methodology (Rice & Essy, 1999), service quality assurance literature (Potter, 1999) and a research study undertaken by the author (Hess, 2003). The chapter concludes by highlighting the impact of this evaluation process on service standards ensuring that they promote positive outcomes for consumers as well as optimal professional education and learning through the CBR Project.

COMMUNITY-BASED REHABILITATION AS A LEAD THEME FOR SERVICE LEARNING

Rehabilitation services in South Africa are in a process of transformation (Department of Health, 2000; Office of the Deputy President, 1997). This requires an increasing willingness on the part of service providers to engage in partnerships with disabled people and local communities in the planning and delivery of services. Social change, legislative initiatives, growing empowerment among consumer groups and changes in service intervention strategies have increased awareness and demands from persons who utilize rehabilitation services. The National Rehabilitation Policy (Department of Health, 2000) emphasizes that CBR, as an integral part of primary healthcare, should ensure accessibility and affordability of appropriate and acceptable services to target communities.

In South Africa, health and rehabilitation services were historically structured according to the ideology of the apartheid government, resulting in the lack of primary healthcare. During the 1980s, non-governmental organizations predominantly took the initiative for CBR as an alternative to the inadequate institution-based services provided by the South African government. After 1994, based on the policies of the new democratic government, changes were made. The World Health Organization (WHO) introduced community-based rehabilitation as an approach for providing services to disabled people, particularly in developing countries. CBR uses a community development approach to achieve equalization of opportunities and social integration of all people with disabilities (WHO, 2003). The broad methods of CBR include the formulation and implementation of policies, encouraging and supporting communities to assume responsibility for the rehabilitation, social integration and equalization of opportunities of disabled people.

Variations of the WHO model can be found (Cornielje, 1993; Miles, 1996; O'Toole, 1988; Werner, 1998) that employ common principles of CBR. Criticism of CBR has focused on rehabilitation being largely medical, therefore detracting attention from aspects of equalization of opportunities and social integration (Miles, 1996; Werner, 1998). Given this criticism, practice learning has had to ensure that students not only understand theories of human development, but also theories of community development, as well as profession-specific CBR policy documents (Kronenberg, 2003; Scaletti, 1999).

A major weakness of CBR is also seen to be the way in which services are delivered. When CBR activities are designed as service-delivery systems rather than development systems, the danger is that it can easily become focused only on physical rehabilitation of children at home, whilst nothing else happens (Coleridge, 1993). David Werner (1998) suggests that a departure point in addressing this weakness would be to encourage disabled people to take over more organizational and service-providing roles in CBR. This has implications for the way in which practice learning is structured and implies that students should be educated to become advocates for change in collaboration with disability activists.

THE UWC COMMUNITY-BASED REHABILITATION PROJECT

This Project is used as a service learning site for third- and fourth-year students fulfilling their practice learning requirements. The quality of learning at the Project is directly related to the quality of service and the 'goodness of fit' that students perceive between the philosophy and principles of CBR and the actions of service providers. This goodness of fit strengthens the quality of both the service and the educational process. Regular evaluation of a service adds to the knowledge base of CBR and allows service providers and educators to identify innovative approaches and methods for future practice learning and service development. Staff of the UWC Rehabilitation Project currently includes two occupational therapists and eight community rehabilitation workers (CRWs). The CRWs work under the direction and supervision of the two occupational therapists.

The next section briefly describes essential demographics of the society that the Project serves. This is followed by an explanation of the implementation, findings and principles of service evaluation and a discussion on how such an evaluation may be used to direct practice learning and service learning.

THE SOCIAL CONTEXT: MITCHELL'S PLAIN AND NYANGA

Mitchell's Plain has a population of 500,000 (Statistics South Africa, 1998). Housing in Mitchell's Plain ranges from informal settlements (shacks) and council houses with poor socioeconomic conditions, to more affluent areas with larger houses and improved standards of living. Most areas in Mitchell's Plain are characterized by high unemployment, crime and gang-related violence. There are shops, schools and churches in the community. Public transport is readily available in the form of mini-bus taxis, buses and trains. Services for disabled people are limited and there is a general lack of awareness of these services in the community. A strong sense of cohesion prevails, especially at times of crisis when the community comes together to fight for a common cause, for example, the safety of their children.

Nyanga is also divided into different geographical areas, but informal settlements are more prevalent here than in Mitchell's Plain. Statistics on the population indicate that there are approximately 60,000 people living in informal settlement areas and 30,000 in formal housing (Statistics South Africa, 1998). Poor socioeconomic conditions include that of high unemployment, poor living standards and poverty. The present infrastructure is generally of a low standard. In some areas there are tarred roads, water and electricity, in others there is nothing. The area is characterized by many political and community-based organizations concerned with issues of health and community development. There is a high presence of non-governmental organizations and community involvement is fairly high.

PILOTING PARTNERSHIP IN SERVICE EVALUATION

The World Health Organization (WHO) defines community-based education (CBE) as a means of achieving educational relevance to community needs (WHO, 1987). CBE provides opportunities for the University to offer services to the community as well as to realize its primary goal of educating professionals in socially responsive ways. Magzoub and Schmidt (1996) warn that a successful partnership between the university and the community requires active community involvement. The community must know that services and programmes, rather than being imposed, should be informed by their self-identified needs.

According to Kisil and Chaves (1994), students are unlikely to understand the community, its health needs and appropriate approaches, unless they have opportunities for repeated contact with its members. 'Community-oriented' means that the objectives of the CBE curriculum are relevant to community health needs. The content of the curriculum is directed towards addressing the priority health and social needs of the local community with which students engage. CBE thus enables students to relate theoretical learning to practice learning and, in turn, for practice learning to inform and assist with theoretical understanding. The reciprocity of CBE ensures that all parties benefit from the partnership between higher education and society (Magzoub, Ahmed & Salih, 1992).

Evaluation may be defined as the systematic collection of information about the characteristics and outcomes of a service to make judgements about its effectiveness and to inform decisions about service development (Patton, 1997). Evaluation, as in the case of the Project, has not been given much emphasis in CBR and disabled people have often been kept silent on issues that affect their lives (WHO, 2001). Twible and Henley (1993) assert that curriculum design often pays too little attention to the needs of society, because of inadequate analysis of the effect of the data on society. Evaluation of services based on data from society can therefore directly inform practice learning because educators can assess if students, during service learning, fulfil rehabilitation and development functions envisaged by society.

In outlining guidelines for the monitoring of CBR programmes, WHO (1996) stresses that it is important to explore whether disabled people feel that their needs are met when rehabilitation programmes are evaluated. According to Mitchell (1999), the features of CBR on which evaluation should focus include service-delivery systems, technology transfer and community involvement. He suggests that the relationship between service providers and consumers, changes in community attitudes towards disabled people, and the role of the community in the management of the programme are specific issues that should be examined.

METHODS OF FORMATIVE SERVICE EVALUATION

Formative evaluation makes use of qualitative methods to document the needs of a purposively selected, representative sample of disabled people in the communities being served by the project under evaluation (Hess, 2003). Formative service evaluation focuses on service development. It aims to gain an understanding of the perceptions, experiences and opinions of service users about benchmark quality assurance indicators in order to identify aspects that need more development. By incorporating consumer feedback on critical domains of service performance, the quality of outcomes achieved may be enhanced creating an optimal learning environment for prospective health practitioners. Qualitative service evaluation methods may include document reviews, participant observation, semi-structured interviews and focus group discussions. These methods yield evaluative feedback in textual format that may be analysed through various processes of thematic, deductive or content analysis (Rice & Essy, 1999).

Analysis of evaluative feedback data aims to provide information about critical performance indicators, such as: the quality of relationships between service providers and consumers; perceived shifts in community attitudes towards disabled people; and the extent to which the voice and power of disabled people are represented in project management structures (Finkelflugel, 1998). Within each of these quality assurance benchmarks are a set of service performance criteria or indicators that may be investigated. Potter (1999) suggests that indicators used should provide evidence of what services actually do, combined with consumer interpretations of their value.

Examples of quality assurance indicators that emerged from formative service evaluation (Hess, 2003) are:

- facilitating social integration
- developing poverty alleviation programmes
- transfer of knowledge and skills
- consumer participation in service management
- empowerment of consumers and communities
- networking and collaboration
- sustainability of service.

The trustworthiness of the evaluative process and its findings may be monitored through triangulation (for example, evidence-based practice literature), reflexivity (for example, critical debate) and checking with members of the community and representatives from the disability sector (Rice & Essy, 1999).

The next section details how the outcomes of an evaluation of the UWC CBR Project, using these methods, were used to hone the practice-learning and service-learning processes at this site.

SERVICE EVALUATION: IMPROVING THE QUALITY OF PRACTICE LEARNING AND SERVICE LEARNING

Five components of the World Health Organization CBR Model were used as indicators for the evaluation of the UWC CBR Project, namely: available resource utilization; transfer of knowledge and skills; community participation; strengthening referral services; and intersectoral collaboration (WHO, 1994). Feedback from consumers is briefly described and the implications for practice learning are highlighted. Examples are provided of ways in which service learning, and by inference the service itself, were modified to promote excellence (bearing in mind that students are amongst the principal providers of the service in collaboration with CRWs and community members).

The formative service evaluation revealed the degree of emotional trauma and deprivation that people with disabilities experience due to physical, social and economic barriers to equal participation in community life. The most marked concerns of participants related to attitudinal barriers caused by a lack of understanding of disability in the broader community. Service learning in this context, therefore, includes theoretical input on the history of the disability movement in South Africa, the social model of disability (Oliver, 1998) and its implications for practice, the principles of CBR, networking, advocacy strategies and self-efficacy building techniques. Service-learning expectations of students expanded to include principles of advocacy and working with disability activists.

The degree of deprivation that the participants experience due to barriers to equal opportunities was evident in the findings. These barriers were related to community attitude (seeing people as objects of pity), economic barriers (poverty and discrimination in the labour market) and physical barriers (inaccessible transport systems). A key issue for participants was financial need. This relates to poor access to employment and discrimination towards disabled people in the workplace. The majority of participants live on a disability grant, which, in most cases, contributes substantially to the overall family and household income. This impoverishes the individual, who already lives in communities where, for many, life is a daily struggle for survival. Research has indicated that barriers to participation in society lead to decreased self-esteem and lack of empowerment (McLaren, Philpott & Mdunyelwa, 2000; O'Toole, 1988). Removal of these barriers is essential in assisting disabled people, particularly women, to overcome feelings of isolation and dependency (Lorenzo, 2001).

The findings highlighted the need for students to work within the full range of problems faced by disabled people in the community during service learning. University practice educators assist students to make a shift from being the professional expert to acknowledging that disabled people could be their partners and must play a more active role in CBR. Students refer to their involvement as intervention or facilitation in order to move away from the medical term 'treatment'. More importantly, in line with occupational therapists' understanding of people as occupational beings and the relationship between occupation and health, students are expected to develop goals for community projects that encompass a vision in which people with disabilities are respected as valuable citizens, who are integrated into community-life and have equal access to social and economic benefits (Kronenberg, 2003). Practice learning, therefore, includes theoretical input on models of facilitating social integration and developing poverty alleviation programmes.

UTILIZATION OF AVAILABLE RESOURCES

The first component of CBR is the utilization of available resources, where people with disabilities and their families are the most important resource of all (O'Toole, 1987). Other than the training and counselling provided during home visits, disabled people and their families rarely have access to any other form of support system. The majority of participants look to their immediate family to solve day-to-day problems. Assisting a disabled person is demanding and many families may not be able to deal with some of the difficulties they experience. The result is that not only disabled people, but also their families, are disempowered by society's failure to ensure adequate support systems. Practice learning thus enables students to explore the utilization of available community resources, such as disabled people themselves, and address accessibility issues where indicated.

TRANSFER OF KNOWLEDGE AND SKILLS

The evaluation of the Project has informed both the UWC curriculum and the facilitation of practice learning in the community. Issues around CBE and helping students to develop a professional identity in community practice have also been addressed. The focus has moved away from encouraging students to perfect a skill by following a particular pattern to achieve a satisfactory end result, to a system of education that facilitates students' personal growth and understanding of practice (Alsop & Ryan, 1996). The focus now is to facilitate the student's ability to use enabling occupation creatively in order to meet individuals', groups' and communities' needs and circumstances (Kronenberg, Simo-Algado & Pollard, 2005). Students learn to adapt and use different ways of working, depending on assessed needs. They learn to explore, to think and to develop clinical reasoning skills. They feel comfortable about modifying their method of working to meet changing needs and circumstances. As professionals, these students will understand historical developments, incorporate government policies into practice, and be sensitive to cultural needs and differences.

The role of occupational therapists and CRWs in home visits and the facilitation of groups were regarded as pivotal to the quality of life of all the participants. The functional activities that participants were now able to perform more independently through the use of assistive devices and the techniques of assistance taught to family members were also apparent. Occupational therapists working in CBR, however, must guard against home visiting becoming an 'institutionalized activity' with people with disabilities being passive recipients (Miles, 1996). As Werner (1998) and Coleridge (1993) suggested, this weakness could be addressed by encouraging people with disabilities to take on service-provider roles.

This suggests that students should be oriented towards the principles of CBR and the social model of disability (Department of Health, 2000), as this would assist them to make a shift from being service providers, working for people with disabilities, to being partners in service provision and working with people with disabilities. Students' service learning objectives, therefore, include objectives related to developing life-skills of disabled people in the community. Students work with Disabled People's Organizations (DPOs) and train their members to be peer-counsellors and to facilitate community awareness raising activities. Examples of practice-learning activities include facilitating workshops on the rights of the disabled and related policies, and training in leadership, organizational management and advocacy skills.

Occupational therapists indicated that factors such as a lack of funding influence their ability to fully achieve facilitation of employment. To relieve this burden, Sharma and Deepak (2001) recommend linking skills development programmes to outside organizations. Research has established that community support of skills-development and intersectoral collaboration are vital to successful integration (O'Toole, 1987; Turmusani, 1999). Collaboration with vocational training programmes and advocacy for employment services should be strengthened (Kent, Chandler & Barnes, 2000; Meyer & Moagi, 2000). Students are therefore expected to foster working relationships with and between DPOs, NGOs, and government departments such as Labour, Transport and Social Services when addressing community and/or disability issues.

It became clear through this service evaluation process that disabled people need to be enabled to take ownership of their own problems so that they can advocate for the resources necessary to solve them. Capacity building is needed so that disabled people can develop positive self-identities and a shared consciousness. In practice learning, students are assisted to appreciate this as part of enabling occupation and an empowering process whereby disabled people are provided with the tools that they need to change their lives.

COMMUNITY PARTICIPATION

Community participation was identified as a major challenge for occupational therapists as awareness-raising campaigns have been relatively ineffective in the broader community. This could be because the occupational therapists' focus has been more on the disabled individual and less on environmental and social barriers. Direct involvement of the community is essential for the sustainability of a CBR programme (Office of the Deputy President, 1997). Enabling occupation results from the dynamic interaction and interdependence between persons, environment and occupation, with occupation emerging from interactions between persons and their environments (Canadian Association of Occupational Therapy, 1997). Krefting (1998) suggests that training provided to community organizations should offer participants a chance to develop new attitudes, beliefs, values and skills to assist disabled people to be included in every sphere of community living. To do this, students need to understand client-centred practice as it relates to CBR and community development. They have to work collaboratively 'with' communities rather than doing things 'for' them. This involves advocating with and for disabled people to equalize opportunities for occupational engagement in society through the notion of occupational justice (Kronenberg, 2003).

STRENGTHENING REFERRAL SYSTEMS AND INTERSECTORAL COLLABORATION

Networking and intersectoral collaboration are vital to ensure successful disability awareness campaigns and for referral systems to be strengthened. This implies that service learning in the context of CBR should be structured to allow students to engage in partnerships with government departments, NGOs and CBOs to promote the concept of disability as a human rights and development issue. In Guyana (O'Toole, 1988) and Bangladesh (Krefting, 1998), such contacts helped to strengthen partnerships and to facilitate efforts that ensured that appropriate attention was given to disability issues in related areas of programme planning and development.

The UWC practice learning curriculum is geared towards producing graduates who understand the ways in which environments support engagement in occupation and how constraints can lead to restriction of health and wellness. The application of the model that students use at the UWC Rehabilitation Project is now described.

CONCLUSION

Occupational therapists have, for a long time, been challenged to learn more about the socio-political factors of communities and their influence on health, to investigate expanding their role from therapist to health agent, and to consider alternative models of practice (Mulholland & Derdall, 2005; Whiteford, Cusick & Strong, 1998). The theory base in occupational therapy that informs community practice has been well-documented (Finlayson & Edwards, 1995; McColl, 1998), whilst literature on the development of occupational therapy curricula stresses that an important outcome should be sound theoretical principles and models of occupational therapy at all levels of care (Watson & Swartz, 2004). This chapter has explained how findings from a partnership in service evaluation could be used practically by occupational therapists to improve services and become more effective in meeting the needs of communities. It has further shown how occupational therapy curricula can prepare students for community service by developing students' professional identity and providing appropriate structures and processes for community practice. It became clear through this service evaluation process that practice learning and service learning could and should enable students to understand theories of community development and to become agents of social change.

REFERENCES

Alsop, A. & Ryan, S. (1996). *Making the most of fieldwork education: a practical approach*. London: Chapman and Hall.

Canadian Association of Occupational Therapy (1997). *Enabling occupation: An occupational therapy perspective*. Ottawa: CAOT.

Coleridge, P. (1993). *Disability, liberation and development*. Oxford: Oxfam.

Cornielje, H. (1993). A local disability movement as part of a CBR programme. In H. Finkenflugel (Ed.), *The handicapped community*. Amsterdam: VU University Press, pp. 17–21.

Department of Health (2000). *Rehabilitation for all. National rehabilitation policy.* Pretoria: Department of Health.

Finkelflugel, H. (1998). Rehabilitation research in South Africa. *Proceedings of the workshop on research informed rehabilitation planning in Southern Africa.* Harare, Zimbabwe, July, 41–60.

Finlayson, M. & Edwards, E. (1995). Integrating concepts of health promotion into occupational therapy practice. *Canadian Journal of Occupational Therapy, 62*(2), 70–75.

Hess, L. (2003). *Consumers' needs and perceptions of a community-based rehabilitation project.* Unpublished thesis for the award of Master of Public Health, Cape Town: University of the Western Cape.

Hocking, C. & Ness, N.E. (2002). *Revised minimum standards for the education of occupational therapists.* Perth, Western Australia: World Federation of Occupational Therapists.

Kent, R.M., Chandler, B.J. & Barnes, M.P. (2000). An epidemiological survey of the health needs of disabled people in a rural community. *Clinical Rehabilitation, 14,* 481–490.

Kisil, M. & Chaves, M. (1994). Linking the university with the community and its health system. *Medical Education, 28,* 343–349.

Krefting, D. (1998). *Implementing CBR: community approaches to handicap and disability.* Bangladesh: Center for Disability and Development.

Kronenberg, F. (2003). *Position paper on community based rehabilitation.* Forrestfield, Western Australia: World Federation of Occupational Therapists. Available at www.wfot.org

Kronenberg, F., Simo-Algado, S. & Pollard, N. (Eds.) (2005). *Occupational therapy without borders: learning from the spirit of survivors.* Edinburgh: Elsevier Churchill Livingstone.

Lorenzo, T. (2001). Collective action for social change: disabled women in the Western Cape. *Agenda, 47,* 89–94.

Magzoub, M.E., Ahmed B.O. & Salih, S.T. (1992). Eleven steps of community-based education as applied at Gezira Medical School. *Anals of Community-oriented Education, 5,* 11–17.

Magzoub, M. & Schmidt, H. (1996). Community-based programmes: what is their impact? *Education for Health, 9*(2), 206–219.

McColl, M. (1998). What do we need to know to practice occupational therapy in the community? *American Journal of Occupational Therapy, 52*(1), 11–18.

McLaren, P., Philpott, S. & Mdunyelwa, M. (2000). *The Disability Information Project (DIP) in the Emtshezi / Okhahlamba district.* Durban: Health Systems Trust.

Meyer, C. & Moagi, S. (2000). Determining priority needs of mothers with disabled children in Winterveldt. *South African Journal of Occupational Therapy, 30*(2), 7–11.

Miles, S. (1996). Engaging with the disability rights movement: the experience of community based rehabilitation in Southern Africa. *Disability & Society, 11*(4), 501–517.

Mitchell, R. (1999). The research-base of community-based rehabilitation. *Disability & Rehabilitation, 21*(10–11), 459–468.

Mulholland, S. & Derdall, M. (2005). A strategy for supervising occupational therapy students at community sites. *Occupational Therapy International, 12*(1), 28–43.

Office of the Deputy President (1997). *White paper on an integrated national disability strategy.* Pretoria: Rustica Press D6078.

Oliver, M. (1998). Theories of disabilities in health practice & research. *British Medical Journal, 317*, 1446–1449.

O'Toole, B. (1987). Community-based rehabilitation (CBR): problems and possibilities. *European Journal of Special Needs and Education, 2*(3), 177–190.

O'Toole, B. (1988). A community-based rehabilitation programme for pre-school disabled children in Guyana. *International Journal of Rehabilitation Research, 11*, 323–334.

Patton, M.Q. (1997). *Utilization-focussed evaluation: the new century text.* Thousand Oaks, CA: Sage.

Potter, C. (1999). Programme evaluation. In M. Blanche & K. Durrheim (Eds.), *Research in practice.* Cape Town: UCT Press, pp. 209–224.

Rice, P. & Essy, D. (1999). *Qualitative research methods – a health focus.* Sydney: Oxford University Press, pp. 40–49.

Scaletti, R. (1999). A community development role for occupational therapists working with children, adolescents and their families: a mental health perspective. *Australian Occupational Therapy Journal, 46*, 43–51.

Sharma, M. & Deepak, S. (2001). A participatory evaluation of a community-based rehabilitation programme in North Central Vietnam. *Disability & Rehabilitation, 23*(8), 352–358.

Statistics South Africa (1998). *Census in brief. The people of South Africa population census 1996.* Pretoria: Statistics South Africa.

Turmusani, M. (1999). The economic needs of disabled people in Jordan: from the personal to the political perspective. *Disability Studies Quarterly, 19*(1), 156–163.

Turmusani, M., Vreede, A. & Wirz, S.L. (2002). Some ethical issues in CBR initiatives in developing countries. *Disability & Rehabilitation, 24*(10), 558–564.

Twible, R. & Henley, E. (1993). A curriculum model for a community development approach to community-based rehabilitation. *Disability, Handicap & Society, 8*(1), 43–57.

Watson, R. & Swartz, L. (Eds.) (2004). *Transformation through occupation.* London: Whurr.

Werner, D. (1998). Nothing about us without us, developing innovative technologies for, by and with disabled persons. *Healthrights, 10.*

Whiteford, G., Cusick, A. & Strong, J. (1998). Dialogue and direction: A new focus for occupational therapy academic programmes in Australia. *Australian Occupational Therapy Journal, 45*, 139–143.

WHO (1986). *Ottawa charter on health promotion.* Geneva: World Health Organization.

WHO (1987). *Community-based education of health personnel: report of a WHO study group.* World Health Organization Technical Report, Series 746.

WHO (1994). *Community based rehabilitation.* Geneva: World Health Organization.

WHO (1996). *Guidelines for conducting, monitoring and self-assessment of community-based rehabilitation programmes.* Geneva: World Health Organization.

WHO (2001). *Rethinking care from the perspective of disabled people: conference report and recommendations.* Geneva: World Health Organization.

WHO (2003). *Report of international consultation to review community-based rehabilitation (CBR).* Helsinki. 25–28 May.

III Enhancing Potential

Introduction to Part III

Part II has offered ideas and strategies for developing students' professional identity through their engagement in different learning scenarios that aim to develop their confidence and competence for their role as occupational therapists. Mechanisms that may be adopted in different contexts to support and promote learning have also been explained. This next part takes *enhancing potential* as its central theme.

Part III addresses the educational processes supporting practice and service learning. Chapter 12 highlights the role of groups and group work in achieving a range of educational objectives in a developing society. It is argued that groups form the social basis of both educational and community contexts, and therefore deserve greater significance in the professional practice curriculum. Chapter 13 explains how students can be guided towards transforming their practice-learning experiences through briefing and debriefing. It is argued that the emotional impact of practice learning in complex contexts may be understood and managed better by students and staff using psychodynamic theory and principles. Chapter 14 presents arguments for promoting competence through assessment and provides practical ideas for adapting assessment methods whilst remaining committed to the principles of rigour. Chapter 15 argues that constructive written and verbal feedback promotes the development of critical thinking and professional reasoning competencies. It is aimed at equipping university practice educators, learning facilitators and students with guidelines for engaging formatively with writing and supervision tasks. Chapter 16 presents a novel approach to student supervision. It describes the structure and principles through which senior students may provide peer supervision to junior students and what both groups may learn in the process. Chapter 17 reaffirms the importance of lifelong learning for ensuring relevant professional growth and Chapter 18 concludes the book by examining the diverse modes of knowledge production that are likely to influence practice education and learning in the future. Reflections on the current status of practice and service learning in the profession of occupational therapy are offered and include suggestions for research as a means for enhancing potential in context.

Practice and Service Learning in Occupational Therapy. Edited by Theresa Lorenzo, Madeleine Duncan, Helen Buchanan, Auldeen Alsop
© 2006 John Wiley & Sons Ltd

12 Group Processes in Practice Education

MADELEINE DUNCAN

OBJECTIVES

The chapter discusses:

- the fundamental principles and processes of groups that may be used in practice education
- group work as an educational strategy for promoting practice learning
- how an understanding of latent group processes enables the educator and the learner to engage creatively with manifest group tasks
- the value of group work for perspective transformation, peer support and community building.

INTRODUCTION

Groups form a natural part of the tertiary education experience and may be used to achieve a range of academic objectives. Students either attend lectures or seminars in large groups; form groups spontaneously to discuss academic matters or they may be expected to work in small groups for specific project-based learning tasks. As a pedagogical tool, the group format enables multiple educational objectives to be accomplished, especially if the latent group processes are harnessed as part of the formal curriculum. The educational group may be seen as an interactional space in which the mutual exchange and dialogue happening between student members in the 'here and now' is aimed at generating professional practice knowledge and gaining personal–professional understanding.

This chapter presents practical ideas for the use of groups as a medium for enhancing practice learning. It explains the use of large, median and small groups to prepare students for, and to support them during, practice-learning experiences. It is argued that, since groups form the matrix (a complex web of

Practice and Service Learning in Occupational Therapy. Edited by Theresa Lorenzo, Madeleine Duncan, Helen Buchanan, Auldeen Alsop
© 2006 John Wiley & Sons Ltd

connections and communications) of society, they may be overtly used in a 'living curriculum' to prepare students for professional practice and for working collaboratively with a range of role-players to bring about social change. The chapter concludes with guidelines for addressing the potential resistances to this form of curriculum and for preparing educators to work creatively with student groups.

FUNDAMENTAL PRINCIPLES AND PROCESSES OF GROUPS

The 'nuts and bolts' of a group, such as its purpose, communication patterns, interaction, goals, norms, culture and roles, impact, in one way or another, on the quality of learning that occurs and on the effectiveness of the group in meeting its educational objectives (Becker & Duncan, 2005). Students are often given group-based learning tasks and expected to 'get on with it'. The 'product' of the group activity, for example, an assignment or project, is then assessed with little attention given to the learning that may occur if the student group is also expected to understand how the latent processes of their interactions influenced their output. If the group is seen as a coherent entity, a system, with properties and dynamics that are independent and more than the whole created by individual members and their various interactions, then the processes of the group itself deserves attention as part of the practice-learning agenda.

At an individual level, students need to acquire three sets of skills in order to participate in, and benefit from, academic group processes:

1. relating skills (for example, finding their voice in the group, accommodating differences of opinion and resolving conflict)
2. thinking skills (for example, generating new ideas and identifying theory in practice through critical group discussion)
3. action skills (for example, making something together or writing a group report).

These three skills may be shaped by getting students to reflect on the internal mechanisms of their academic group processes. At a meta-level, the student 'group-as-a-whole' (a cohort of students following a professional programme together for an extended period of time) is likely to express, and be influenced by, broader sociocultural discourses, such as gender, race and power (de Maré, 1998). These discourses may also become the focus of exploration in order for students to gain a deeper understanding of the society (or organization) within which they are situated. A group-based approach to curriculum, therefore, offers scope for achieving learning outcomes associated with appropriate community entry, understanding organizational and social dynamics, promoting cultural sensitivity and advancing professional socialization.

GROUPS: THE MATRIX OF ACADEMIC AND SOCIAL COMMUNITIES

Groups constitute the matrix within which social and learning communities operate. People live, work, play and learn in small and large groups, thereby creating a multi-facetted web of social connectedness. They find individual and collective meaning, support and a sense of belonging (or alienation) through linking with (or distancing themselves from) a network of 'others' in culturally or contextually determined ways. Group work is likewise embedded in the education process. Students invariably learn in either small or large group formats, especially if a problem-orientated or problem-based learning approach is followed (Savin-Baden, 2000). Novice professionals, therefore, require:

- knowledge of relevant group theories and group-work skills for promoting community or organizational development (Smit, 2005). For example, students doing service learning at non-governmental organizations need to discern how the management structures operate in order to engage through the appropriate channels
- awareness of group and social phenomena, such as power and politics as these play out in the dynamics of small groups, organizations and systems. For example, understanding more about social discourse helps students recognize the dynamics of stigma and power that leads to the marginalization and exclusion of disabled people (Baworowska and Schick 2000; Marks, 1999)
- attitudes and values that contribute to a progressive realization of human rights in communities disenfranchized during apartheid or other instances of social oppression (Baldwin-Ragaven, de Gruchy & London, 1999)
- group-work techniques and methods for the attainment of a range of health and development objectives. For example, forum theatre may be used as a group-based, health promotion strategy and large groups may be used to facilitate the adjustment of communities in transition (O'Brien, 2005).

A distinction is made here between group work as an education strategy within an undergraduate health professional curriculum and training students in group-work skills as an intervention method in practice. The former use of groups prepares and contains students for and during practice learning. The latter refers to training in group-work methodology for professional practice with groups of clients. Groups, in both scenarios, create opportunities for learning that enhances the outcomes of practice education.

GROUPS: CONNECTING WITH COMMUNITY

Words, such as 'service', 'meeting community needs' and 'civic responsibility', imply a set of attitudes that are aligned with social justice and with proactive participation in activities that contribute to social change. Attitudes, such as other centeredness, connectedness and mutuality, suggest an orientation towards promoting the good of the group or society through responsible, goal-directed collaborative action. The actions and involvement of health professionals in community development are sanctioned by the community within which, for whom, and in collaboration with whom, they work. Health professionals must be good team players. They must understand how groups and organizations work in order to build the necessary connections through which change may occur. Student health professionals are not only learners 'from' others (for example, patients/clients, disabled persons, community members, health team colleagues), but also, as knowledgeable citizens, a valuable resource 'giving to' and 'working with' others in finding solutions for mutually identified, meaningful concerns.

A collaborative (as opposed to prescriptive) approach to the design of a practice-learning curriculum requires that attention be paid to community entry processes and to organizational and social dynamics. Understanding more about group principles and processes is one way of managing the relationship between the academic institution that is negotiating access for students to practice learning opportunities on the one hand, and site representatives on the other hand. Students also gain a deeper understanding of community entry dynamics once they appreciate the latent processes against which people need to defend themselves during times of change, stress and pain (for example, unconscious mistrust leading to the defence of splitting between 'the university' and 'the community'). Group work provides a valuable educational medium for exploring and learning about social processes that impact on the practice contexts in which students work.

Community Entry

It has been suggested thus far that community entry is, for all health professionals including the learner therapist, a privilege and not a right that may be assumed by virtue of their professional expertise and level of education. The responsibility for knowing how to behave and for displaying appropriate attitudes that are sensitive to local cultural norms rests with the professional. In delivering community-based services, the student health professional is essentially an outsider who has to seek permission to enter what may be considered the sacred spaces of people's private lives and circumstances. The learner, as an outsider, has to enter the community humbly, with a deep respect for its diversity. Community entry requires the willingness to listen and learn rather than zeal to 'make things better' because of an assumed authority situated in academic knowledge and professional expertise.

This kind of awareness and social sensitivity may be shaped through enabling students to learn from the 'underground' processes of their own group experiences. Community members are usually keen to collaborate with trainee health professionals and service providers in anticipation of benefiting in some way from the mutual exchange. Practice education should therefore shape professional attitudes and values that convey commitment to partnership, social development, transformation and lifelong learning.

One avenue for attaining these curriculum outcomes is through maximizing the educational potential of the dynamics, structures and processes of small, median and large groups throughout the undergraduate programme. For example, the ethics of community entry affirm diversity, endorse human rights and promote justice, equity and participation. By grouping a cohort of students into 'class-as-community', they begin to discover how they conduct their lives in each other's presence. The class becomes a microcosm of society, offering some insights into community dynamics (for example, subgrouping according to ethnicity); social discourse (for example, gendered nuances in the use of language); and participatory ethics (for example, democratic decision making). Group work enables the curriculum to come 'alive', because it creates opportunities for stepping back from established ways of thinking about the world in order to ponder and, if indicated, embrace alternative perspectives and behaviours. Groups provide a forum for bringing the tacit, attitudinal and moral-ethical dimensions of professional practice to the surface progressively and iteratively throughout the formative educational programme.

GROUP PROCESSES AS 'LIVING CURRICULUM'

Slattery (1995, p. 56) suggests that a curriculum is more than 'a tangible object or the implementation of planned lessons or course guides, it is a process of running the lifelong learning racecourse'. Professional socialization occurs through 'living curriculum'; that is, through the process of becoming competent in a particular interpretation of reality. By creating a culture of community amongst a cohort of students, transformation moves out of the textbook into a lived experience of professional values and ethics in the mainstream of the educational process. Group work provides an educational strategy for students to learn about themselves as members of a practice community.

GROUPS AND PERSPECTIVE TRANSFORMATION

Perspective transformation has been described as freeing the self from the taken-for-granted ideology of social conventions, beliefs and modes of operation in order to view the world and its possibilities for affirming human diversity differently (Duncan, 2005). Group work offers an ideal medium, a 'living curriculum' as it were, through which attitudes, values and beliefs may be addressed, especially if attention is paid to the latent social discourses about power, race, gender and ability that underpin discussions about manifest curriculum topics. Students may, for example, do small group projects on income-generating occupations with disabled persons and, during the course of planning, identify the numerous barriers faced by disabled women in particular. They may use this opportunity to learn about the social discourses associated with gender oppression, or the ethnocentric beliefs about the roles of women and the impact that cultural values may have on occupational deprivation, alienation and development. Students come to a deeper appreciation of the potential that role diversity plays in the development of new forms of knowledge and understanding. This appreciation is made possible through an exploration of alternative world-views that exist amongst students from different ethnic backgrounds within the student group itself.

GROUPS: A SPACE FOR COLLECTIVE REFLECTION

Groups raise awareness about the phenomenology of 'the other', and thereby create opportunities for the shared exploration of dominant social discourses, ideologies and values (Blackwell, 2000). By structuring a cohort of students into 'class-as-community', the large group, so constituted (usually 45–55 in size), may be viewed as a microcosm of society, which, on considered reflection, offers rudimentary insights into community dynamics, social discourse and participatory ethics. In this way, group work enables the curriculum to come 'alive' because it creates opportunities for stepping back from established ways of thinking about the world in order to ponder and, if indicated, embrace alternative perspectives and behaviours. Figure 12.1 depicts a layered approach to group work in practice education. The various levels are nested

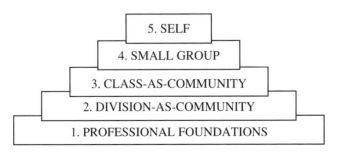

Figure 12.1 Levels of group work in practice education

in each other creating a seamless infrastructure for reflection within the curriculum.

LEVEL 1: PROFESSIONAL FOUNDATIONS

The practice education curriculum is built on the foundations of professional philosophy, values and theory. It is suggested throughout this book that when the philosophy of occupational therapy is experienced as a way of life during the professional socialization process; then students become transformed in much the same way as clients do who discover their potential through purposeful and meaningful occupation. Adult education is more than grasping knowledge; it involves actively transforming knowledge and being transformed by it through the praxis or dynamic engagement between educators, learners and learning systems in a reciprocal process of exploration, action and reflection. Groups provide a forum for these kinds of critical reflection.

LEVEL 2: DIVISION-AS-COMMUNITY

Arising from collective deliberations between students, staff and community representatives, a Statement of Intent aims to reinforce professional socialization. It sets the tone for interactions amongst staff and students and between the Division and practice learning sites by, for example, guiding how written feedback is given to students; the tone and content of handouts; or ensuring that academic discussions remain vigilant about oppressive language practices. Here is an example of a Statement of Intent:

> One of the cornerstones of our therapeutic approach is a value for human relationships. Occupational therapists meet many different people through their work. Past experiences influence the relationships we form. We believe that our attitude to any human condition that is different from what we ourselves are familiar with is usually based on assumptions, stereotypes, prejudice and personal values. It is our personal and professional responsibility as staff and students to explore and deal with these biases on a individual and organizational level. Forms of discrimination that occupational therapists encounter relate to resistance against the diversity of disability, age, gender, class, sexual orientation and religion amongst others . . . We are committed to raising awareness about diversity and trying to address all issues that lead to discrimination. The richness of shared experience and group process will be used in strategies to promote learning and develop skills to address discrimination in constructive and creative ways. Together we want to unlearn prejudice, foster awareness of human rights and celebrate diversity.
> Dated 1999, Division of Occupational Therapy, UCT.

(Watson, 2002)

The Statement of Intent may be supported by a set of perspective triggers that alert students and staff to ways in which diversity may be affirmed and a sense of community built:

- **Language**: do we use language in ways that perpetuate racism, ageism, disabilism, sexism and other isms? Do we reinforce stereotypes about gender, class, ability, religion or other dimensions of difference by our choice of words or attitudes?
- **Culture**: what prejudices do we hold towards people who are different from us and how may these lead to the unintentional oppression of others?
- **Educational preparedness**: what assumptions do we make about people who have different educational histories to our own? How do these assumptions influence the reciprocity of knowledge sharing amongst us?
- **Status**: what impact do our stereotypes about social status have on the balance of power in relations between people? Do our attitudes affirm or negate human dignity?
- **Knowledge**: how may we affirm the indigenous knowledge of different social groupings? In what ways do our biases marginalize the voices of other perspectives?
- **Power**: in what ways can the direction and force of influence be equalized?

Perspective triggers pose rhetorical questions that challenge taken for granted assumptions about the way things should or ought to be done within a group or community. They also act as potential reference points for reflection in median groups (see below) and help in the affirmation of indigenous world-views.

Application

'Division-as-community' large group gatherings focus on promoting inclusive organizational behaviour amongst staff and students. These gatherings, held once or twice a year, aim to establish an ethos of collegiality within the Division and to create opportunities for the Statement of Intent to be revised. In the spirit of transformational leadership, students take responsibility with staff for the development the Division transformation agenda. Large group experiences act as intermittent reminders for the Division-as-community that transformation is an ongoing, lifelong learning agenda worthy of attention in the interest of nation building, professional development and social relevance.

One gathering, for example, discussed the annual social event that is usually held in honour of the graduating class. Historically, it took the form of a dance and meal at an expensive restaurant. Group dialogue focused on inclusion and exclusion; many students acknowledging that it had 'never entered our minds' that the venue, time, dress, food, alcohol, dancing and late night transport from township areas excluded a number of students. Our assumptions were unpacked and an alternative, more inclusive event was planned. This learning was taken forward into an exploration of community processes, cultural practices and the need for students to be vigilant about their assumptions when entering culturally unfamiliar contexts.

LEVEL 3: CLASS-AS-COMMUNITY

Each cohort of students develops a class constitution soon after they enter the undergraduate programme and revisit it at strategic points throughout the ensuing four years of professional education. A class constitution is a working, one-page document guiding the activities of the 'class-as-community'. It consists of a set of norms that guide collegiality during the knowledge construction process within a particular class and smaller working groups.

Application: Class Constitution

Typically a class constitution may consist of a purpose statement; an analysis of current strengths and challenges amongst the cohort of students; and a series of guidelines for class interaction and interdependence in the knowledge construction process. The constitution is 'workshopped' against the backdrop of relevant literature, anti-bias exercises and group discussions about pertinent issues, such as historical influences on professional values and ethics. Substantial reference is made to the contexts of practice learning, current political agendas influencing health practices and the ways in which power manifests in organizations and social systems.

Application: Median Groups

Typically a median group consists of 15–35 people who meet formally for social learning through an exploration of the internal events of group behaviour and thought. The group is the object of discussion, not the individual (Lyndon, 1995). The emphasis is on the 'the work of the group itself . . . to humanize the group rather than to socialize the individual' (Lyndon, 1995, p. 40). There is no attempt at using the group to gain insight into how the unconscious mind of the individual student operates or to use the group as a therapeutic space for students.

The University of Cape Town (UCT) Division of occupational therapy has been running median groups since 1995 (Duncan, 2005). Two members of the academic staff act as constant facilitators with a particular cohort of students from first through to fourth year. There are two teams of facilitators in the Division who meet for in-service training and to review the educational benefits of the process without compromising group confidentiality. Students are informed about the anticipated learning outcomes for median groups (for example, enhanced reflective practice and cultural competence) and are encouraged to engage with relevant literature in making theoretical sense of their group learning (Baworowska & Schick, 2000; Lyndon, 1995; Maxwell, 2000).

The 'cultural context' of the class-as-group becomes the foreground of dialogue within the median group. 'Cultural context' in this instance refers to the diversity amongst students within the class as well as the sociocultural environments of the practice learning sites where they work. The 'life-world' (here-and-now) in the classroom and in the practice-learning context becomes the landscape against which the group explores alternative interpretations of socially constructed attitudes and assumptions. It is the commonly shared ground that ultimately determines the meaning and significance of all events brought to the groups' attention through individual practice learning stories.

Collective assumptions, attitudes and ideologies become identified when individual concerns, such as discomfort in dealing with poverty or social injustice, are raised. Students come to appreciate, through exploration of intra-group phenomena, how their attitudes, values and beliefs are situated, on the one hand, in social discourses about difference in all its forms (for example, gender, race, ability) and, on the other hand, in professional philosophy. Their unfolding professional identity and growing sense of social responsiveness enables them to clarify, for example, how it may have been possible for clinicians during the apartheid era to become complacent or apathetic in the face of pervasive oppression.

Median group discussions, interspersed by reflections or interpretations from the facilitators, offer students containment for the emotions and questions that arise during practice learning in complex social environments. By listening for the unconscious group mind as it tells a social story, facilitators are able to offer possible 'outsights' (reflections that may point to shared assumptions operating through attitudes, ideologies and group culture) at appropriate times and in affirming ways, always seeking to trust the groups' capacity for interdependence in the knowledge construction process (Lyndon, 1995). 'Outsights' promote an understanding that 'what we know in our lived experience is shaped through the cultural weave of community discourse' (Madigan, 1996, p. 49).

As time progresses, the group starts to venture its own interpretations of 'group mind as culture' (de Mare, 1991). Students learn during the first year how to dialogue in generative, supportive ways during the median group space and to use the time to consider their personal development from 'individual', to 'social being', to 'health professional with social responsibilities'. The group is free to explore its own intra-group communication; the content of which changes over the years as students mature and are able to identify praxis between theory, experience and personal/professional development. Minorities in the group start finding their voice when there is evidence that the student cohort in which they find themselves is committed to understanding and redressing prejudicial, biased or complacent attitudes. This is always an exceptionally humbling and enriching space to witness; a space when people from different world-views, experiences and social histories find meaning in their common humanity or gain an understanding of the 'other' perspective.

LEVEL 4: PEER GROUP

Global trends in curriculum design favour the use of group-based learning (Wenger, 1998). Small group (5–8 students) dynamics influence how and what people learn. Groups open up the possibility for students to construct knowledge together, whilst also learning how to work as members of a team and, in so doing, to become sensitized to alternative visions of society. Educators therefore have to be skilled, not only in identifying subject specific triggers for group learning, but also in enabling study groups to reflect on their particular group dynamics. Understanding how the internal processes of the group impact on the progression of learning through inclusion and accommodation of diverse perspectives promotes professional socialization. This in turn equips students with skills to use during practice learning with small and large groups of clients.

The pressure of getting through curriculum content often means that the tacit dimensions of the learning process in groups and the concurrent conscientisation of the participants about issues of diversity are either not addressed or not deemed relevant to professional socialization. Valuable opportunities for effecting attitudinal shifts are therefore lost. Optimizing the educational benefits of groups requires academic staff to be informed about group theory, methods and processes irrespective of their discipline specific expertise.

Application

Task and maintenance functions may be fulfilled by any person in the group; in fact, the aim is for the group members to share these functions flexibly amongst themselves.

The ideal is for the facilitator to model these leadership functions during the initial phase of the group and to create opportunities for members to acquire and exercise these functions as the group unfolds. In this way the responsibility for learning lies with the students as they come to appreciate the various ways in which they may use these group leadership functions in the field. Examples of the task and maintenance leadership functions that small group learning facilitators may use to promote group interaction and learning (for example, during tutorials) are given below (adapted from Johnson & Johnson, 1975).

Task functions:

- **Information and opinion giver**: offers facts, opinions, ideas, suggestions and relevant information/principles/core concepts/to help group discussion. Didactic input is kept to a minimum.

- **Information and opinion seeker/prober**: asks for facts, information, opinions, ideas and feelings from other members to help group discussion.
- **Starter**: proposes goals and tasks to initiate action within the group.
- **Direction giver**: develops plans on how to proceed and focuses attention on the task to be done.
- **Summarizer/linker**: pulls together related ideas or suggestions and restates them by paraphrasing major points discussed.
- **Coordinator**: shows relationships among various ideas by pulling them together and harmonizes activities of various subgroups and members.
- **Diagnoser**: figures out sources of difficulties the group has in working effectively and the blocks to progress in accomplishing the group's goals.
- **Energizer**: stimulates a higher quality of work from the group.
- **Reality tester**: examines the practicality and workability of ideas, evaluates alternative solutions, and applies them to real situations to see how they will work. Introduces an Afrocentric perspective to Eurocentric literature.
- **Evaluator**: compares group decisions and accomplishments with group standards and goals.

Maintenance functions:

- **Encourager of participation**: warmly encourages everyone to participate, giving recognition for contributions, demonstrating acceptance and openness to ideas of others, affirms and is responsive to differences in group members.
- **Harmonizer and compromiser**: persuades members to analyse constructively their differences in opinions, searches for common elements in conflicts, and tries to reconcile disagreements.
- **Tension reliever**: eases tensions and increases the enjoyment of group members by joking, suggesting breaks, and proposing fun approaches to group work.
- **Communication helper**: shows good communication skills and makes sure that each group member understands what other members are saying.
- **Evaluator of emotional climate**: asks members how they feel about the way in which the group is working and shares own feelings about climate of group.
- **Process observer**: watches the process by which the group is working and uses the observations to help examine group effectiveness.
- **Standard setter**: expresses group standards and goals to make members aware of the direction of the work and the progress being

made towards the goal and to get open acceptance of group norms and procedures.

- **Active listener**: listens and serves as an interested audience for other members, is receptive to others' ideas, goes along with group and trusts the group process when not in disagreement.
- **Trust builder**: accepts and supports openness of other group members, reinforcing risk taking and encouraging/affirming individuality.
- **Interpersonal problem solver**: promotes open discussion of conflicts between group members in order to resolve conflicts and increase group togetherness.

LEVEL 5: SELF

Practice learning equips the student for practice. It also shapes the professional as a person. Service learning in particular requires independent, critical and reflective thinkers who have a strong sense of personal power. Students who experience disjunction between their current knowledge and skills and the demands of practice may carry their anxieties into tutorials and median groups. They may also resist engaging with the demands of practice learning, feeling that the cost of changing their perspectives and world-views is more than what they are able to deal with at this stage of their professional development.

Resistance as a defence against change has to be respected, especially given that the average age of undergraduate students in South Africa is between 18 and 22 years. As young adults some may not yet be developmentally ready to engage with the extent of introspection and reflection required by practice and service learning in historically disadvantaged and socially disorganized contexts. Defence mechanisms such as isolation, projection or splitting may be used to protect repressed feelings from becoming overwhelming. Different defences may surface in tutorials and median groups (or on site) depending on the time of year (for example, prior to exams). Contextual circumstances at practice learning sites, such as political unrest and high incidence of violence, may also trigger resistance. For example, a monologue by one student about some perceived injustice towards a client may lead to dialogue about 'expert' and 'incompetent' clinicians, or a comparison of the quality of supervision received by students during practice learning similar to siblings competing for parental attention. The task of the facilitator is to recognize the defence and to honour its function in containing the group's or individual student's anxiety. Some interpretation of the defence may be indicated. When the defences prevent the student from learning, action needs to be taken, such as referral to appropriate support structures such as counselling.

FUTURE POSSIBILITIES

Strategies, processes and challenges in the use of groups to prepare students for, and to contain them during, practice learning have been described. Groups provide a mechanism for understanding more about social responsiveness. No education is politically neutral and it is therefore incumbent on educators to structure learning experiences that respect the social reality of all groups in society as these are represented amongst a particular cohort of students. Groups as 'living systems of dialogue' (de Maré, 1991) offer numerous possibilities for the achievement of a range of educational purposes, including laying a foundation from which practice learning may proceed.

REFERENCES

Baldwin-Ragaven, L., de Gruchy, J. & London, L. (1999). *An Ambulance of the Wrong Colour: Health Professionals, Human Rights and Ethics in South Africa*. Rondebosch: University of Cape Town Press.

Baworowska, H. & Schick, H. (2000). Culture as group mind: a summary of the acheivements of Patrick de Maré in understanding median groups. *Group Analysis, 33*, 21–27.

Becker, L. & Duncan, M. (2005). Thinking about groups. In L. Becker (Ed.), *Working with groups*. Cape Town: Oxford University Press, pp. 31–51.

Blackwell, D. (2000). And everyone shall have a voice: the political vision of Pat de Maré. *Group Analysis, 33*, 151–162.

de Maré, P. (1991). *Koinonia: from hate, through dialogue to culture in the large group*. London: Karnac.

de Maré, P. (1998). The development of the median group. *Group Analysis, 23*, 11–27.

Duncan, M. (2005). Groups for perspective transformation in health professional education. In L. Becker (Ed.), *Working with groups*. Cape Town: Oxford University Press, pp. 185–203.

Johnson, D.W. & Johnson, F.P. (1975). *Joining together: group theory and group skills*. New Jersey: Prentice-Hall.

Lyndon, P. (1995). The median group: an introduction. *Group Analysis, 28*, 251–260.

Madigan, S. (1996). The politics of identity: considering community discourse in the externalizing of internalized problem conversations. *Journal of Systemic Therapies, 15*, 47–61.

Marks, D. (Ed.) (1999). *Disability: controversial debates and psychosocial perspectives*. London: Routledge.

Maxwell, B. (2000). The median group. *Group Analysis, 33*, 35–47.

O'Brien, C. (2005). Community groups and peace building from below. In L. Becker (Ed.), *Working with groups*. Cape Town: Oxford University Press, pp. 52–65.

Savin-Baden, M. (2000). *Problem-based learning in Higher Education: untold stories*. Buckingham: The Society for Research into Higher Educatioin and Open University Press.

Slattery, P. (1995). *Curriculum development in the post-modern era*. Garland Press.

Smit, A. deV. (2005). Groups and organisational life. In L. Becker (Ed.), *Working with groups.* Cape Town: Oxford University Press, pp. 66–81.

Watson, R. (2002). Competence: a transformative approach. *World Federation of Occupational Therapists Bulletin, 45*, 7–11.

Wenger, E. (1998). *Communities of practice: learning, meaning and identity.* Cambridge: Cambridge University Press.

13 Transforming Experience into Learning: Briefing and Debriefing for Practice Learning

LINDSEY NICHOLLS and ALICE MACKENZIE

OBJECTIVES

This chapter discusses:

- the concept of experiential learning
- the relative merits of briefing and debriefing in conjunction with practice learning
- the nature of transformation through experience.

INTRODUCTION

There was a wise man who asked his student to observe a fish and tell him what he saw. After five minutes the young man returned and said it's just a fish. The sage asked the student to look again.

After half an hour the sage interrupted the student and asked what he thought. The young man said it would probably take him the rest of his life to describe all he saw.

(Story from the account by Doris Lessing of having her portrait painted, National Portrait Gallery, London)

This chapter aims to explain the role of briefing and debriefing within the practice learning modules that are embedded within the three-year undergraduate degree programme at a university in the United Kingdom. The World Federation of Occupational Therapists (Hocking & Ness, 2002) specifies that any recognized occupational therapy qualifying programme must incorporate a minimum of 1000 hours of practice experience to enable students to develop essential professional skills. It also creates a foundation for reflective practice (Alsop, 2002).

Practice and Service Learning in Occupational Therapy. Edited by Theresa Lorenzo, Madeleine Duncan, Helen Buchanan, Auldeen Alsop
© 2006 John Wiley & Sons Ltd

Learning in practice is a highly complex activity and involves the student's capacity to learn from experience. This chapter explores the challenges that students face in learning from their practice experiences and describes the current framework used at the university to facilitate the transformation of the students' practice learning into meaningful reflection. An exploration of the role of experience in learning should be pertinent to any practice learning endeavour.

Firstly, some of the difficulties in learning from experience are discussed, taking account of how new learning might pose a challenge to students' values and/or assumptions about the world. The realities and complexities of practice learning will also be explored. A brief description of the modularized university curriculum that embraces practice learning will be given. Lastly, the models of briefing and debriefing used with students will be described and explored as a means to transforming the students' experiential learning from practice. The process of debriefing, which is described in the final part of this chapter, draws on Mackenzie's (2002) work on briefing and debriefing of student fieldwork experiences. The model originally used with a large group was modified in an attempt to assist students to make sense of their experiences during practice education so that that learning was available to them when they engaged in the theoretical scholarship that forms part of the academic course.

LEARNING FROM EXPERIENCE

Learning from experience is a complex process that does not have an 'outcome based' sureness as the following illustration shows. The scenario is based on the personal experience of one of the authors.

> My introduction to the difficulty of anticipating the results of experiential learning was in 1982, whilst I was working with clients who abused alcohol. It was one of my tasks to run a group that looked at the physical effects on the body of drinking alcohol after taking an 'antabuse' tablet. Having shown a film to the clients that explained the chemical pathway of the antabuse tablet and answered questions from the group about their concerns, I asked if any client had drunk alcohol after taking an antabuse tablet. A client volunteered to give a full and dramatic description of his experience of the physical results of drinking alcohol after swallowing an antabuse tablet. He went on to reassure the group he had learnt a great deal from the experience, in particular, never to take such a tablet again.

This introduction to the role of experience in learning was a sobering one! It sparked thoughts about what people learn from their experiences particularly if those experiences are noxious or novel ones. To what extent do the experiences we have reinforce what we already think and believe? If a person is faced with an unexpected or entirely new situation, can they assimilate all that they see and feel, or do they fall back on previous knowledge and deny (unconsciously) the experience, thereby avoiding the potential challenge of new learning? It could be argued that this is due to the person, unconsciously avoiding what is occurring (psychically) between themselves and the 'other', be it another person or the learning environment.

In the novel *Oranges are not the only fruit* (Winterson, 1985, p. 45), the main character, Jeanette, gives a critical description of her school needlework teacher as being unable to learn from any new (novel) situation.

> My needlework teacher suffered from a problem of vision. She recognised things according to expectation and environment. If you were in a particular place, you expected to see particular things . . . if there was an elephant in the supermarket, she'd either not see it at all, or call it Mrs Jones and talk about fishcakes.

Learning may be a product of what we are able to remember or emotionally manage but it also occurs within a social and cultural context. Although the example of elephants in supermarkets is humorous, it also draws our attention to the sociocultural nature of experience, in other words what a person may expect from a certain place. We may wonder whether a schoolteacher from the town of Victoria Falls in Zimbabwe would be quite as shocked at seeing an elephant in the middle of the town as a suburban wife in Huddersfield, England. Nonetheless, the examples of the patient who drank on top of his antabuse tablet and the needlework teacher in Jeanette Winterson's novel reveal to us phenomena about learning from experience; namely that we cannot predict what can be learnt, or be reinforced by the experience, and that we tend to respond to, or learn from, things that are familiar to us. In other words, our experiences (potential new learning) can simply reinforce what we already know, that is, that we have not learnt anything at all.

Difficulty in learning from experience is articulated by Palmer (1999) who draws on the work of Bion (1990) and Bateson (1973) to highlight the barriers to learning from experience that exist within people. Palmer uses Bateson's theories about our capacity to learn, and the different levels of learning through which we may move, beginning with trial and error learning (level 1 learning). This can result in habit formation (known as zero level learning). Table 13.1 attempts to tabulate Bateson's different levels of learning.

As our learning evolves, we reach 'level 2' learning. At this stage we have a fair amount of knowledge, gathered through trial and error learning and through the absorption of current sociocultural and/or professional knowledge. This acquisition of knowledge is influenced by our personality and our ability to question the assumptions that we make about the events that befall us. Bateson's argument is that, at this point, many people stop learning as the comfort of seeing what they know prevents them from questioning their assumptions within the experience and this can then lead to self-fulfilling prophecies.

Table 13.1 Outline of a hierarchy of learning

Level of learning	Stage of learning	Example of learning
Zero	Habit	Taken for granted knowledge, no longer required to think about it, e.g. taking a certain route to work; tying your shoe laces, preparing a snack – the things we can do without thinking.
Level 1	Trial and error	Learning about the way of the world through immediate response and reinforced by results. Finding a route to work, driving a car, ironing a shirt for the first time, using a computer mouse.
Level 2	Self-fulfilling prophesy	Framing new situations into previously identified categories experiences, or values, e.g. colleagues are often unhelpful, older people are unable to remember detailed information, dogs always bite, OTs who work in mental health are a bit mad themselves, etc.
Level 3	Taking responsibility	Challenging the personal assumptions made about events. Interrogating the 'facts', one's beliefs and feelings. Reflection and reflexivity encouraged, e.g. considering how you may have provoked a client's anger or envy from a colleague.

Source: adapted from Bateson, 1973, *Steps to an ecology of mind*, St Albans: Paladin.

Palmer (1999, p. 169) identified behaviour that he termed 'apperceptive habits' that operate in level 2 learning. These are behaviours that encompass the specific skill and knowledge acquired over time and include our personal orientation to the world, such as optimism, pessimism, or idealism. What Palmer is suggesting is that our learning is influenced by our ability to incorporate new knowledge based on what we anticipate we will find. This process, which he calls 'level 2 learning', potentially creates a self-fulfilling prophesy. An example would be a somewhat mistrustful person who believes that he is constantly belittled by others. However, on closer analysis it appears that his manner with colleagues or friends, such as being overly sensitive to jokes or off-the-cuff comments, appears to elicit that very behaviour from colleagues. Although many of us may be aware of these dynamics in the behaviour of others (friends, colleagues, partners and children), we are seldom able to see them operating in our own modus operandi.

Social construction theorists (for example, Burr, 2003) maintain that knowledge is a product of our social and personal values and only has significance as a relative truth. What Palmer and the social construction theorists are suggesting is that we cannot learn from experience simply by having the experience. Learning from experience may require a deeper reflexive process that involves questioning our assumptions and feeling responses to situations. Reflexivity, as a method of engaging with qualitative research material by questioning one's taken for granted knowledge, has been well described by Finlay (1998) and Finlay and Gough (2003). This questioning of our experience is an ever-deepening reflective process and may involve conscious and unconscious processes.

Learning from experience is neither a simple nor comfortable process. The enthusiasm that has commonly been shown for 'experiential learning' in academic institutions could be misguided as it belies the difficulty we all have in allowing ourselves to learn something new. Bion (1990, p. 95) stated that he 'was interested in the contrast between learning "about" things, and being able to learn from the experience of the-self-in-the world'. Bion (1962) a psychoanalyst and prodigious thinker on learning from experience, believed we all have a natural hatred for learning new things because it exposes us to a potential void of 'not knowing'. He also suggested that this experience of frustration in not knowing something can help us to learn it at a deeper level, not by memorizing it, but by understanding it for ourselves.

This learning for understanding and for developing a sense of self in the world commences in childhood, continues throughout our lifespan (Belenky, Clinchy, Goldberger & Tarule, 1986; Waddell, 1998), and so can be applied to adult learning. In the process of learning, Lawrence (2003) invites us to explore the unknown without coming to any immediate conclusions and to experience mystery, doubts and uncertainties without worrying about fact or reason. He suggests that it is our ability not to know something that allows us to discover it.

Students, whilst on a practice placement, are potentially learning for every moment of their working day. This learning process is supported by supervision with a practice educator or learning facilitator. In dialogue with the educator who, in the UK, is normally the occupational therapist based at the practice learning site, the student reflects on experiences by thinking about assumptions, thoughts, feelings and associations. The debriefing session at the end of practice learning experience, described more fully below, aims to extend this process of reflection.

THE PREMISE OF PRACTICE LEARNING: THE KNOWING, THE DOING AND THE NOT KNOWING

Occupational therapy requires the practitioner to use both scientific knowledge and creative skills and knowledge when working in complex and demanding environments (Crabtree & Lyons, 1997; Creek, 2003). Consequently, much of a student's learning in practice will focus on the development and integration of knowledge and skills, some of which will already be known to the student, whilst some will be new.

Titchen and Higgs (1999) suggested two categories of knowledge: propositional knowledge, which is the knowledge of facts acquired through research and scholarship; and non-propositional knowledge, which emanates from 'knowing how' to do something. They call this type of knowledge 'professional craft knowledge' (Titchen & Higgs, 1999, p. 181). It includes tacit, rational or intuitive ways of knowing; it is developed through work experience; and is linked with the person's own understanding of life. This is not dissimilar to the understanding a person can reach through the experience of not knowing something.

Practice learning is multifaceted and the learning experience is neither predictable nor pre-determined. When occupational therapy students undertake practice learning they work with a variety of clients in a range of different health or social care settings. Unlike the university, in which the student has clear delineated times and tasks for lectures and seminars, practice learning can feel more uncertain and unstructured. The priority of a university is to further the individuals' scholarly knowledge, whereas the priorities for the health or social care practice setting are set by the needs of clients, and these may not always be pre-determined and clear-cut. In addition, the work a student undertakes with a client may be straightforward, for example, text book style, or, it may be complex and uncertain (Blackwell, Bowes & Harvey, 2001; Boud and Edwards, 1999; Crabtree & Lyons 1997). Consequently, given these aspects of the learning environment the student may well experience the anxiety and uncertainty of 'not knowing' in practice and fall back on previously held knowledge and assumptions.

As the authors have implied, learning most often takes place within a relationship and within this relationship conscious and unconscious processes will occur. (This relationship takes place between student and client, carer, or learning facilitator.) The psychoanalytic concepts of transference, counter-transference and projective identification can be useful in helping us to understand these unconscious and potentially complicated processes. For example, when observing a particular situation or when engaged in a situation the observer, be they the practitioner and/or student, may experience comfortable or uncomfortable feelings or a mixture of emotions, some of which may be familiar, some of which may be not. What the 'observer' is experiencing may be reactions transferred on to them [or in to them] from the 'other', which the person (i.e. other) is unable to articulate or is unaware. The observer's feeling state may also be an internal highly personal one that is triggered by the experience in which they are engaged. These experiences in themselves can be part of the 'not knowing' that the student can go through during their practice learning. Having the time and space to discuss and think about these emotional responses to people and situations can help the practitioner and/or student to understand what is occurring with their client and within the care environment. This reflective time can allow the student or practitioner to develop their 'professional craft knowledge' (Mackenzie & Beecraft, 2004; Terry, 1997).

The student is encouraged during practice learning to reflect on and develop knowledge from their experiences but, as already suggested by Bateson (1973), to move from a 'level 2 learning' to a 'level 3 learning' requires the learner to engage in deeper reflection, and to question their immediate assumptions about events and experiences. As stated earlier, access to this knowledge is often difficult because it involves questioning oneself and the things that are assumed as being 'true', so this stage of learning may occur more easily in dialogue with another person, such as a learning facilitator or within a group context with fellow learners. It could be suggested that it is this experience that enables the student to start to develop their 'professional craft knowledge', and the process through which both propositional knowledge and professional craft knowledge become integrated. This process is a task for all professionals, not just students. It was as a result of wanting to enable students to begin, and/or to notice, this process, and move to transform their practice learning into meaningful reflections, that a culture of briefing and debriefing was introduced into the curriculum.

THE CONTEXT OF PRACTICE LEARNING

Occupational therapy students at our identified university, in common with many other occupational therapy students in the UK, undertake practice learning modules as part of their three-year undergraduate degree programme. The modules are spread throughout the three years of the course. The practice education modules are set between academic modules, which cover the informing sciences, concepts of occupational therapy practice, theoretical aspects of occupational therapy interventions and research methodology. Practice and therapeutic skills are normally developed during practice learning.

In order to achieve a pass for each practice learning module the student must demonstrate competence in five domains: communication and professional relationships; management and organization; professional development; professional conduct; and the occupational therapy process. Learning is developmental, occurring over the designated weeks in practice and is supported by weekly supervision with a practice educator. As part of this process, the student brings written reflections on their experiences from the previous week and, together, the student and educator develop learning objectives for the following week. These will be based on the opportunities for learning offered by the practice setting and the student's individual learning needs. Prior to practice learning, however, it is important for students to be orientated to how they might prepare for and best learn from practice experience (Alsop & Ryan, 1996).

BRIEFING PRIOR TO PRACTICE LEARNING

Students are prepared for practice learning on campus through lectures and seminars that centre on the theme and module aims for the coming practice experience. The lecture and seminars are held approximately a week before the student enters the practice setting. Seminar topics are relevant to the module objectives, for example, how to use supervision, how to determine learning needs through reflecting on previous practice experiences, how to manage challenging client/patient interactions and ethical dilemmas. Additionally, students are given a practice handbook that aims to guide and support their learning. A university-specific web-based programme provides an e-learning facility for students to enable them, whilst outside the university, to access module information through the internet and participate in student discussions, share their learning experiences and get advice from each other.

Although briefings commonly preceded each practice experience, no debriefing had been scheduled to take place at the end of the practice learning experience. However, it became apparent that the students were returning from practice with a range of different experiences but with little opportunity to share these events with each other and thereby enhance their learning from each other. Consequently, a regular debriefing session for each year group of students was established at the end of every practice learning experience.

DEBRIEFING

The explicit aims of the debriefing are to provide an end-point to practice learning and allow students to share their learning experiences with each other and with the staff. Once the whole group has been welcomed back to the university and the module aims have been reviewed, each student is given a sheet of paper on which there are two statements:

> I found my placement a useful learning experience because . . .

> It was difficult for me to learn during my placement because . . .

These are intended to encourage the student to reflect on their learning experience. Students are asked individually to consider the two statements for themselves and then to share their responses with each other.

In groups, students are then asked to consider the common themes from their discussions that can be shared with the whole cohort and to reach a consensus on five points that reflect 'useful learning', and a further five points that reflect 'difficulties in learning'. They are then asked to write these up on flip chart paper and present them to the whole cohort. It is an important feature of the debriefing sessions that students work within groups with colleagues with whom they have already worked before. The hope is that students will feel comfortable enough in the group to be able to share experiences openly and honestly.

The period of debriefing is often an intense time for talking within each group. Tutors are also present to facilitate the discussion as needed. The students in each group will have been working in different settings and with different client groups in practice. The session encourages students to share not only their experiences but also their understanding of the role of occupational therapy in the different areas. The final phase of the debriefing is the time when the students begin to see common threads in their learning. Tutors also identify areas of difficulty that seem to run across the whole class group.

Table 13.2 shows some general themes that have arisen from debriefing sessions from across all four practice learning experiences. The emerging themes are also the issues that are eventually presented as feedback to the practice educators.

Table 13.2 Examples of themes from the debriefing session

Useful learning	Difficulties in learning
Practice learning 1 The placement provided a confirmation of their choice of career through the chance to observe the role and scope of OT	Practice learning 1 Feeling overwhelmed by the clinical environment and emotional burden in working with clients
Practice learning 2 Having contact with clients, being valued as a multidisciplinary team member and practising assessment skills	Practice learning 2 Feeling unsure of OT role within generic teams, struggle to understand technical/clinical terms and record interventions in client notes
Practice learning 3 Being able to apply theory to practice and work in the 'real world'. Experience which increases confidence in clinical role and the ability to take responsibility in practice setting	Practice learning 3 Difficulty in gaining access to appropriate information or direct contact with clients and/or difficulties in the supervisory relationship leaving student feeling unsupported
Practice learning 4 Opportunity to address gaps in knowledge and consolidate previous learning, take responsibility for case load and have time to reflect on practice	Practice learning 4 Feeling unprepared for client group and unsure of theoretical underpinning for specific client group. Insufficient supervisory support. Time constraints on learning and pressure to perform

TRANSFORMATION

The debriefing provides an occasion for all the students to reflect on the learning that occurred overall in practice. It also provides a space for the students to speak in an uncensored environment to gain insights and support from their peers. In this way, it serves as a valuable opportunity for the students to start the process of moving from describing the actual experiences to transforming them into deep personal learning. The debriefing can also offer some opportunity for a process of deep reflection and learning within the context of a known relationship within a group. The students tell each other their stories from practice, and in so doing are hopefully able to gain a deeper or broader perspective on their experience by listening to the feedback, comments or questions from other students. This process is enhanced through each student listening to each other's story and comparing their learning and understanding. Students are given a brief introduction to the idea that 'points of view' can alter depending on where and how you view a situation or class colleague's narrative. They are asked to consider the different accounts from the point of view of the client, the student and the learning facilitator, as well as to consider how they may have viewed the same event a year earlier or a year later. With these ideas as a starting point, students are asked to give honest and helpful feedback to each other about the experiences that they shared.

FURTHER THOUGHTS

Although this chapter has focused on a specific strategy that has been developed to encourage a reflexive learning style amongst the large class cohorts, it is suggested that the use of small group discussions within the larger class cohort can enhance student learning. Learning from practice is complex; it can be uncertain and not easily captured in the usual assessment process adopted for practice learning. The authors recognize that the action of the assessment process within practice learning may prevent students from describing the full extent of their feelings as they may fear that these feelings may be seen as being 'unprofessional'. Therefore, opportunities that are created to enable students to speak openly to their peers about their experiences may allow for an acknowledgment of the experience that can lead to a critical questioning and the development of further insights that can allow for new learning.

At the start of the debriefing process some of the groups can be taken up with students comparing their grades with each other and sharing stories of learning facilitators who may have been seen as harsh and/or 'unhelpful' towards the students. In anticipating these comparisons the students are often told before the debriefing begins that the mark they receive will never be an accurate measurement of all that they have learnt, and the experience that they have in practice learning will most likely remain with them for most of their professional lives.

Students are also asked to reflect in their groups on whether the practice learning was affected by social and intuitional pressures of which they may not have always been fully conscious at the time of their learning. These institutional pressures may relate to the wider social and healthcare environment (e.g. the cutting of posts, or the reorganization of care facilities for a particular client group, etc.), or they may relate to staff stress and burn-out as a result of multiple (or unclear) role demands.

Debriefing for practice learning can give the students an emotional space to review what impact working with clients has had on them. This use of 'debriefing' as a mechanism of working through the events which occurred during the placement learning is similar to the processes used with emergency and rescue personal following a critical incident (Michell & Everly, 1995).

CONCLUSION

Universities that encourage students to use journalling, peer review and/or supervision groups and the recording of 'critical incidents' during practice learning may be facilitating a reflexive practice within the student. The role of the group debriefing (alongside these other processes) allows the students to 'tell it as it is' in the non-judgemental supportive atmosphere of their fellow learners. It is within the relationship with the other students that the individual student may be able to make sense of their experiences, transforming the experience into knowledge and an understanding that they can draw on in their future education.

REFERENCES

Alsop, A. (2002). Portfolios: portraits of our professional lives. *British Journal of Occupational Therapy*, 65(5), 201–206.

Alsop, A. & Ryan, S. (1996). *Making the most of fieldwork education*. Cheltenham: Stanley Thornes.

Bateson, G. (1973). *Steps to an ecology of mind*. St Albans: Paladin.

Belenky, M.F., Clinchy, B.M., Goldberger, N.R. & Tarule, J.M. (1986). *Women's ways of knowing: the development of self, voice and mind*. New York: Basic Books.

Bion, W.R. (1962). *Learning from experience*. London: Heinemann.

Bion, W. (1990). *Second thoughts*. London: Karnac Books.

Blackwell, A., Bowes, L. & Harvey, L. (2001). Transforming work experience in higher education. *British Educational Research Journal*, 27(3), 269–285.

Boud, D. & Edwards, H. (1999). Learning for practice: promoting learning in clinical and community settings. In J. Higgs & H. Edwards (Eds.), *Educating beginning practitioners: challenges for health professional education.* Oxford: Butterworth Heinemann, pp. 173–179.

Burr, V. (2003). *Social constructionism,* 2nd edn. Lewes: Routledge.

Crabtree, M. & Lyons, M. (1997). Focal points and relationships: a study of clinical reasoning. *British Journal of Occupational Therapy, 60*(2), 57–64.

Creek, J. (2003). *Occupational therapy defined as a complex intervention.* London: College of Occupational Therapists.

Finlay, L. (1998). Reflexivity: An essential component for all research? *British Journal of Occupational Therapy, 61*(10), 453–456.

Finlay, L. & Gough, B. (2003). *Reflexivity, a practical guide for researchers in health and social sciences.* Oxford: Blackwell Publishing.

Hocking, C. & Ness, E.N. (2002). *Revised minimum standards for the education of occupational therapists.* Perth, Western Australia: World Federation of Occupational Therapists.

Lawrence, W.G. (1999). *Exploring Individual and Organisational Boundaries,* London: Karnac Books.

Lawrence, W.G. (2003). *Experiences in social dreaming.* London: Karnac Books.

Mackenzie, A. & Beecraft, S. (2004). The use of psychodynamic observation as a tool for learning and reflective practice when working with older adults. *British Journal of Occupational Therapy, 67*(12), 533–539.

Mackenzie, L. (2002). Briefing and debriefing of student fieldwork experiences: Exploring concerns and reflecting on practice. *Australian Occupational Therapy Journal, 49,* 82–92.

Michell, J. & Everly, G. (1995). *Critical incident stress debriefing.* USA: Chevron.

Palmer, B. (1999). Learning and the group experience. In W.G. Lawrence (Ed.), *Exploring individual and organisational boundaries.* London: Karnac Books, pp. 169–192.

Terry, P. (1997). *Counselling the elderly and their carers.* London: Macmillan.

Titchen, A. & Higgs, J. (1999). Facilitating the development of knowledge. In J. Higgs & H. Edwards (Eds.), *Educating beginning practitioners: challenges for health professional education.* Oxford: Butterworth Heinemann, pp. 180–188.

Waddell, M. (1998). *Inside lives, psychoanalysis and the growth of the personality,* Tavistock Clinic Series. London: Duckworth.

Winterson, J. (1985). *Oranges are not the only fruit.* London: Pandora Press.

14 Promoting Competence through Assessment

MADELEINE DUNCAN and ROBIN JOUBERT

OBJECTIVES

This chapter discusses:

- the nature and importance of rigour in assessment practices
- critical issues of performance and competence assessment in complex practice learning environments
- domains of competence that may be addressed in an integrated assessment suite
- principles for developing and implementing formative and summative assessments.

INTRODUCTION

Assessment essentially consists of taking a sample of what students do, and making inferences about and estimating the sophistication of their actions, knowledge and understanding against a set of predetermined criteria. The primary task of assessment is twofold. On the one hand, assessment should enable students to transmit evidence of their performance competence in professional processes and procedures and, on the other hand, it should enable them to construct understanding that is progressively mature and responsive to the demands of a particular practice context (Shepard, 2000). Whilst assessment is meant to ascertain the depth and quality of a student's learning, it should also promote continuous development of their professional knowledge, skills and attitudes. An integrated approach to assessment ensures that the tacit, 'underground' dimensions of student learning (their reasoning and reflections in-and-on action) (Mattingly, 1991), as well as their manifest, visible performance skills and professional behaviours, are equally valued during assessment events. Different methods of assessment are indicated for assessing different domains of performance and competence.

Practice and Service Learning in Occupational Therapy. Edited by Theresa Lorenzo, Madeleine Duncan, Helen Buchanan, Auldeen Alsop
© 2006 John Wiley & Sons Ltd

The twofold task of assessment may be achieved through the integrated use of formative and summative assessment methods (Luckett & Sutherland, 2000). Formative assessment serves the learning needs of students through continuous feedback on progress being made in critical learning domains. Formative assessment methods may include case studies, logs, portfolios, journals and interim performance appraisals, the use of which are aimed at promoting continuous learning through written and verbal feedback. Summative assessment occurs at a point in time along the developmental continuum. It is concerned with making a judgement about the student's achievements against professional standards and learning outcomes set by external stakeholders. Summative assessment usually involves structured examination events (for example, a formal case presentation, demonstration of practice competence or any of the above formative methods). It signals the termination of a particular stage of professional development or practice learning experience.

This chapter highlights how assessment methods and criteria may be structured to promote learning, whilst allowing evidence to emerge of a student's progress in key performance and competence areas. It argues that the complexity of assessment in complex practice and service learning contexts can be managed by using diverse and rigorous assessment approaches (Brown, 1999). Examples of assessment methods are suggested and ways of helping students structure their thinking so that their evolving competence may be discerned are described.

PRINCIPLES OF ASSESSMENT

Assessment should be a beneficial learning opportunity for both the student and the assessor. Understanding more about the theory of assessment enables both parties to engage proactively with the assessment process. Expert practitioners do not automatically know how to use their own, intuitive thinking and professional actions as benchmarks or 'gold standards' against which to gauge a student's level of skill and competence (Wolf, 1995). Practitioners, who act as student assessors, therefore benefit from in-service training in the principles and processes of assessment. Students likewise benefit from knowing how the assessment process works, what the benchmarks for competence are and how to utilize the learning opportunities embedded in assessment tasks. The next section briefly reviews the assessment theory that substantiates the practical examples of assessment methods that follow later in the chapter.

COMPLEMENTARY ASSESSMENT APPROACHES

The complexity of occupational therapy requires the complementary use of performance and competence-based assessment approaches. The performance approach makes use of direct measurement or observation. It assesses a skill or objective behaviour, such as making a splint, running a group, naming the principles of balance retraining or doing a mental state examination. The competence approach makes use of professional judgement in discerning the sophistication of understanding that the student has achieved (Wolf, 1995). It assumes that, when assessing complex outcomes such as the ability to reason clinically, use needs to be made of intuitive judgement based on expert opinion.

The performance assessment tradition describes learning as the aggregation of content. To be a good practitioner is to know more; it means to have quantity of declarative or procedural knowledge (South African Universities Vice-Chancellors Association, 1999, p. 28). Performance assessment is usually easier to execute and less resource intensive because there are standard answers or ways of executing a skill that are either correct or incorrect (Biggs, 1996b). The competence tradition of assessment describes learning as the act of 'making meaning' by 'thinking about thinking'. To be a competent practitioner is to arrive at a reasoned understanding of the pathways of critical interpretation used to find and implement solutions to complex problems (Kinsella, 2001; Youngstrom, 1998). The degree or level of competence can be inferred when tacit reasoning processes are made accessible for scrutiny through dialogue (for example, a verbal presentation followed by a viva) or writing. In this approach there is no single 'right' answer or way to practice. There is only the learner's ability to defend a theoretical position or an approach to practice based on their interpretation of evidence and understanding of a range of variables (Biggs, 1996b). The structural coherence of the student's reasoning and acting thus becomes the focus of assessment; that is, the extent to which integration of understanding and discernment results in intuitive yet well-reasoned action (Biggs, 1996a).

ASSESSMENT RIGOUR

Assessment rigour refers to the exactitude of, or adherence to, the rules of validity, reliability and trustworthiness in the development and use of assessment methods and grading systems. Fair, objective assessment is promoted when assessors are able to discern the sophistication of a student's knowledge, skills and attitude using assessment indicators that comply with the principles of rigour. Validity is concerned with the accuracy and truthfulness of the assessment indicator. It should assess what it is supposed to assess. Concern about validity means that educators are clear about what they want students to learn and how that learning may be demonstrated in 'performances of understanding' or 'competencies of practice' (Biggs, 1996a, p. 360). Reliability addresses the stability and objectivity of the assessment indicator as well as the assessor's ability to be consistent over repeated assessments of the same phenomenon (Luckett & Sutherland, 2000). Trustworthiness is concerned with

Table 14.1 Dimensions of assessment

Criterion	Qualitative	Quantitative
Truth value	Credibility	Internal validity
Applicability	Transferability	External validity
Consistency	Dependabilty	Reliability
Neutrality	Confirmability	Objectivity

Source: adapted from Lincoln & Guba, 1985, Naturalistic inquiry. Beverley Hills, CA: Sage.

the qualitative dimensions of assessment rigour. It strives to achieve 'goodness of fit' between the type of assessment method used; the domain of professional performance being assessed and the indicators used to determine the quality or internal coherence of the student's understanding and reasoning.

QUANTITATIVE AND QUALITATIVE DIMENSIONS OF ASSESSMENT RIGOUR

Table 14.1 depicts the dimensions of rigour that may be considered in designing and applying an integrated assessment suite.

TRUTH VALUE: CREDIBILITY AND INTERNAL VALIDITY

The truth value of an assessment method or grading system addresses credibility and internal validity. Students should be able to showcase their best practice using the most applicable assessment method for a particular context. For example, the traditional approach to practice learning assessment usually involves one or two extensive 'case studies' done over a set period of days, followed by a verbal presentation and 'treatment demonstration'. This method of assessment no longer has truth value beyond hospital-based settings. Individual 'case studies' may also be inappropriate in other practice settings where students work in groups with community rehabilitation workers, mothers of disabled children, employers or disability activists. The most credible and internally valid forms of assessment are those that closely approximate the actual working patterns, processes and models of practice appropriate to the context. Students need to be assessed using their everyday means of practice. A series of shorter case reports using a flexible case story guide, or video recordings, followed by tutorial presentations and peer reviews (see below) may be more appropriate.

APPLICABILITY: TRANSFERABILITY AND EXTERNAL VALIDITY

The applicability of an assessment method or grading system addresses transferability and external validity. The assessment task(s) should elicit sufficient 'thick' evidence of the student's performance and competence so as to enable the assessor to anticipate the student's capacity to apply these abilities elsewhere under different circumstances. The skill of making a splint may be deemed transferable when the student is able to demonstrate and justify making an appropriate splint for a particular hand on a particular day for a particular person with a particular health condition. Well-defined, criterion-based structural indicators enable the assessor to make these kinds of distinctions between skill and understanding at various stages of professional development.

CONSISTENCY: DEPENDABILITY AND RELIABILITY

The consistency of an assessment method and grading system addresses dependability and reliability. The student must know what is valued in assessment, and the examiners what is evaluated. Concerted effort should be made to define and describe the indicators of structural coherence (level of sophistication attained in the construction of knowledge) that correspond with different grading bands (Biggs & Collis, 1982). The use of standard criterion across assessment methods, events and contexts ensure that assessors and students are 'on the same page' thereby increasing the dependability and reliability of assessment results.

NEUTRALITY: CONFIRMABILITY AND OBJECTIVITY

Neutrality is enhanced when assessment is objective and results are confirmed across a range of assessment events. This means that the student's results are relatively consistent across assessors and learning sites and there is evidence of developing competence during a particular stage of practice learning. Demonstrating competence in the field is difficult and complex especially for novice practitioners who are still in apprenticeship. Working with real people with real problems means anything can and should be able to happen, that is real life, and the student's response to emerging events and reflexivity is what matters most. This is the reliable focus of competence-based assessment because it brings the student's intuitive abilities, that is thinking, clinical reasoning, reflection-on-action, to the surface (Mattingly & Fleming, 1994).

Rigorous assessment practices should yield evidence of good fit between what is being assessed in one student and many others without imposing 'recipes' for the occupational therapy process or prescribed formats according to which students are expected to present evidence of their learning. Independent thinking and clinical reasoning is stifled when too much structure is imposed in an attempt to be rigorous. The occupational therapy process and human condition is far too complex to fit formative and summative evaluations into rigid, prescribed formats. The next section of the chapter presents a few practical examples of ways in which rigour may be enhanced.

PROMOTING RIGOUR IN ASSESSMENT

USING PARADIGM NEUTRAL LANGUAGE

Language has the power to convey a particular philosophical or attitudinal stance (Marks, 1999). Terminology used in various learning and performance assessment guidelines, such as case study guides or performance assessment forms, should be as 'paradigm neutral' as possible. Words such as 'patient', 'treatment' and 'intervention' point to the medical paradigm of practice and may be replaced with paradigm neutral language, such as individual/group/community' and 'action', thereby ensuring that assessment forms and student writing guidelines are relevant across practice learning sites.

Students should be encouraged to identify appropriate words; select relevant change strategies and follow action processes based on the practice paradigm of a particular learning site and the needs of the person(s) with whom they are working. For example, in health-promoting schools in socially disrupted communities, where there is high incidence of gang-related violence, drugs or child abuse, students work with at-risk 'learners' in an 'occupational enrichment programme' using a 'participatory-action process'. An example of how paradigm neutral language is used in a marking guideline for assessing procedural practice competence is presented below:

- **Information-gathering and interpretation:** use of formal and informal data gathering or investigative procedures; interpretation of findings to guide action; discernment of and collaboration in identifying critical focus for action
- **Planning:** sets priority aims with due consideration of outcomes and/or evidence-based practice; selects appropriate change modalities and strategies; incorporates motivational aspects; considers impact of context and diversity
- **Acting:** use of self and selected change modalities in action; considers safety and ethics; monitors progress; responds to emerging needs and dynamics; adapts-in-action; terminates/refers/collaborates
- **Evaluating action and outcomes:** reflects in and on action; integrates theory and feedback; critical self-appraisal of competence; demonstrates relevant level of clinical/population reasoning for stage of professional development

ALTERNATIVE PRACTICE PROCESSES

The 'biopsychosocial practice process' (Stein & Cutler, 2002, p. 187) has guided occupational therapy intervention to date. Originating from the medical model it continues to be the most appropriate process in therapeutic and remedial programmes with individuals or groups. Alternative practice processes are indicated as the profession moves towards an occupational perspective of public health. For example, the action learning process is most suited to health promotion and prevention programmes or community-based social development projects. The hermeneutic process facilitates self-directed learning and may be used to direct action across a range of contexts because of its attention to the phenomenological dimensions of the participant/facilitator interaction. Any one of the three processes or a combination may be used in the individual, group or community case stories that students are expected to submit in partial fulfillment of learning requirements.

Table 14.2 depicts three processes that may be used in various combinations depending on the context and the negotiated objectives of the exchange between the client/group/community and the health practitioner.

Deciding how and what to record when gathering data about an individual, group or community in order to plan appropriate action must be guided by the requirements of a particular practice learning site, the people with whom students are working, models of practice being followed, the amount of time available for the student to work with the identified person(s) and the student's stage of learning. A 'one-size-fits-all' guideline for recording case material is not useful because it invariably endorses a particular paradigm of practice. Table 14.3 provides an example of a flexible case story guideline. It consists of four key domains that may be the focus of a student's practical experience, that is, an individual, a group, a community or an organization.

Each client/group/community/organization will require a different combination of information to be recorded in order for appropriate action to be described. Students and supervisors identify the ideal combination and sequence of sections (much like building a jigsaw puzzle) from the flexible guideline at the beginning of the practice learning placement. A flexible approach to the construction of writing tasks enables the student to be very focused, efficient and effective during data gathering and recording of their proposed actions and anticipated outcomes.

FLEXIBLE PRESENTATION GUIDELINES

As with the flexible case story guide, students self-select what aspects they want to cover during verbal presentations prior to practical demonstrations.

Figure 14.1 suggests an outline for the content of a verbal presentation that may be applied across contexts and stages of the student's development. It provides the student with a structure for thinking about what to address in a verbal case story presentation without imposing rigid formats. It enables the student to demonstrate competence in both clinical and population reasoning, for example, convergent (with a focus on the individual/group and action) and divergent thinking (with a focus on context, policy and politics impacting on the participants and action). These forms of professional reasoning and critical thinking are considered crucial for effective engagement with the demands of generalist, primary healthcare practice.

Table 14.2 Examples of alternative practice processes

Hermeneutic process (adapted from White, 1991; Schön, 1983)	Biopsychosocial process (Stein & Cutler, 2002, p. 189)	Action learning process (adapted from Hope & Timmel, 1995)
Naming the issue(s): • identifying and describing core issue(s) of concern • mapping the history of, and influences on, the identified priority issues	**Referral** • interpret referral **Initial Interview** • establish contact • identify need for intervention	**Establish Relationship** • participants build rapport **Exploration** • 'real-talk' (sharing of lives), i.e. participants uncover what they collectively experience as oppressive and marginalizing, and what capacity they share • identify collaborators and support structures
Framing the action • negotiating co-authorship of solution generating actions • identifying contributions to a shared process of creating an alternative, hopeful story	**Assessment** • identification of problems and assets **Establish goals** • long-term goals (LTG) address function and participation • short-term goals (STG) address impairments	**Identify patterns** • seek commonalities and differences; • identify critical actions for change; • negotiate roles and responsibilities.
Acting • 'doing' to achieve selected outcomes • continuous detection of clues indicating potential avenues for exploration	**Implement treatment** • operationalize STG and LTG **Re-assess/evaluate**	**Supply information** • add new knowledge/educate for transformation • draw on analytic ability of participants • generate ideas
Evaluating • collecting evidence to serve as a record of progress • adapting action in response to feedback • iteratively re-enter process	**Re-adjust treatment** **Termination/Follow up** • ensure gains are maintained	**Enable action learning** • practice skills in action, • develop a learning/doing culture **Reflection** • Iteratively re-enter process

Source: modified from Duncan, 2005, *Occupational therapy in psychiatry and mental health*, London: Whurr, p. 464.

ENHANCING THE MARKING PROCESS

Gipps (1999, p. 370) suggests that 'we are social beings who construe the world according to our values and perceptions, thus biographies are central to what we see and how we interpret. Similarly in assessment, performance is not "objective", rather it is construed according to the perspectives and values of

Table 14.3 Example of structure and content of a flexible case story

Cover sheet	Individual	Group	Community	Organization
Student information Site detail	Demographic data Health and occupational history Occupational strengths and concerns	Rationale for group-based service Structure of group-based programme Group planning grid	Population demographics Occupational geography Human geography Service infrastructures Comprehensive programme(s)	Purpose, vision and objectives Stage of development Management systems Organizational dynamics

the assessor'. Expert practitioners are technically skilled and usually function at unconscious competence themselves (Hager, Gonczi & Athanasou, 1993). They intuitively employ a 'way of perceiving' their work and take the best actions that are deemed appropriate at a point in time (Mattingly & Fleming, 1994). Expert practitioners are therefore able to recognize the best possible options available to a student and can make inferences about the degree of cognitive sophistication that the student has attained in a particular domain of practice. The structural coherence or sophistication of the student's understanding can be described making use of a set of structural indicators ranging in complexity from pre-structural (the student has not got the point) to extended abstract (the student thinks, acts and understands at a meta-cognitive level) (Biggs, 1996a; Biggs & Collis, 1982)

INDICATORS OF STRUCTURAL COHERENCE

Indicators of structural coherence may be used as benchmarks for awarding grades across a range of practice contexts, thereby reducing subjectivity in the marking process; increasing inter-rater reliability; and enabling students to identify the level of integration they have attained based on expert, external professional opinion. Table 14.4 captures the quality of learning and structural integration that may be associated with a particular marking band, such as first, upper second, fail, etc. The marking bands correspond with the current national secondary and tertiary education grading systems in South Africa.

A set of unifying features (that is, critical factors for consideration that promote an integrated approach to assessment) assists assessors to discern current progress or competence in a particular performance area. Competence in a particular key performance area may be attributed through discerning the degree of integration that exists (with regards to the domain that is being assessed) in terms of professional knowledge; understanding and reasoning;

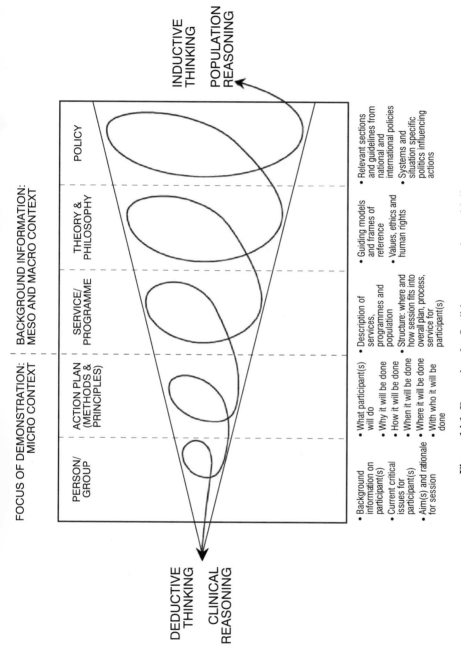

Figure 14.1 Example of a flexible presentation guideline

Table 14.4 Example of a generic marking guide

Classification	Percentage	Grade	Descriptors	Indicators of structural coherence
Fail	0–47	F	Empty: Very poor, clear fail, does not meet minimum requirements for stage of learning	Fundamental flaws; significant gaps in knowledge, skills and attitudes; fragmented and inaccurate reproduction of information; unaware of unsafe practice; may pose danger to others and self due to unsafe practice
Fail-Sup	47–49	FS	Weak: Just meeting threshold standard, barely satisfactory with significant weaknesses, sup exam may be needed	Reproduces with limited understanding of inter-relatedness of concepts; some unsafe practice but has awareness; sparse understanding of fundamental principles; rudimentary attempts at linking constructs
Third	50–59	3	Shallow: Basics present but shallow, obvious weakness in certain in certain areas	Develops structure using external frames of reference; begins to interpret evidence; uses unsupported personal rather than professional or academic beliefs; beginning to substantiate with reference to theory
Lower Second	60–69	2–	Sound: Basics intact and integration beginning to be evident; good across most domains, some aspects are strong	Grasps key issues; appreciates and uses essential principles; well-developed concrete arguments; some consideration of meta theories and starting to apply critical thinking
Upper Second	70–74	2+	Strong: Consistently good integration; some aspects are excellent	Applies relevant theory to represent personal and professional insights but misses finer points; attempts to transfer emerging insights to wider contexts; integrates evidence into practice
Lower First	75–84	1	Excellent: Consistently integrates and excels across most domains	Well grounded in professional paradigms; applies and critiques theory in practice; interpretive, reflective and intuitive implementation; modifies judgement using objective and intuitive evidence
Upper First	85–100	1+	Brilliant: Far exceeds expectations; absolutely outstanding for stage of learning/professional development; excels across all domains	Exceptional coherence, integration of and abstraction from theory and practice; formulates new constructs; high order interrogation and reconceptualization of practice

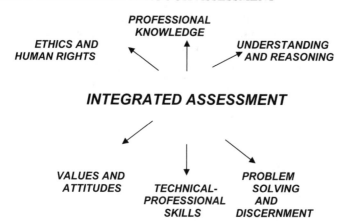

Figure 14.2 Unifying features of integrated assessment (adapted from Hager et al., 1994, *The development of competency-based assessment strategies for professions*, Canberra: Australian Government Publishing Service)

technical professional skills; problem solving and discernment; attitudes and values; and ethics and human rights (see Figure 14.2).

Integrated assessment should be based on performance indicators that are negotiated with the students at the start of the practice so that they are active participants in the assessment process based on clearly articulated learning goals under each key performance area. For example, assuming a final-year student is placed at a psychosocial rehabilitation facility for persons living with chronic mental illness. An integrated assessment of the student's competence in the key performance area of 'interpersonal relationships' (with service users) may include discernment by assessors of the student's:

- professional knowledge about psychiatric diagnoses; the impact of mental illness on the ability of individuals to form and maintain interpersonal relationships and professional theories supporting client-centred practice
- understanding of and reasoning about the psychodynamics of the interpersonal behaviours of clients
- solving of interpersonal problems that arise whilst working with this client group and discerning appropriate actions
- professional and technical skills involved in handling idiosyncratic illness behaviours such as hallucinations, compulsions and paranoid thinking
- values and attitudes that display professionalism and sensitivity to issues of power and diversity
- awareness of ethics and human rights, for example recognizing beneficent and non-maleficent interpersonal actions and the rights of people with mental illness.

It has been suggested thus far that the rigour of assessment may be promoted, not through the standardization of the content of assessment tasks but in the principled use of indicators that assist assessors in discerning the sophistication of a student's thinking and acting. A range of innovative, contextually relevant assessment methods may then be implemented, creating opportunities for students to showcase their best practice under conditions that are optimal for learning and professional socialization.

ASSESSMENT METHODS

This section explores some methods through which formative and summative assessment may occur in contexts where there is a shortage of assessors, time and other resources. Shepard (2000, p. 10) suggests that

> we have not only to make assessment more informative, more insightfully tied to learning steps, but at the same time we must change the social meaning of evaluation. Our aim should be to change our cultural practices so that students and teachers look to assessment as a source of insight and help instead of an occasion for meting out rewards and punishments.

The methods highlighted here were selected because they facilitate the efficient, effective collection of evidence about academic progress.

LOGS, JOURNALS AND PORTFOLIOS

It is widely recognized that the process of writing promotes reflection; facilitates sense making and influences subsequent action in unique ways (White, 1994). Writing requirements also present objective formative and summative material for student assessment (see Chapter 15). Writing methods may include the following:

- *Practice logs:* the daily/weekly record of intended professional actions taken with a particular individual/group/community and evaluation of subsequent outcomes, which may be used in formative assessment through structured feedback (Buchanan, Moore & Van Niekerk, 1998).
- *Journals:* an ongoing, personalized account of experiences, feelings and subjective insights gained during the developmental process of becoming a health practitioner. Journals should ideally be private but this does not mean they cannot be used for assessment purposes. Well-written journals contain descriptive, qualitative data that may be used, in quote format, to support the content of developmental portfolios. Students may be equipped with journalling

skills through writers' workshops and encouraged to make journalling a part of their ongoing professional development. Knowing
that their journalling will not be assessed or reviewed liberates students to use their journals for debriefing; clarifying feelings and processing personal issues that are affected by their practice learning
experiences.

- *Developmental portfolios:* a collection of a student's work that
  represents their learning over time. Portfolios yield substantive
  evidence of the structural coherence of a student's overall learning
  over a period of time (see Chapter 15 for portfolio assessment criteria). Portfolios may be constructed by self-selecting and motivating
  a collection of excerpts from a cycle of actions taken, or interventions made during a period of practice learning that provides
  evidence of longitudinal professional development and learning
  based on reflection-in-hindsight (Buchanan, Van Niekerk & Moore,
  2001; Crist, Wilcox & McCarron, 1998). Portfolios also yield substantial evidence for curriculum evaluation and quality promotion
  (Shay, 1998).

SELF-ASSESSMENT

Gipps (1999) suggests that self-assessment increases the student's responsibility for their own learning and that the assessor, by sharing assessment tasks
with students, fosters greater student ownership, less distrust and more appreciation so that grading standards are not arbitrary. Students may be invited to
award themselves a grade and to substantiate their self-assessment either in
writing or verbally. Assessors may moderate this self-assessment through discussion about finer points (see Figure 14.2) that the students may have over-
looked in either over- or under-evaluating themselves.

PARTNERSHIP ASSESSMENT

The people with whom students work are entitled to evaluate the quality of
the student's contribution to their recovery and/or development. Whilst informal feedback is useful (in that it can be used to confirm an assessor's
observations of a student's progress or areas that need attention), the
implementation of formal feedback from the persons with whom students
work is advisable because it provides objective information on which practice
competence reports can be based. Use may be made of multi-lingual check-
lists (such as Lickert scales that are aligned with the generic marking guide),
covering a range of key performance areas, such as interpersonal relationships,
time use, quality of problem solving and information that was made available.
Partners in the practice and service learning process may also be invited to

attend and participate in their case story presentations, thereby equalizing the power between the novice health practitioner, learning facilitator and person with whom the student has worked and learnt from.

PEER-ASSESSED TUTORIALS

Tutorials refer to a period of instruction given to an individual or small group of students by an 'expert' or informed tutor. The aim is to facilitate integration of theory with practice; expand knowledge about an identified topic of current interest to participants and to promote learning through debate; clarification of ideas and interrogation of supporting literature. Tutorials, run by a student tutor with their peers working in a similar practice learning domain (for example, pediatrics or mental health), provide a forum for achieving learning objectives, whilst simultaneously allowing the assessment of the student tutor on a range of predetermined performance areas, such as knowledge about the topic, group handling and ability to facilitate adult learning. An academic tutor, who is an 'expert' in the domain of practice, participates in the tutorial as a resource and as moderator of the anonymous peer assessment.

VIDEO

Whilst video equipment is expensive and requires substantial security from theft and abuse, the initial financial investment is worthwhile in the long run. Video recordings can capture the student 'in action', showing an example of their practice competence without the threat of feeling 'examined'. Following negotiations between the training institution and relevant site authorities, permission may be granted for students to video record themselves working. Participants must give written informed consent for the recording to be used for assessment and learning purposes. Recordings are erased after the assessment event for confidentiality purposes. The recording may be used in a number of different ways suited to a particular assessment and learning agenda of a student. For example:

- view the tape and write a report on observations and reflections-on-action
- self-select a ten-minute clip that demonstrates a particular incident of good practice or critical learning and do a verbal presentation on the clip
- use clips from the tape as triggers for a peer-assessed tutorial
- use a self-selected collage of clips from recording as part of a summative examination presentation or portfolio
- use the recording for offsite academic supervision.

POSTER

A poster, constructed to comply with standard conference specifications, whilst making use of recycled or cost saving materials, is a method for assessing a student's conceptualization of a particular point of praxis between theory and practice. A well-constructed poster demonstrates the student's ability to achieve 'goodness of fit' between an identified problem and actions taken for example a novel game for HIV/Aids education developed in collaboration with youth.

The poster should contain sufficient information to convey the student's interpretation of investigative findings about client/group needs; theoretical evidence to substantiate the actions taken; agency (solutions used to address critical issues arising from the investigation of need); context (principles for accommodating or regulating the impact of the environment) and learning (evidence of reflective practice).

The content and design of the poster may be structured to achieve any number of assessment objectives, for example, students may do presentations of their poster followed by an oral examination on the content, or posters may be used as triggers for peer-assessed tutorials.

CONCLUSION

This chapter has argued that, apart from assessing the extent to which a student's knowledge has increased as a result of exposure to practice opportunities, assessment is also concerned with determining the competence with which the student is able to apply knowledge, skills and attitudes in response to the dynamics of a particular learning experience. Attention to the quantitative and qualitative dimensions of rigour ensures that assessment methods and processes are student friendly whilst matching the demands of the practice learning context. Principles for developing an assessment suite that is flexible enough to be useful and relevant across a range of practice paradigms (medical, social and occupational) and contexts (comprehensive primary healthcare and multi-sectoral services) have been suggested. The role of assessment for the promotion of professional socialization has also been emphasized, as has the importance of using assessment methods that accommodate diverse learning styles and indigenous, culturally relevant ways of self-expression.

REFERENCES

Biggs, J. (1996a). Enhancing teaching through constructive alignment. *Higher Education*, *32*, 347–364.

Biggs, J. (1996b). Assessing learning quality: reconciling institutional, staff and educational demands. *Assessment and Evaluation in Higher Education, 21*(1), 5–16.

Biggs, J.B. & Collis, K.F. (1982). *Evaluating the quality of learning: the SOLO taxonomy.* New York: Academic Press.

Brown, S. (Ed.) (1999). *Assessment matters in higher education: choosing and using diverse approaches.* Buckingham: Society for Research into Higher Education and Open University Press.

Buchanan, H., Moore, R. & Van Niekerk, L. (1998). The fieldwork case study: writing for clinical reasoning. *American Journal of Occupational Therapy, 52*(4), 291–295.

Buchanan, H., Van Niekerk, L. & Moore, R. (2001). Assessing fieldwork journals: developmental portfolios. *British Journal of Occupational Therapy, 64*(8), 398–402.

Crist, P., Wilcox, B. & McCarron, K. (1998). Transitional portfolios: Orchestrating our professional competence. *American Journal of Occupational Therapy, 52*(9), 729–736.

Duncan, M. (2005). Three approaches and processes in occupational therapy with mood disorders. In R. Crouch & V. Alers (Eds.), *Occupational therapy in psychiatry and mental health.* London: Whurr, p. 464.

Gipps, C. (1999). Socio-cultural aspects of assessment. *Review of Research in Education, 24*, 355–392.

Hager, P., Gonczi, A. & Athanasou, J. (1993). *The development of competency-based assessment strategies for professions.* National Office of Overseas Skills Recognition research paper no 8. DEET. Canberra: Australian Government Publishing Service.

Hope, A. & Timmel, S. (1995). *Training for transformation: a handbook for community workers* (Books 1–3). Gweru, Zimbabwe: Mambo Press.

Kinsella, E.A. (2001). Reflections on reflective practice. *Canadian Journal of Occupational Therapy, 68*, 3195–3199.

Lincoln, Y.S. & Guba, E.A. (1985). *Naturalistic inquiry.* Beverley Hills, CA: Sage.

Luckett, K. & Sutherland, L. (2000). Assessment practices that improve teaching and learning. In S. Makoni (Ed.), *Improving teaching and learning in higher education.* Johannesburg: Witwatersrand University Press, Chapter 4.

Marks, D. (Ed.) (1999). *Disability: controversial debates and psychosocial perspectives.* London: Routledge.

Mattingly, C. (1991). What is clinical reasoning? *American Journal of Occupational Therapy, 45*(11), 979–986.

Mattingly, C. & Fleming, M.H. (1994). *Clinical reasoning: forms of inquiry in a therapeutic practice.* Philadelphia, PA: FA Davis.

Schön, D. (1983). *The reflective practitioner: how professionals think in action.* New York: Basic Books.

Shay, S. (1998). Portfolio assessment for curriculum inquiry and quality promotion. In S. Angelil-Carter (Ed.), *Access to success: academic literacy in higher education.* Cape Town: University of Cape Town Press, pp. 160–177.

Shepard, L. (2000). The role of assessment in a learning culture. *Educational Researcher, 29*(7), 4–14.

South African Universities Vice-Chancellors Association (1999). *Facilitatory handbook on the interim registration of whole university qualifications.* Pretoria: SAQA Action Group.

Stein, F. & Cutler, S.K. (2002). *Psychosocial occupational therapy – a holistic approach.* Delmar: Thomson Learning.

White, E. (1994). *Teaching and assessing writing.* San Francisco, CA: Jossey Bass.

White, M. (1991). Deconstruction and therapy. *Dulwich Newsletter*, *3*, 21–40.
Wolf, A. (1995). The case for competence based assessment. In A. Wolf (Ed.), *Competence-based assessment*. Buckingham: Open University Press.
Youngstrom, M.J. (1998). Evolving competence in the practitioner role. *American Journal of Occupational Therapy*, *52*(9), 716–721.

15 Engaging with Student Writing: Using Feedback to Promote Learning

MADELEINE DUNCAN and HELEN BUCHANAN

OBJECTIVES

This chapter discusses:

- the educational value of writing for developing critical thinking and reflection-on-action
- the functions and focus of written feedback from learning facilitators on the written work of students
- four levels at which student writers and writing assessors may engage with the praxis between theory and practice.

WRITING FOR LEARNING

Writing in the form of case studies and progress reports on clients, daily logs detailing action plans and outcomes and reflective journalling about personal–professional experiences in the field are an integral part of under-graduate professional practice learning (Buchanan, Moore & Van Niekerk, 1998). Writing becomes particularly relevant as an educational resource and means of communication between students and learning facilitators/university practice educators in resource constrained contexts where contact between professional role models and students may be sporadic. Students, in writing about their work, are able to clarify ideas, develop critical thinking and objectify progress in their professional reasoning and learning. The discipline of writing is seen to achieve a range of educational objectives, such as the integration of theory with practice and the advancement of critical thinking and clinical reasoning (Neistadt, 1995; Tryssenaar, 1995). These outcomes are dependent, in part, on the quality of written work done by the student and on the specificity of formative (developmental) feedback given to students about

Practice and Service Learning in Occupational Therapy. Edited by Theresa Lorenzo, Madeleine Duncan, Helen Buchanan, Auldeen Alsop
© 2006 John Wiley & Sons Ltd

the content of their writing. In discussing the use of daily logs, reflective journals and developmental portfolios, Buchanan, Van Niekerk and Moore (2001, p. 294) suggested that 'constructive feedback practices need to be more widely fostered, reflecting commonly understood educational goals in the local occupational therapy community'. They suggested that feedback must be student centred and aligned with the academic needs of the individual learner. This is particularly relevant in contexts where the language of instruction is not the first (home) language of the student who may grapple, not only with mastering language syntax, but also with capturing the complexity of practice in written form.

This chapter identifies four levels at which educators may engage with student writing in the form of either written or verbal comments, or questions aimed at fostering learning and deeper reflection-on-action. It argues that comments on writing should help students gain a more integrated sense of what they are doing; to 'know what they know' and where to look for answers if they 'don't know'. Formative comments should aim to expand the student's understanding or trigger deeper reflection depending on which one (or all) of the four levels deserves attention. This requires the assessor to engage at multiple levels with 'the what' and 'the how' of student writing in order to discern and affirm where progress is being made or where change may be indicated.

WRITTEN FEEDBACK AS DELIBERATIVE PROCESS

Students articulate, in written form, their propositions about practice and their perceptions of actions taken and subsequent outcomes. The sophistication of their propositions should increase over time as they continue to test and acquire personal–professional knowledge and skill. Higgs and Titchen (2001) believe it is essential for beginning practitioners to develop their own professional judgement (as opposed to following prescribed or 'recipe' ways of working) in order to become autonomous, efficient practitioners. For this to occur their thinking needs to be facilitated and their reflection-on-action guided through feedback that provides direction without imposing prepositional knowledge as absolute knowledge.

Written feedback is essentially a deliberate intervention during the process of knowledge construction that promotes deliberation and reflection about practice. Knowledge is never separate from practice; it arises from and within practice. Knowledge relating to, and arising out of, practice can therefore be facilitated through focused comments from learning facilitators. Written (and verbal) comments should aim to:

- help the student identify areas of practice that need special attention
- promote the student's ability to evaluate their performance

- facilitate effective engagement with the construction of knowledge
- motivate students to learn by pointing out areas worthy of exploration and meaning making
- enable the student to map practice into existing knowledge or theoretical schema.

FUNCTION OF WRITTEN FEEDBACK

The function of feedback on written work is to objectify the dialectical relationship between knowledge and practice. Higgs and Titchen (2001, p. 527) suggest that a dialectical relationship occurs when 'the contradictions of experience in relation to two phenomena (for example, differences between practice and knowledge) are reconciled in a higher synthesis'. Higher synthesis is made possible for the student by paying close attention to the quality of feedback (written or verbal) given on written work. Critical issues for consideration are identified through questioning or pointing out alternative interpretations, thereby facilitating the connection between theory and action.

According to Vygotsky (1978, p. 79) 'the essential feature of learning is that it creates a zone of proximal development (ZPD) that is, internal developmental processes that are able to operate only when the learner is interacting with people in his/her environment and in co-operation with peers. Once these processes are internalised they become part of the learner's independent developmental achievement'. Deliberative feedback expands the learner's ZPD (see Figure 15.1). This is the space within which a learner engages with the active construction of knowledge through a dynamic interaction between their innate capacity (mind of learner) and the external sociocultural environment or 'more knowledgeable other', for example the university practice educator/learning facilitator who is giving feedback. Vygotsky pointed to the importance of assessors as tools and aids in human learning, for example when educators and students interact and reflect on the content of student writing (Gipps, 1999).

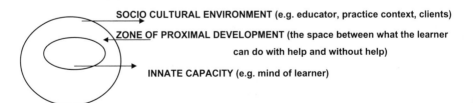

Figure 15.1 Focus of feedback: expanding the zone of proximal development (adapted from Vygotsky, 1978, Mind in society: the development of higher psychological process, Cambridge, MA: Harvard University Press)

Students and learning facilitators engage with practice epistemology (knowing how practice knowledge is created), through the dialogue that ensues between them from written and verbal feedback on the student's written work and practical performance. This chapter focuses exclusively on the former. Dialogue about a student's written work happens at two levels for the student, either with the self as in 'reflection-on-practice' and thinking through comments made by the university practice educator, or through deliberation with another observer (peer or learning facilitator) who offers a critical appraisal of knowledge and skill demonstrated in practice. This dynamic interaction is facilitated, according to Vygotsky, by the introduction of organizing frameworks or units of analysis. He suggests that human activity cannot be studied or evaluated apart from creating the very tools with which to study or evaluate it. Practical-critical activity in the ZPD is seen to be human practice that is self-reflexive, dialectical, continuously emergent and transformative of the totality (Newman and Holzman, 1993). Critical appraisal of praxis leads to understanding theory in practice and increased confidence in action. It also leads to the generation of theory through practice. The act of 'making sense' through 'thinking about thinking' helps the student expand their ZPD. Feedback helps students to 'know what they know', to appreciate that 'knowing' is always relative and to understand that 'not knowing' is often a place of great learning. It should set in motion the possibilities of inquisitiveness, understanding and intuitiveness.

GIVING AND RECEIVING FEEDBACK

Expert practitioners give feedback from an intuitive grasp of situations. Expertise as a practitioner, however, does not necessarily translate into expertise as a learning facilitator or expertise in engaging with student writing. Supervision is a dynamic interaction between a senior member of a profession and a junior member or student of the same profession. It is a supportive activity, the purpose of which is to enhance the professional development and functioning of the junior member. Both parties should assume responsibility for the way in which they seek, receive and respond to feedback and for acquiring skills in doing so (Sweeney, Wembley & Treacher, 2001). Learning facilitators should provide a safe, non-judgemental learning environment for students, whilst students should learn how to incorporate feedback into their practice.

Giving formative written feedback is both time consuming and challenging as it requires the university practice educator to engage actively, not only with the learners' perspectives on practice, but also with their personal interpretation of practice. Students producing weak or shallow written work may require substantive feedback. This can be very time consuming and is considered one of the disadvantages of substituting verbal, face-to-face supervision with writing. A series of ticks or comments, such as 'good idea', do not suffice in advancing the ZPD. Shallow comments may indicate to the student that their action plans, evaluations and reasoning are strong enough to warrant inclusion in a portfolio (a self-selected compilation of logs over a period of time), when in fact this may not be the case when reviewed from an objective, 'outside' perspective (Buchanan et al., 2001). The quality of feedback therefore influences not only how deeply the student learns but may also determine how effectively the student evaluates the development of their professional competence over time.

Shallow comments or a series of ticks could indicate a number of concerns. For example, the assessor:

- may not have been sufficiently trained in marking student writing
- has not had exposure to theoretical models of supervision
- has not had (or made) sufficient time to engage with the written work
- lacks specific knowledge to pass on to the student.

The selection of supervisors should, therefore, also receive attention as a quality assurance measure in education. Perkins and Blythe (1993, p. 351, cited in Biggs, 1996) suggested 'that teachers say they "teach for understanding" but that few do so in any sustainable way . . . To do so they need a framework of some kind to help them operationalise what "understanding" might mean in their particular case'.

A framework for engaging critically with professional writing for learning and for giving structure to formative feedback and student writing is suggested below. It aims to enhance the quality of feedback and student writing by honing in on four possible levels at which reflection and learning about practice may occur. Students often anticipate the evaluative dimension of feedback as potentially threatening and exposing of their incompetence. Formative feedback should not lead to resistance or demoralize the student. It should help the student to identify areas that need working on whilst promoting their ability to evaluate progress against a set of criteria representative of patterns in professional practice. Specificity in the feedback process helps students learn by pointing out dimensions for exploration, for meaning making and for mapping into existing knowledge schema. This is where the framework for levels of feedback becomes particularly useful. It aligns and specifies feedback in accordance with the student's progressively sophisticated constructions of knowledge as well as signalling to the student those dimensions of practice that deserve attention in the process of writing.

ASSESSMENT OF STUDENT WRITING

Consistent criteria and processes for feedback and assessment are important given the range of learning facilitators working with students in different contexts. The levels of feedback proposed here enable both learning facilitators and students to know what is valued in the curriculum and what will be assessed in student writing at various stages of professional development. Criterion-referenced assessment attempts to unearth the tacit dimensions of professional practice. It makes transparent the kind of knowledge that deserves attention in the process of becoming a competent practitioner as well as the dimensions of practice that will be assessed (Luckett & Sutherland, 2000; Shepard, 2000). The use of a feedback framework, such as the one suggested here, increases inter-assessor reliability, consistency and internal moderation because it facilitates uniform approaches to feedback and assessment.

Criterion-referenced assessment usually tracks a student's progress along a continuum of competency from novice through advanced beginner, competent therapist, proficient therapist to expert practitioner (Westcott & Rugg, 2001). This progression is supported by the increasing complexity of the four levels of feedback. Shepard (2000, p. 11) suggests that 'we take it for granted that providing feedback to the learner about performance will lead to self-correction and improvement. For the most part, however, the existing literature on feedback will be of limited value to us in reconceptualising assessment from a constructivist perspective, because the great majority of existing studies are based on behaviourist assumptions'. Competency-based assessment and the development of reflexivity in practice may be enhanced by structuring the specificity of feedback according to the four levels described in the next section of the chapter.

FOUR LEVELS OF FORMATIVE FEEDBACK

Different stages of student learning and professional development, practice or service contexts, client needs and a range of other variables, such as availability of time to engage with student writing, will determine at which level the assessor gives feedback (see Table 15.1). They may approach student writing using all the levels as a lens, or may elect to use a different level for giving feedback on different logs.

LEVEL ONE FEEDBACK: MANIFEST PRACTICE

The junior student learns to write at *level one* by following prescribed guidelines for writing an intervention log or action plan. Level one serves as an organizing framework for the student to chart in stepwise, procedural fashion the dimensions of practice that they have to attend to in using particular stages of the occupational therapy process. Level one feedback addresses critical dimensions of the selected professional process, such as how to formulate an aim as opposed to an outcome or how to decide which theory best matches the needs of the client at a particular stage of recovery or development.

Table 15.1 A framework for formative written feedback

Formative written feedback	Level 1 (Manifest practice)	Level 2 (Latent practice)	Level 3 (Integrated practice)	Level 4 (Meta-practice)
Purpose of comments	To guide students to write sections of an intervention or action log, i.e. step-wise approach to observable action	To prompt students to think and reason professionally; to uncover underground practice	To alert students to see the coherence of their practice over time, i.e. to make longitudinal links	To prompt constant awareness and vigilance about professional values, attitudes and ethics
Focus of comments	Monitor procedural processes and stages of practice and an OT process, e.g. assess, plan, act, evaluate	Identify instances in student writing that point to presence or absence of different types of clinical (or population) reasoning	Elucidate patterns and components of practice that contribute to overall coherence of OT in that specific context	Instances of moral understanding, deliberation and self-regulation as an ethical practitioner; issues of attitude, values and beliefs

By posing a reflective question or making an affirmative remark that points out new directions for thinking and investigation, the learning facilitator/ practice educator sets in motion a train of thought about dimensions of practice that may have remained inaccessible to the learner had it not been brought to their conscious awareness. Engaging with level one feedback is important for progression in competence. Specific, clear and balanced comments, aimed at triggering the creation or critique of practice knowledge, enables the student to claim and internalize legitimate knowledge about a selected process and to uncover prepositional knowledge as it unfolds in the telling of their practice story.

Practice learning may commence with individual case stories of selected clients, collective case studies of a group of clients, or a systematic review of a service, a programme or an organization. From this baseline of data, the student is able to plan and report on daily sessions using the log writing guideline outlined below (adapted from Buchanan et al., 1998).

1. **Planning:** Interpretation of investigative findings, formulating aims in collaboration with client(s), identifying possible outcomes based on evidence and selecting theoretical principles. Criteria for selection of action methods and/or modalities and occupational rationale. Criteria for guiding appropriate relationship(s) with client(s) and other role players. Criteria for structure of context or micro/meso/macro environment as indicated. Indicators for use of

self and any other relevant details appropriate to the setting and/or planned action.

2. **Report on action:** A brief record of what actually happened during the action, noting any important deviations from the plan.

3. **Evaluation:** An analysis of critical incidents within the action session. Comments on problems experienced, progress made (were the stated aims and outcomes achieved or not and why?) and implications for future actions.

4. **Reflection:** Thinking about thinking during the session and what was learnt. Interpretation of what happened between theory and practice and vice versa (personal sense making of the influences at stake during the session). A deeper look into the *interactional dynamics* of the session (how the session progressed in terms of personal initiatives and competencies in response to client(s) actions and reactions and contextual influences).

5. **Follow-up planning:** Revision or modification of planning done in 1 above.

Examples of level one comments:

- Which criteria guided your selection of this particular activity for this client at this stage of recovery?
- How might you rewrite this aim as an outcome for participants?
- How about considering principles from Max-Neef's work to guide your entry into this community? I suggest you read up on *Human Scale Development* (Max-Neef, 1991) to learn more about the dimensions of poverty before planning your next session.

LEVEL TWO FEEDBACK: LATENT PRACTICE

The challenge of level two feedback is to recognize instances of emerging clinical reasoning in the text. To do this, the learning facilitator needs to be familiar with how the various types of reasoning manifest and how to unfold dormant capacity for professional reasoning by giving feedback that challenges 'thinking about thinking'. The assessor needs to 'think about the student's thinking' and then give feedback aligned with various types of clinical reasoning (Mattingly, 1991; Neistadt, 1995). Of particular importance here, is the distinction and overlap between clinical reasoning and population reasoning. The former has been documented as the convergent thinking processes that occur during direct client (individual or group) and therapist exchanges usually within a biopsychosocial paradigm. Population reasoning usually occurs during indirect service delivery within a public health paradigm.

Level two feedback should strengthen the student's understanding of how to reason about practice, that means, their ability to act and think about action in ways that address the unique needs of client(s) as these emerge at any point in time during the interaction. The assessor has to read deeply into the student's sense making of practice with particular reference to the range of reasoning domains listed below (adapted from Mattingly, 1991; Neistadt, 1995).

- **Procedural reasoning**, e.g. student's ability to assess and define client/group/context needs; choose principles; identify aims and possible outcomes; select appropriate interventions or identify relevant actions; provide rationale for choices; implement selected actions via systematic gathering and interpretation of appropriate data.
- **Narrative reasoning**, e.g. student's ability to tell the client/group/ context story, i.e. life, health and/or occupational history of an individual, group or community; ability to anticipate a prospective story about how the client's/group's preferred activities, habits, roles and/or occupations and resources may be translated into action to build a meaningful future.
- **Interactive reasoning**, e.g. student's understanding of, and response to, emerging interpersonal phenomena during interactions with significant role-players, i.e. client/group/community representatives (ability to interpret the processes and content of interpersonal relationships between self and others).
- **Conditional reasoning**, e.g. student's ability to implement and revise their responses moment to moment, or day by day, to meet the client's/group's emerging needs 'in action', as well as student's understanding of this revision in the light of the client's/group's current and possible future needs or the emerging requirements of the context.
- **Pragmatic reasoning**, e.g. student's ability to consider the practical and systemic issues that affect the session or service, i.e. ability to decide what is possible and feasible for the client/group/ community in a given context at a given point in time with due consideration of extraneous factors impacting on outcomes.
- **Ethical reasoning**, e.g. student's ability to think critically about human rights, the ethics of care and participatory ethics. Evidence of using principled ethics, i.e. deontological (set of codes and guidelines, such as confidentiality, veracity, beneficence, non-maleficence and justice) and teleological (considering the long-term consequences of moral decisions and seeking greatest good for the largest number of people) reasoning in response to moral and ethical dilemmas in the field. Recognition of and responsiveness to rights and responsibilities.
- **Population reasoning**, e.g. student's occupational perspective of public health, i.e. ability to conceptualize the epidemiological distribution of health needs and the socio-political, economic and

geographical factors that impact on the occupational well-being and/or justice of representative populations of people.

There are many other forms of reasoning but these six are considered core in most occupational therapy literature. These forms of reasoning are used simultaneously in tacit, highly imaginistic and deeply phenomenological ways, whether working with an individual, a group or a community/population.

Examples of level two comments:

- (Procedural reasoning) Why are these particular activity requirements indicated to achieve this aim at this stage of the clients recovery?
- (Conditional reasoning) If you were to change the sequence of the activity demands what would happen? What changes need to occur in the dynamics of this group before it will become more goal directed and proactive?
- (Ethical reasoning) Your actions demonstrate sensitivity to patient rights. Which ethical principles informed your decisions, which will guide your further actions and how?
- (Interactive reasoning) Why may the community rehabilitation worker be treating the client in this way and how may she be enabled to adopt a client-centred approach? How has your relationship with her changed over time and why?

Level two feedback may pose a particular challenge to English second-language students as their command of English may not reflect the depth of their understanding or integration of theory with practice and vice versa. To enable such students to showcase their reasoning skills the assessor may:

- encourage the student to tell the story of those critical dimensions of practice that they have difficulty conveying in written English
- request that the student mind map (as opposed to write) their insights and then talk through their thinking with the assessor
- use metaphors to explain concepts
- let the student video record self in action followed by discussion
- refer the student for specialist writing instruction
- make use of a translator so that the student can convey understanding in their home language (this has cost implications).

LEVEL THREE FEEDBACK: INTEGRATED PRACTICE

Level three feedback addresses integrated practice over time; evidence of which is usually captured in a self-selected collection of writings, for example a portfolio of a series of logs (Buchanan et al., 2001). This feedback takes a step up from the whole to comment from a 'bird's eye view' on the integration of professional practice evident in the selected writings. It takes into account the longitudinal development of the student's thinking and reasoning about the patterns and processes of occupational therapy with a particular client, group or community in a specific context. As such it attends to the 'extended abstract'; the integrated whole that enables generalization to other cases, contexts or service domains to emerge. Listed below are possible criteria for assessing integrated practice and giving level three feedback (adapted from Buchanan et al., 2001).

- **Uncovering client/group/community needs and capacities:** Competence in investigative data gathering, i.e. screening, assessment and ongoing evaluation of the specific circumstances/needs/problems as well as capacities and assets of this client/group/community/ organization. Responsiveness to the dynamic and evolving nature of client/group/community needs and development potential.
- **Theoretical constructs:** Evidence of praxis between theory and action. Ability to draw on theory to make sense of the various dimensions of practice. Ability to apply theory in action and to recognize theory emerging during action.
- **Context:** Student's recognition of and responsiveness to significant factors (tangible and intangible) in the micro (immediate action space) and macro (systemic, topographical) environment that impact on the process and outcomes of occupational therapy.
- **Agent:** Effectiveness and efficiency of selected change agency, i.e. activity/occupation; modality; therapeutic method or development action. Use of self and ability to develop/apply/adapt or modify actions and strategies in effecting change.
- **Learner:** The ability to capture what was learned and how this learning could be generalized to other situations.

Examples of level three comments:

- Have you noticed that the principles you selected at the start of this learning experience no longer apply to the rationale for action you suggest here?
- How are the principles of community-based rehabilitation being/not being operationalized by this service?
- In which ways have politics and organizational dynamics affected the outcomes of community action and what proposals can you make to address these?

LEVEL FOUR FEEDBACK: META-PRACTICE

Level four feedback addresses the moral and ethical dimensions of student writing. Very little has been published about the qualitative dimensions of ethical and moral experiences of undergraduate health professional students, how these experiences are reflected in their writing and how educators may engage with the moral and ethical development of students through written feedback. Occupational therapy literature usually focuses on the principles that regulate clinical encounters of occupational therapists with individual or groups of clients and on the rules that guide the resolution of ethical dilemmas that arise within a disease paradigm or between individual practitioners and the public or colleagues (Barnitt, Warby & Rawlins, 1998). Professional codes of conduct and ethical guidelines specify 'what to do' and 'how to behave', yet despite such comprehensive background information, therapists have to rely on their own resources, reflections and problem-solving ability when faced with ethical and moral dilemmas in the field. Therapists, however, 'are human and, inevitably "bad" decisions will be made at times because duty or consequences of actions have either been ignored or are in conflict' (Barnitt et al., 1998, p. 56). The same applies to students – their writing will inevitably reveal their attitudes, moral dilemmas and their evolving ethical reasoning, especially if reflection on such dilemmas is an explicit writing expectation. Formative feedback should guide the possible reasoning processes that students may use in reaching moral and ethical judgements. The aim of such feedback is always to advance ethical self-regulation.

The quality of self-regulation is, in essence, enhanced by the quality of moral imagination, deliberation and reflection. This is a skill that has to be consciously developed and nurtured. Students do not overtly emphasize the moral dimensions of their actions in the field, neither do they consciously engage metaphors to describe the moral tensions that surface whilst working with clients. In writing, however, the use of metaphor may become apparent. Writing is an important educational method for shaping moral understanding and professional self-regulation. Reflective logs, learning journals and portfolios should ideally create the space into which the student can project their moral deliberations. Student narratives become imbued with moral significance when they are invited to share their stories.

THE IMPORTANCE OF SELF-REGULATION

Students enter undergraduate training programmes with established worldviews and well-developed moral values (usually based on cultural/religious norms and ethics). However, Seedhouse (1991, p. 281) argued that the grounding question of ethics is 'how best to conduct one's life in the presence of other lives'. Students need to learn how to conduct themselves within a professional identity with due consideration of the lives being served. Educators should help them in knowing 'where and how to find ways ahead for themselves' in the often confusing gap between personal beliefs, service expectations and the concrete realities of life.

For example, students in South Africa have to grapple with the legacy of human rights abuses following the demise of apartheid. They may tend to see professional ethics as supplementary to law. However, according to Koniak (1996) a contemporary account of ethics requires substantial regard for the influences of personal moral values and relationships. She argued for a new conception of the relationship between law and ethics and suggested that instead of the common perception that ethics takes over when the law is deemed inadequate, that the law should be seen as being informed and challenged by ethics and morality. The problem with the commonly understood approach to ethics for members of the professions (a set of rules and codes of conduct) is that it is inconsistent with the self-regulation associated with professionalism. Personal morality must, in other words, regain a place in meeting legal and professional demands. Law, ethics and personal morality must all speak equally to professional conduct. Students must be invited to bring their consciences to bear in describing the inevitable moral and ethical dilemmas of working in complex social environments.

Christakis and Fendtner (1993:254) argued that 'ethics presented as moral theory or a set of principles can go only so far: personal problems, culled from the daily events of students' lives and rooted in the complex social situation of the ward [*learning site*], more thoroughly capture their consciences. It is making decisions and living with their consequences that ethics ceases to be only a theoretical discipline and begins to become a professional code of conduct'. If students are not given the opportunities to discuss and think through the anxieties associated with the ethical issues that face them in day-to-day practice they will most likely, as qualified practitioners, adopt stereotyped and limited responses to the ethical aspects of their work. Every available opportunity should be used to develop self-regulation by alerting students to the interface between law, ethics and personal morality in the course of their daily experiences in the field. They should be encouraged to write about how their consciences are aroused in response to what they are witnessing or doing, and how they create understanding of themselves as moral beings in the face of ethical dilemmas.

ENGAGING WITH THE MORAL DIMENSIONS OF STUDENT WRITING

Moral understanding and deliberation is highly imaginative and only marginally self-conscious. According to Johnson (1993, p. 242) 'acts of imagination allow us to see that, and how, things might be better and done differently'. Morality is not obeying a set of rules – it is the imaginative exploration of possibilities with due consideration of consequences. Imaginative activity is a means for assuming different perspectives or taking different actions and then tracing how each may develop. According to Johnson, morality is central to students' search for promoting the well-being of their clients. Their motivation is instinctively to do good. This inherent principled morality will surface, unconsciously, in their writing through the use of images and metaphors that convey how they experience a moral dilemma, for example 'I hit a brick wall when . . .' or 'I felt down in the dumps after . . .'. They will likewise use opinions or views to explain their actions, usually with reference to professional rules and regulations, for example 'I think it is in the client's best interest to tell him the truth about . . .', or 'I didn't consider the implications of confidentiality when . . .'. The challenge for assessors is to bring this inherent, principled moral sensitivity to the fore by alerting students to instances of moral imagination in their narrative.

A student's choice of words, images and the attitudinal nuances of the narrative will reflect their notions of action, purpose, rights, law and duty (Fairbairn, 2002). The way a student frames a given event or situation indicates what they think they ought to do about it and the probable consequences of the proposed action, that is, how others will be affected, how it may change their future actions and so forth. Morally, sensitivity and ethical behaviour is increased to the extent that they are able or encouraged to envision or imagine the consequences of their (and others') actions and attitudes. According to Fairbairn (2002, p. 23) 'our moral imagination is formed in the lives we lead. It is because our moral understanding is limited that if we want to be ethical in our professional practices, we need to rehearse decisions, reasons and justifications'. Feedback should facilitate such rehearsal.

Extract from student log:
As I walked along the main corridor of the hospital I passed a porter pushing an elderly man in a wheelchair in the opposite direction. The patient looked as if he had had a stroke. The porter was talking to another porter and did not notice that the patient's flaccid arm was dangling in the wheel of the wheelchair. The patient was slumped in the chair and the front of his pyjamas was open revealing his genitals. The corridor was full of visitors and I was very embarrassed for the patient's sake and cross with the porter for being so negligent. I felt helpless because I did not know the porter or the patient and I did not want to make a scene in front of everyone. I wondered why the porter paid so little attention to the patient he was supposed to be caring for and how the patient was feeling because he couldn't talk and help himself. I spoke to my clinician about this and she said she would talk to the chief porter.

Example of comment:
I have underlined some words in the log that describe your moral sensitivity during this event. Do you notice how your feelings may be giving voice to the patient's experience? How may this awareness of your moral imagination help you in future to act more boldly based on principled ethics? Which ethical principles will guide your actions and why?

CONCLUSION

This chapter suggests four different angles from which student writing may be viewed and responded to by learning facilitators and university practice educators. It offers a set of guidelines for giving written (and verbal) feedback with increasing complexity in response to the evolving professional competence of the novice practitioner. Giving formative feedback according to these levels is both time consuming and arduous and may be considered idealistic given the workload of learning facilitators and university practice educators. Focused, well-structured feedback may, however, compensate, in part, for the shortage of on-site practitioners and role models. Whilst this is not the ideal, the judicious use of writing and formative feedback is one avenue for containing students in complex contexts and for attaining a range of learning outcomes, not least the development of reflective, interdependent and ethically responsible practitioners.

REFERENCES

Barnitt, R., Warby, J. & Rawlins, S. (1998). Two case discussions of ethics: editing the truth and the right to resources. *British Journal of Occupational Therapy*, *61*(2), 52–56.

Biggs, J. (1996). Enhancing teaching through constructive alignment. *Higher Education*, *32*, 347–364.

Buchanan, H., Moore, R. & Van Niekerk, L. (1998). The fieldwork case study: writing for clinical reasoning. *American Journal of Occupational Therapy*, *52*(4), 291–295.

Buchanan, H., Van Niekerk, L. & Moore, R. (2001). Assessing fieldwork journals: developmental portfolios. *British Journal of Occupational Therapy*, *64*(8), 398–402.

Christakis, A. & Fendtner, M.A. (1993). Ethics in a short white coat: the ethical dilemmas that medical students confront. *Academic Medicine*, *68*(4), 249–254.

Fairbairn, G.J. (2002). Ethics, empathy and storytelling in professional development. *Learning in Health and Social Care*, *1*(1), 22–32.

Gipps, C. (1999). Socio-cultural aspects of assessment. *Review of Research in Education*, *24*, 355–392.

Higgs, J. & Titchen, A. (2001). Rethinking the practice-knowledge interface in an uncertain world: A model for practice development. *British Journal of Occupational Therapy*, *64*(11), 526–533.

Johnson, M. (1993). *Moral imagination.* Chicago, IL: University of Chicago Press.

Koniak, S. (1996). Law and ethics in a world of rights and unsuitable wrongs. *The Canadian Journal of Law and Jurisprudence*, *9*, 1–32.

Luckett, K. & Sutherland, L. (2000). Assessment practices that improve teaching and learning. In S. Makoni (Ed.), *Improving teaching and learning in higher education.* Johannesburg: Witwatersrand University Press, pp. 96–130.

Mattingly, C. (1991). What is clinical reasoning? *American Journal of Occupational Therapy*, *45*(11), 979–986.

Max-Neef, M.A. (1991). *Human scale development: conception, application and further reflections*. London: The Apex Press.

Neistadt, M.E. (1995). Teaching strategies for the development of clinical reasoning. *American Journal of Occupational Therapy*, 2(8), 676–684.

Newman, F. & Holzman, L. (1993). *Lev Vygotsky: revolutionary scientist*. London: Routledge.

Perkins, D. & Blythe, T. (1993). Understanding up front: a performance approach to testing understanding. Paper presented to Annual Meeting, American Educational Research Association, Atlanta, April.

Seedhouse, D. (1991). Against medical ethics: a philosopher's view. *Medical Education*, 25, 250–282.

Shepard, L. (2000). The role of assessment in a learning culture. *Educational Researcher*, 29(7), 4–14.

Sweeney, G., Wembley, P. & Treacher, A. (2001). Supervision in occupational therapy, Part 3: Accommodating the supervisor and the supervisee. *British Journal of Occupational Therapy*, 64(9), 426–431.

Tryssenaar, J. (1995). Interactive journals: An educational strategy to promote reflection. *American Journal of Occupational Therapy*, 50, 676–684.

Vygotsky, L.S. (1978). *Mind in society: the development of higher psychological process*. Cambridge, MA: Harvard University Press.

Westcott, L. & Rugg, S. (2001). The computation of fieldwork achievement in occupational therapy degrees: measuring a minefield? *British Journal of Occupational Therapy*, 64(11), 541–548.

16 The Student as Supervisor

**LANA VAN NIEKERK, MADELEINE DUNCAN and
KAREN PRAKKE**

OBJECTIVES

This chapter discusses:

- the rationale for a student-led supervision structure
- the principles and processes of peer supervision
- the experiences of senior student supervisors and junior student supervisees
- the ethics of a peer supervision structure.

INTRODUCTION

In contexts where resources and skilled supervisors are scarce, alternative strategies are required to afford students the experience of positive practice learning through appropriate supervision. The undergraduate occupational therapy programme at the University of Cape Town (UCT) has implemented an alternative supervision structure, one that makes use of senior (fourth-year) students as supervisors of junior (first-year) students. This structure provides a pragmatic solution to the shortage of occupational therapy clinicians, who can supervise students. Research evidence indicates that the peer supervision structure produces positive learning outcomes for both groups of students (Brauteseth, Bluck, Prakke & Schou, pers comm; Rau, 2002). Senior students have the opportunity to develop and practise managerial and supervisory skills, whilst junior students benefit from the role modelling that senior students provide and the opportunity to understand more about their chosen profession through practical experiences that are carefully structured by their senior peers.

This chapter is based on the findings of a qualitative research study into peer supervision that was conducted by, and with, students in the Division of Occupational Therapy at the University of Cape Town during 2004

Practice and Service Learning in Occupational Therapy. Edited by Theresa Lorenzo, Madeleine Duncan, Helen Buchanan, Auldeen Alsop
© 2006 John Wiley & Sons Ltd

(Brauteseth et al., pers comm). It commences with a brief description of the peer supervision structure and a rationale for its implementation. The theory of supervision is briefly reviewed, after which the perspectives of senior and junior students are described and principles for implementation extrapolated. The chapter concludes with a set of guidelines to promote positive outcomes for peer supervision as a practice learning activity.

A PEER SUPERVISION STRUCTURE

Final-year students at the University of Cape Town have been supervising first year students since 2000. Students have particular educational needs in each stage of professional development. Practice learning is therefore structured to allow both final-year and first-year students to achieve appropriate learning objectives. Service learning is considered too complex for junior students and they are therefore placed at selected practice learning sites at which final-year students can safely and competently oversee them. Practice educators and site learning facilitators supervise senior students to ensure that ethical and educationally sound learning experiences are provided for the first-year students.

Senior students, usually working in pairs at selected practice learning sites, supervise a small group of junior students who visit the same site once a week for a three-hour session for five consecutive weeks. Junior students complete three such practice learning experiences during their first year of undergraduate studies. The responsibilities of a senior student as a peer supervisor of junior students include:

- orientation to the practice learning setting
- planning and structuring appropriate practical learning tasks
- monitoring the execution of the learning tasks, and
- evaluating individual and group performance.

A two-hour joint workshop with first- and fourth-year students is held at the beginning of the academic year to prepare students for their respective roles within the peer supervision structure. Learning objectives are made available to the students in a practice learning manual, which includes supervision, performance assessment and evaluation guidelines. Supervisees are given an opportunity at the end of a placement to comment on their own performance before senior student supervisors add their comments on the performance assessment form. The first-year performance report form has the same structure and requires similar evaluation processes as the form that is used for third- and fourth-year students in subsequent years. Senior students, therefore, have a good understanding of the components of professional competence being assessed, the processes used during performance assessment (including self-assessment) and the grading criteria used for determining progress (see Chapter 14). Senior students, in turn, are assessed by university practice educators and site learning facilitators with particular reference to their managerial competencies in dealing with the first-year supervisory processes. Managerial components include administration, planning appropriate entry level practice learning experiences, dealing with interpersonal issues within the first-year group and giving feedback.

RATIONALE FOR A PEER SUPERVISION STRUCTURE

Literature indicates that new graduates have to demonstrate proficient clinical skills as well as a range of managerial skills, including supervision, in order to meet the needs of a changing healthcare environment (Adamson, Cant & Hummel, 2001). Proficiency in the supervision and guidance of support staff and mid-level workers, such as community rehabilitation workers and home-based carers is a skill required by occupational therapy graduates in the South African public health context. However, it is inappropriate for final-year students to be practising their supervision skills on qualified, and often very experienced, support staff or mid-level workers.

The peer supervision structure discussed here provides final-year students with rudimentary experience in supervision and human resource management. First-year students also gain from being supervised by their senior peers. They value the opportunity of observing senior students in action, especially since there are few qualified role models in the public sector. First-year students are encouraged by the evidence of who they also may become in a few years time as they watch senior students work with apparent confidence and competence.

THE NATURE OF SUPERVISION

Supervision has been described as a dynamic interaction between a senior and a junior member of the profession, with emphasis on the educative, evaluative and monitoring functions inherent in the professional socialization process (Sweeney, Webley & Treacher, 2001a). The supervisory relationship is evaluative in nature, extends over time, and has the simultaneous purpose of enhancing the professional practice competence of junior colleagues. It monitors the quality of the professional services offered to clients and serves a gate-keeping function to determine who enters the particular profession (Bernard & Goodyear, 1992). According to Morris (1995), supervision provides support and a strong sense of professional identity for the supervisee, whilst Farrington (1995) suggests that it improves professional autonomy.

Supervision is not equivalent to performance review, counselling or monitoring; it is a relationship concerned with accountability for work carried out.

This is an important distinction when considering the involvement of senior students in the practice education of junior students. It could be argued that students should not be allowed or expected to take responsibility for fellow students because of ethical and pedagogical reasons. If, however, the emphasis is developmental and adequate guidance is provided, the academic benefits are worth pursuing.

The supervision process may result in anxieties for both supervisors and supervisees. These feelings can contribute to unsatisfactory supervision and impact negatively on subsequent learning outcomes (Skoberne, 1996; Sweeney, Webley & Treacher, 2001b). Supervision is hard work. It takes time, effort and commitment from the supervisor (Farrington, 1995). Practice competence does not necessarily imply competence as a supervisor (Sweeney et al., 2001 a,b,c). Senior students may therefore resent the additional demands on their time due to the commitment involved with planning for and monitoring first-year students especially considering the extent of their own practice learning requirements.

First-year students enter practice learning with many assumptions, fears and expectations about the kind of role modelling and guidance they will receive. They have to negotiate their needs with senior students who may not be adequately equipped to deal with the demands of supervision. Literature points to the need for educational programmes to support the training and development of practice educators (Bonello, 2001). The supervision of junior students is therefore likely to enhance the skills of senior students for future supervisory roles. Whether first-year students gain as much from learning experiences that are structured and monitored by senior students as they would from qualified practitioners remains an unanswered question in the literature and points to the need for further research into the value of peer supervision.

Martin (1996) criticized the fact that supervision subject matter is not taught in the majority of undergraduate education programmes, and is often only briefly covered in practice educator courses. Paucity of training could lead to first-time supervisors feeling inadequate and lacking in direction. Hall (1998) noted that occupational therapists should extend their knowledge of supervision further, especially with regards to its implementation and its benefits. Novice supervisors should consult with more experienced supervisors about their performance because supervised supervision helps to lessen crises of competence and confidence (Rau, 2002). Successful supervision involves moving away from the perception of being an expert with specialized knowledge to being a collaborator who helps the supervisee develop professional competence and confidence. It may be argued that student peer supervision potentially sets this notion of supervision as collaborative learning into motion. By including peer supervision into the undergraduate practice education curriculum, students are better orientated to the values, attitudes and skills of supervision once they are practising clinicians.

SUPERVISION AS PRACTICE LEARNING

The next section of the chapter describes the principles of supervision as practice learning. The following five themes, emanating from the UCT research findings (Brauteseth et al., pers comm), capture the essence of peer supervision as practice learning. The themes reflect the experiences of senior students as peer supervisors of junior students, namely: being a role model; maintaining a 'give and gain' balance; constructing a 'just-right' challenge; meeting both emotional and practical needs; and reflection on personal growth. Each of these themes is briefly discussed and guidelines are extrapolated to promote supervision as practice learning.

BEING A ROLE MODEL

Peer supervision requires that senior students become a role model, someone the first years could aspire to be like. This expectation places pressure on senior students to portray characteristics that are at a desired level of competence and performance. They feel compelled to perform in ways that give a good and lasting impression of occupational therapy. Senior students place these expectations on themselves based on their own previous role models, such as their perceptions about, and experiences of, supervisors when they were junior students. Those who had positive supervision experiences in the past want to emulate their own role models, whilst those who had negative experiences want to avoid being viewed in the same way.

To deal with these and other internalized expectations, senior students may sometimes need to 'wear a mask'. At some stage during the supervision process they may feel the pressure to pretend or 'fake it' in order to give a good impression of occupational therapy, or to appear more competent than they actually are or perceive themselves to be. This tendency is compounded when senior students are struggling with their own practice learning demands. It is particularly difficult to be a positive role model when they actively dislike working in a particular domain or have unresolved past issues with practice educators or learning facilitators. These internal struggles highlight the difficulty of simultaneously being a supervisor and a student. One student described this experience as follows:

> I think also though that there's a negative aspect to that, because, um, if you're in a fieldwork block, that you yourself are really battling with, and that you, um, are not enjoying, and that, and a block where you don't see the point of OT, um, to be able to try make the first years feel, or have a positive experience and feel that yes OT is fabulous in this setting, or whatever, whatever, I found that really difficult because I was battling to try and make it sound all positive, when I didn't feel that way myself.

Qualified practitioners may have less difficulty in 'being a role model' because they have already developed a sense of self-efficacy, professional competence, autonomy and identity. 'Being a role model' can, however, be considered a valuable practice learning experience because it challenges senior students to explore and develop their professional identity and autonomy, even if it is emotionally difficult. Practice education should therefore put adequate learning and support structures in place to help students process the dynamics of their internalized professional ideals.

MAINTAINING THE 'GIVE–GAIN' BALANCE

Peer supervision is described as a 'two-way value, mutual learning' experience. Senior students tend to oscillate between 'giving' to the learning process of first-year students and 'gaining' personal learning from the giving process. Reciprocal learning is ensured by maintaining a give–take balance in meeting the practice development needs of both supervisor and supervisee. Qualified supervisors do not necessarily need the same degree of reciprocity. When senior students value and enjoy their contribution to the learning of fellow students, supervision is experienced as worthwhile and a reciprocal give–gain balance can easily be created. The supervision process is then described as 'mutually beneficial'. The learning of senior students may be enhanced by a number of processes inherent in the supervision process itself:

- The opportunity to witness the growth and learning of junior students.
- Increased awareness of personal–professional growth and learning needs.
- Reflection on occupational therapy practice from different perspectives and being challenged to justify various assumptions, methods and approaches.
- Learning about group dynamics; human motivation and adult education.

The tasks and responsibilities of being a supervisor are demanding and require additional effort on the part of senior students. This is similar to the nature of supervision for qualified supervisors. The process of planning, selecting and structuring the appropriate learning environments, giving input and organizing opportunities to observe occupational therapy in practice is time consuming and emotionally taxing.

Senior students may feel compromised when their investments of time and effort are not reciprocated with equal 'gains' in learning, assessment rewards and acknowledgement. Those students who are unable or unwilling to optimize the learning potential of the supervision process may not experience the same personal and professional rewards. This is likely to be the case with senior students who have personally unfulfilled needs in terms of evaluation and supervision. Attention should therefore be given to regulating the demands placed on senior students through considered negotiation of site-specific learning objectives and practice expectations.

Senior students are able to empathize with what first-year students are going through as novice professionals because of their own recent first-year experiences. They can offer appropriate peer support and encouragement by pointing to the growth that will take place in the future and by helping first-year students to put their future learning and current challenges into perspective. Senior students gain personal rewards that make the work, time and energy invested during supervision worthwhile. These rewards include verbal acknowledgement of work done, affirmation from the final-year students' own supervisors, feedback from clinicians, and having the first years aspire to them as role models. A considerable amount of time and energy, however, needs to be put into the supervision infrastructure to reap these rewards.

CONSTRUCTING A 'JUST-RIGHT' CHALLENGE

Senior students are responsible for identifying appropriate practice learning opportunities for first-year students. They may, for example, identify a child with whom the first-year student is expected to do a particular play activity, using a plan of action that they prescribe or develop in collaboration with the first-year student. The prescribed activity is matched to the child's needs with due consideration of the first-year student's competence. Through structuring various learning activities, senior students demonstrate occupational therapy in practice and facilitate an understanding of the occupational therapist's role in various settings. They enable junior students to put theory into practice by finding the 'just-right challenge', through which learning may occur that is simultaneously beneficial to the patient or client. The supervision process becomes less than optimal when senior students lack sufficient time or an effective structure within which to plan for first-year students.

Senior students are able to create 'just-right' learning opportunities by following written guidelines and structured practice requirements that are provided to all students as part of the practice learning curriculum. Supervision guidelines, developed by practice educators using appropriate pedagogical principles, help students understand the educational expectations that may lead to relevant learning outcomes. The level of learning required by junior students may be anticipated and addressed by selecting appropriate learning environments, clients and opportunities to assist in professional activities. Constructing the 'just-right' challenge includes the ethical responsibility of ensuring non-maleficence in the actions of inexperienced first students. Senior students, who are able to reflect on their own experiences as first years, are able to anticipate and mediate the cultural and social challenges that are faced by junior students in the implementation of occupational therapy.

Senior students need reassurance and affirmation that they are doing 'the right thing' and that they are successfully facilitating the learning of junior students, whilst meeting the needs of the clients in their care. They seek validation from junior students that they are, in fact, meeting their educational needs. Opportunities for validation, evaluation and feedback from their own clinicians and supervisors on their performance as supervisor are also valued. One senior student remarked:

> I think in some way it should also be part of our, I don't know how it could be possible, like part of our evaluation . . . as fourth year students, like how well did you support [because] you, there's definitely an amount of input you can put into your first years or not.

MEETING BOTH EMOTIONAL AND PRACTICAL NEEDS

The burden of being a supervisor places an emotional load on senior students who may feel as if they are carrying the feelings of their supervisees. They may experience supervision as being 'more emotional than practical' at times. One senior student shared the following:

> On that Thursday when the first years left, I just cried that night [because] I was so, like you just feeling all of their issues and all of their like emotions are coming in, like that's kind of yours . . . I mean, all that emotional stuff does get loaded onto you as well, like as a supervisor, that's the sort of stuff you need to like debrief from, and I mean, we didn't really have that . . . but like, like you really do feel that emotional stuff.

Being a supervisor and a student can be emotionally draining when students struggle to maintain an objective distance and to differentiate between their own processes of learning and those of their supervisees. This is not very different from maintaining a therapeutic distance and managing issues of transference and counter-transference when working with clients. As one student stated:

> It's not a huge thing that makes or breaks you, but you do talk to each other about it, it's quite nice though, even something like this [referring to the research focus group], where you get to just chat to other people about it, and the experiences we've had with the first years, [because] we don't have any outlet then to go to.

It is therefore important to find and provide avenues such as support groups to 'unload the load' in order to deal with the emotions associated with providing supervision.

REFLECTION ON PERSONAL–PROFESSIONAL GROWTH

The supervision experience gives senior students an opportunity to reflect on their evolving personal–professional identities and practice competence. This reflection may be described as standing in 'a room full of mirrors'. Two processes are involved in this reflection. In the first process, students come to appreciate how far they themselves have come along the professional development continuum. In the second process, they face themselves; they appraise their personal abilities and weaknesses. One student shared:

> I think the biggest thing for me, which I loved about supervising first years, was that it showed me how much I knew and how much I'd learnt and where I'd come from, and it really it, sort of, was just so incredible to see that journey that I'd taken.

The experiences, reactions and abilities of junior students highlight for senior students just how far they have come since they started their training. Self-reflection brings them full circle from a place where they were once insecure to a place where they have gained confidence. One student reported:

> . . . it does give you that confidence, it makes you feel good about yourself sometimes, because you really do see where you're at, . . . to know like that you actually reached this place, you know, so its like, it's the, it builds you up as a person, sometimes you can surprise people.

PERSPECTIVES OF FIRST-YEAR SUPERVISEES

The practice education curriculum of first-year students traditionally involves orientation visits to various occupational therapy departments with little 'hands on' work with individuals or groups. The peer supervision structure described here is based on the belief that first-year students can make a meaningful contribution to the well-being of selected individuals or groups if they are given ample guidance, structure and adequate supervision. The following section of the chapter briefly describes the challenges and potential benefits of peer supervision for first-year students.

AN INFLUENTIAL RELATIONSHIP

First-year supervisees experience being supervised by their senior peers as 'a learning relationship that really influenced me'. This learning relationship impacts on their feelings of competence, what they learn about their role as a student and about the role of qualified occupational therapists, and the development of their clinical reasoning skills. It also influences whether they continue studying occupational therapy or not. The nature of the learning relationship is determined by the attitude of the fourth-year supervisor, not only to the domain of practice but also to the supervision task itself. The more committed the senior student is to the relationship and the more organized they are in planning and guiding the activities of the supervisees, the more they are likely to gain from the supervision process and the practice learning experience.

First-year students feel uncertain, incompetent and anxious when entering a new practice learning placement for the first time. These feelings are compounded when the senior student is unprepared, apparently uncommitted to creating an optimal learning environment or when expectations are not clearly explained. A comprehensive induction and orientation, coupled with effective planning and implementation of activities provides first-year students with a clearer understanding of occupational therapy, which in turn leads to a growing sense of competence and confidence. This raises questions about the ethics of exposing first years to 'hands on' practice when their competence and confidence is limited, and what risk this poses to the people with whom they work. The beneficence of what first-year students are able to offer individuals and groups is directly dependent on the vigilance and ethical sensitivity of senior students and indirectly on the supervision given to them by practice educators and site learning facilitators. The activities that the first years implement with individuals and groups (for example, a soccer match with forensic patients or a baking activity with orphans) must be appropriately selected and monitored to ensure compliance with patient rights and ethical standards. First-year students make a collective statement of intent prior to starting practice learning for the first time. This statement is a precursor to the professional oath they take on graduating and sensitises them to the various ethical requirements of working, as student professionals, with members of the public.

ESSENCE OF OCCUPATIONAL THERAPY

Encouragement and approval of their actions influences the extent to which first-year students are able to grasp the 'essence of OT', a concept which is central to a positive professional identity and conceptualizing future roles. Practice learning highlights the reasons why they entered the profession. Feelings of success or frustration in applying new found knowledge and skill influences their decisions around continuing in the profession. The question of 'is OT for me?' is answered by exposure to a range of practice domains. The attitudes of senior supervisors and their teaching methods contribute to the clarity with which first-year students become socialized into the philosophy and values of the profession.

EXPERIENTIAL LEARNING

Whilst there was a need for guidance, direction and clear explanation, junior students respond well and are clearly empowered through the adult education, 'experiential learning' approach that some senior student supervisors are able to adopt. By being involved in a problem-posing, action-reflection process of adult learning, supervisees feel that they contribute to, and participate in, their own learning process. Students who are given too much freedom and too little direction feel very overwhelmed.

An overly supportive relationship, on the other hand, is experienced as 'friendship'; 'closeness'; 'an intimate, trusting thing'; and 'comfortable'. This nurturing type of supervision relationship is seen to be analogous with a 'mother hen caring for her young chicks'. Whilst supervisees appreciate this kind of support from their supervisors, it raises the question about the extent to which professional boundaries need to be maintained in the peer supervision relationship and the influence this has on mutual learning. These questions require further research.

GUIDELINES FOR SUPPORTING LEARNING THROUGH SUPERVISON

Since peer supervision may be seen as an 'identity-building' experience, particular attention needs to be paid to the academic structures that are put in place to support the practice learning of both senior and first-year students. Learning through peer supervision may be promoted when:

- formal preparation and training on how to supervise and how to use supervision is provided as part of the practice learning curriculum
- clear learning objectives for both senior and junior students are provided and modified according to emerging needs
- structures, such as support groups and individual mentoring, are readily available
- discussion groups and tutorials to facilitate reflective learning
- student-supervisors have easy access to an experienced supervisor who can assist them as needed, especially for emotional support and feedback on performance
- reasonable expectations are placed on junior students. They should not be expected to participate in techniques or modalities for which they have not been adequately prepared in lectures and practical seminars
- supervising is done in pairs by senior students to share the work load
- a reward system such as academic grades to acknowledge the additional responsibility placed on senior students is incorporated into their performance assessment
- accomplishments are validated and acknowledged through formal feedback and evaluation mechanisms involving all parties.

CONCLUSION

The skills of a supervisor are best developed through opportunities to gain experience in the role. The advantage of providing this experience during undergraduate training is that the learning can be structured as part of the formal practice education curriculum. Novice supervisors can reflect on and learn through 'hands on' experience, thereby equipping them with an important professional skill. Using adequately prepared senior students to supervise junior students is essentially beneficial to all concerned: clinicians have more time to do their work; fourth-year students gain supervisory experience; and first-year students gain the necessary experience for their stage of professional development.

ACKNOWLEDGEMENTS

This chapter is based on the final-year research project conducted by Kerryn Brauteseth, Lauren Bluck, Karen Prakke and Jenna Schou. This project won the national student research award from the Occupational Therapy Association of South Africa in 2004.

REFERENCES

Adamson, B., Cant, R. & Hummel, J. (2001). What managerial skills do newly graduated occupational therapists need? A view from their managers. *British Journal of Occupational Therapy, 64*(4), 184–190.

Bernard, J.M. & Goodyear, R.K. (1992). *Fundamentals of clinical supervision.* Boston: Allyn and Bacon.

Bonello, M. (2001). Fieldwork within the context of higher education: a literature review. *British Journal of Occupational Therapy, 64*(2), 93–99.

Farrington, A. (1995). Defining and setting the parameters of clinical supervision. *British Journal of Nursing, 4,* 874–875.

Hall, D. (1998). Supervision and the occupational therapy profession. *Mental Health Occupational Therapy, 3,* 10–13.

Kautzmann, L.N. (1990). Clinical teaching: fieldwork supervisors' attitudes and values. *American Journal of Occupational Therapy, 44,* 835–838.

Martin, M. (1996). How reflective is student supervision? A study of supervision in action. *British Journal of Occupational Therapy, 59*(5), 229–232.

Morris, M. (1995). The role of clinical supervision in mental health practice. *British Journal of Occupational Therapy, 58,* 886–888.

Rau, D.R. (2002). Advanced trainees supervising junior trainees. *The Clinical Supervisor, 21,* 115–124.

Skoberne, M. (1996). Supervision in nursing; my experience and views. *Journal of Nursing Management, 4,* 289–295.

Sweeney, G., Webley, P. & Treacher, A. (2001a). Supervision in occupational therapy, part 1: the supervisor's anxieties. *British Journal of Occupational Therapy*, *64*(7), 337–345.

Sweeney, G., Webley, P. & Treacher, A. (2001b). Supervision in occupational therapy, part 2: the supervisee's dilemma. *British Journal of Occupational Therapy*, *64*(8), 380–386.

Sweeney, G., Webley, P. & Treacher, A. (2001c). Supervision in occupational therapy, part 3: accommodating the supervisor and the supervisee. *British Journal of Occupational Therapy*, *64*(9), 426–431.

17 Enhancing Potential through Lifelong Learning and Research

AULDEEN ALSOP

OBJECTIVES

This chapter discusses:

- personal responsibility for professional updating in line with changes in healthcare practice
- lifelong learning and research as ways of enhancing personal and professional effectiveness
- the implications of professional isolation
- support mechanisms that can promote professional growth.

EMBRACING CHANGE

Many of the chapters of this book have identified just how important it is for occupational therapists to embrace and work with political and organizational changes and related developments. They must do this in order to survive and thrive within an environment that, as it evolves, continuously impacts on the profession's work not just at a national but also at an international level. It has to be recognized that occupational therapy is a fast moving and evolving profession globally. It is thus important for occupational therapists to recognize the influence of context and to critically evaluate emerging ideas, concepts and frameworks from other countries and to make informed decisions about the potential application of global perspectives to the local scene.

Ryan, Esdaile and Brown (2003) observed that change has always been present in healthcare but now, rather than settling down, the pace was gaining momentum. In healthcare, new ideas were emerging so fast that the ideas could eventually outstrip the abilities of many of those trying to implement them. This suggests that occupational therapists must continuously appraise new ideas but learn to discriminate carefully in favour of those that will clearly benefit the service. Additionally, they must be prepared to engage in ongoing

Practice and Service Learning in Occupational Therapy. Edited by Theresa Lorenzo, Madeleine Duncan, Helen Buchanan, Auldeen Alsop
© 2006 John Wiley & Sons Ltd

learning activities to keep apace of service developments within an ever-changing socio-political context as well as to fulfil their obligations for updating themselves as professionals and for ensuring their continuing competence to practise.

PROFESSIONAL RESPONSIBILITIES

Higgs et al. (2004a) remarked that practice in the health sciences was a challenging responsibility. It required health professionals to have a rich array of knowledge and skills in order to work in complex situations and environments. Occupational therapy, wherever it is practised, has been deemed complex (Creek, 2003), the complexity being situated in the occupational therapist's thinking and doing in a dynamic relationship with each individual in each unique and complex context (Butler, 2004). Even at its simplest, occupational therapy can be classed as complex. It follows that occupational therapists must engage in learning through critical thinking to develop competence for complexity. Learning that just develops a sound knowledge base is not enough. Occupational therapists must also develop their reasoning skills to the highest level in order to maintain their capacity to practise in contexts that are not just complex but constantly evolving and changing. But 'thinking is not easy; it can be a painful process that involves challenge, upset and uncertainty' (Butler, 2004, p. 289). As a responsible professional, occupational therapists must learn and be prepared to manage uncertainty in difficult situations in everyday practice.

Professional education and professional development assist the process, but competence attained at the time of qualification is not competence for life. Swartz (2004) clearly stated that professionals registered with a statutory body to practise their profession must keep up to date with developments in their field. It is a professional obligation often specified in a profession's Code of Ethics, an obligation to which Eraut (1994) drew attention. Eraut claimed that the professional status conferred on health professionals at the point of qualification created an expectation that they would continue to learn and develop. This is a necessity so that professionals can be judged at any time as delivering the best available service to the people with whom they work. Butler (2004), however, suggested that codes of ethics could be viewed simply as guides to behaviour. The ethical principles within the codes may not be situated within an individual's personal beliefs. Personal ethics that guide behaviour concern integrity and morality and these underpin personal commitment to professional behaviour, and the consequential need for professional updating.

Being a professional required an ongoing commitment to education and also to the generation of new knowledge (Higgs, 2003). As Barnett (1997) professed, professionals have a responsibility to develop themselves and to contribute proactively to developing the knowledge base of their profession so as to bring about professional growth. Barnett further claimed that the transactions with clients did not define the limits of a professional's responsibility. Professionals also had a duty to maintain and develop their critical powers so that they could ask radical questions and contribute to debates in their professional world as a prerequisite to being able to practice effectively in a changing environment. Building capacity in research and practise and pushing the boundaries of practice will enhance the potential of a profession and enable others to benefit from that new knowledge (Swartz, 2004).

Dahlgren, Richardson and Kalman (2004, p. 15) reinforced Barnett's contention suggesting that there was a need for professionals to develop 'practical and discursive consciousness' and a capacity for reflecting not only in and on practice, but also *about* practice as a condition for shaping the future of their profession. Reflection, they claimed, 'conveys the continuity of change, which is intrinsic to an epistemological perspective of knowledge being contextual and unfolding' (Dahlgren et al., 2004, p. 28). Practitioners should thus take responsibility for suggesting areas of research that could be undertaken to create or further develop the evidence base for practice. In order to do this, practitioners must foster a reflective and critical stance in an effort to 'uncover premises and presuppositions underlying everyday practice that are not currently articulated in research or articulated in practice knowledge discourse' (Dahlgren et al., 2004, p. 21).

Higgs, Fish and Rothwell (2004b) reinforced the expectation that practitioners, in their everyday role, should critically evaluate their own performance in order to become aware of emerging issues in practice. The importance of articulating practice knowledge verbally is the first step towards 'being able to scrutinise critically the rationale for the choices and decisions' made in the clinical encounter (Richardson, Dahlgren & Higgs, 2004, p. 204). Prospective research ideas can be generated in this way. These observations suggest that it is important to enhance the potential of the profession to enable it to contribute to the health and social care of the population through modes of critical enquiry. It means enhancing the potential of individuals so that they can offer best practice to service users through skilled professional reasoning. It means enhancing the potential of students by supporting them, modelling for them, engaging them, and promoting best practice so that they can become autonomous practitioners, able to contribute effectively to the provision of services both in institutional environments and out in communities.

Students, as developing therapists, assume a professional role and associated responsibilities as soon as they enter professional education. Engaging in practice and service learning exposes them to the realities of professional practice where they observe, question and seek rationales for the ways in which qualified staff address their professional responsibilities. Here, the foundations of students' learning are formed. From the point of their engagement with professional practice, students learn to learn, learn to make judgements, develop their knowledge and develop the reasoning skills that underpin aspects of practice. They observe and critique the practice of their educators, learning facilitators and mentors, and shape their own practice according to their personal interests, values, beliefs and professional preferences. Professional education thus provides the medium for setting the course of students' professionalism and lifelong learning, but the extent to which this is successful depends on how far those attitudes are modelled and reinforced in practice. By engaging fully in their own professional agenda, qualified staff will ensure that their practice affirms the professional's responsibility for lifelong learning, personal and professional development and professional growth. This will be addressed in different ways, dependent on the context of practice.

Many occupational therapists work as members of a team. Others work in isolation. Those who work both in isolation and in deprived areas find themselves with many challenges, a significant proportion of which may be influenced by complex environmental issues. Whatever the environment, professional responsibilities create expectations that occupational therapists will engage with ongoing learning that will help them to develop knowledge and skills and so enhance their potential in practice. Learning can occur at any time and through everyday events. It is not always planned and not always apparent until revealed through reflection. The art is to recognize that learning has occurred by raising it to consciousness. Opening up reflective debates with colleagues and students about unintended learning from experience can assist everyone's development and model good practice that contributes to the lifelong learning agenda.

WHAT IS LIFELONG LEARNING?

Longworth and Davies (1996, p. 22) coined a useful definition of lifelong learning as:

> the development of human potential through a continuously supportive process which stimulates and empowers individuals to acquire all the knowledge, values, skills and understanding they will require throughout their lifetimes and to apply them with confidence, creativity and enjoyment in all roles, circumstances and environments.

Griffin (2001) raised questions about whether lifelong learning related to the lifetime or just to the time frame of working life. The definition above, however, seems to capture the features of learning in its widest sense. The emphasis is clearly placed on the individual to engage in the learning process, but to be effective it has to be an active process. The process allows the individual's potential to be enhanced so that they can engage in roles and contexts that are personally meaningful and important both to the present and to future development. It could also be suggested, however, that the individual's enhanced capacity as a result of learning might also be of benefit to others with whom that individual comes into contact. Hence, colleagues and the service may also benefit from those endeavours and, if individuals within a team collectively engage in lifelong learning, the benefits to all could be magnified.

According to Brownhill (2001, p. 78) lifelong learning is a 'process of discovery', reinforcing the notion of learning not just as an active process but also as an evolutionary process. Jarvis (2001) expressed concern, however, that there was little or no emphasis on criticality in much of the lifelong learning literature. He advocated that learners needed to be encouraged to evaluate the nature of society and be free to think and make their own judgements about their experiences. As Brownhill (2001, p. 71) suggested, we become what we are by experiencing the culture in which we exist by interacting with others, and by reflecting on those experiences and interactions. These comments reinforce the importance of reflection and critical engagement in the learning process, but Eraut (2005) also noted how difficult it was for practitioners to find time for reflection. Goodfellow, McAllister, Best, Webb and Fredericks (2001) asserted that personal practical knowledge required reflective thought in and about practice in the process of engaging in life's learning journey. Reflection is thus not an option but an integral feature of competent practice to which time must be allocated.

Griffin (2001) pointed out that some models reduce the concept of lifelong learning to measurements of participation in learning events or to qualifications and credentialism. Others would see this as a fairly limited view, suggesting that lifelong learning could embrace a wide range of both formal and informal learning opportunities (Alsop, 2000; College of Occupational Therapists, 2004). According to the College of Occupational Therapists (2004), lifelong learning should necessarily be concerned with raising aspirations about learning of all occupational therapy staff, at pre-registration level, for continuing professional development and with regards to scholarship and research. The College's vision is that all occupational therapy personnel should be encouraged to take advantage of both formal and informal learning opportunities, in a variety of situations, in order to maintain and enhance competence, knowledge and expertise. At a glance, the websites of several other occupational therapy professional bodies across the world indicate that this is a global expectation.

Learning, it seems, has an important function in that it is perceived to be the process whereby individuals develop a sense of self and identity, biography and personal history. 'It is the process of internalising the external world and being able to locate ourselves within it' (Jarvis 2001, p. 201). For practitioners, this external world can comprise both practice and academic settings but as Eraut (2005) concluded, whilst evidence had shown that there was a strong connection between education and practice, neither practitioners nor educators paid sufficient attention to this link. No one disputed that effort focused on different goals in the two settings, but the power of a strong theoretical basis for practice seemed to be ignored. In healthcare in particular, practitioners could survive without theory. Patients' needs could adequately be met through fluent practice. Yet Eraut (2005) contended that there was a danger in neglecting the theoretical side of practice as theory was strongly aligned with research, evidence-based practice and with professional status. Abandoning theory meant relinquishing potential power and this could reduce a group's sense of agency. As Higgs (2003, p. 151) asserted,

> Expertise is a journey towards professional artistry, the essence of which is the ability to bring together technical competencies, the humanity of people-centred practice, the grounding of experience in the reality of practice and in the evidence from both practice and science, to support and give credibility to practice

Richardson et al. (2004) suggested that departmental managers had an important role to play, not just in the day-to-day delivery of healthcare, but also in establishing a culture of a community of practice to help ensure interaction of the profession with the social world of which members form a part. They had a responsibility to promote ongoing learning and engagement in research so as to contribute both individually and collectively to the growth of the profession. Through detailing practice activities and analysing them together, new knowledge could be identified and old knowledge could appropriately be abandoned as no longer relevant (Richardson et al., 2004, p. 208). Barnett (1994) claimed that professionals had to abandon outdated practices as an essential prerequisite for the development of the profession, but many find it hard to do.

CULTURAL SENSITIVITY

Joubert (2003, p. 2) made a plea for occupational therapy education to reflect the needs of the service in which newly qualified staff would be working. She was commenting particularly from a South African perspective where policies had emerged that required higher education to address 'the diverse problems and demands of the local, national, southern African and African contexts'. The challenge to the profession was to devise and implement culturally relevant and sensitive models and practices that reflected local needs and working methods. It was all too easy to import practices that had been tried and tested in the Western world and to adopt them without a critical evaluation of their relevance to the South African context. But this was inappropriate. New versions were required to meet the specific needs of occupational therapists working in South Africa and students needed to develop competence in their use.

Michael Iwama (2003) made similar claims. Western occupational therapy models and practices were perceived to be inappropriate for the Asian culture as viewpoints of the two populations differed considerably. The Japanese philosophy focused on harmony and embraced values and beliefs around adaptation and accommodation. These were completely different to those of a Western society that valued empowerment and control. Educational and professional practices needed to identify and adopt culturally relevant practices that were informed by research. Cultural borders could be transcended if occupational therapists thought creatively beyond the usual frameworks and models and their underlying assumptions (Iwama, 2005).

Occupational therapists, therefore, have a responsibility to enhance their practice by taking full account of the cultural context of their work and to recognize the need for empirical work to determine best practice relevant to the situations in which they find themselves working. This notion has been endorsed by Garbett (2004), who advocated practitioner research grounded in case studies of professional practice, and by Crossley (2000), who promoted bridge-building and reconceptualization through research practices across cultures. This could mean evaluating critically and systematically the models and approaches emerging from other societies to determine relevance or to explore possible modifications. It could also mean undertaking research that would allow uniquely appropriate models to emerge for use in defined geographical areas or cultures. Educational programmes would then need to enable their students to become well-versed in the new approaches as preparation for practice. Occupational therapists thus needed to enhance their potential by acquiring research skills and by engaging in research as a feature of their everyday practice after qualification.

THE RESEARCH AGENDA

The world of practice is complex, uncertain and ever changing (Barnett, 2000) and as changes occur, from time to time, the value of professionals and the contribution they make to society are called into question, often for economic reasons. Occupational therapy is one profession where research into practice in order to demonstrate its contribution to society is crucial to survival, yet the history of research within the profession might still be said to be in its infancy. There is a desire, however, for the profession to be viewed as a learning society, a society that makes progress, a society that takes a critical stance towards its practice (Barnett, 1997). Serious, systematic research must therefore be on the agenda to establish the foundations of effective practice and to support decisions to withdraw from practices that are demonstrated as ineffective or uneconomic.

Institutes of higher education, professional bodies and health organizations all have a vested interest in research even though the rationale for research might be different for each of them. The responsibility for engaging in research is often placed with practitioners so it is vital that professionals, as part of their learning agenda, consolidate and develop their research skills by engaging in research. The research could be collaborative or single-handed, but it should be informative, of current interest and methodologically sound so that it stands up to scientific scrutiny (Walker, 2003). The more that qualified practitioners engage in the research process, the sooner it will become custom-and-practice within the profession. As Walker (2003, p. 341) advocated: 'The ideal future scenario would be to expect clinicians to become research "doers" as part of their professional development'. This position would enable students to see research as an everyday part of their practice and an activity that contributes not just to their personal lifelong learning agenda but also to the overall growth of the profession itself.

Practitioners should thus acknowledge how they can model good practice by engaging in research. It should feature in the practice education curriculum, with opportunities for students at least to be able to discuss 'live' research, if not engage in some aspect of it by exploring literature, generating data or contributing to the data analysis process. As service learning expands, so should research into practice and the service learning agenda expand also. Research is certainly needed now. But even if students ensure that they understand the principles of research so that they can explore and debate possible research ideas with some degree of reality, then strategies for undertaking the research might ensue. It is important as a feature of the professional agenda to move to a position where, instead of the minority of practitioners being involved in research, it is the majority. Those who have advanced practitioner status have even more of a responsibility for contributing to that agenda.

THE ADVANCED PRACTITIONER

It is worth considering here the relationship between enhancing potential of the individual and the concept of advanced practice. Madill and Hollis (2003, p. 32) presented their thoughts on the essence of advanced practice, which are embedded in the list below. The term 'advanced practitioner' may be attributed to someone who has:

- breadth and depth of professional knowledge
- an appreciation of the environment and wider context of practice
- ability to think critically and engage in critical analysis

- ability to contribute extensively to one or more areas of practice
- commitment to quality and quality enhancement
- commitment to the development of personal knowledge and skills
- advanced qualifications or at least evidence of serious continuing professional development.

McAllister (2003) drew conclusions from her research that advanced practitioners were individuals with a clear sense of self. They seemed to be people who had the capacity to manage the work environment, tasks and roles, self and others and they brought heightened levels of awareness to their work. Having a sense of self included having self-awareness and self-knowledge, self-acceptance and self-identity, being aware of one's level of need to control people, time and events and seeing oneself as a lifelong learner (McAllister, 2003, p. 234). Esdaile and Roth (2003) maintained that becoming an advanced practitioner not only took time and effort, but also required emotional investment.

WAYS OF ENHANCING PERSONAL POTENTIAL

Alsop (2000), in an earlier text, and later Brown et al. (2003), described many different ways in which personal potential could be developed, taking particular account of individual preferences in learning styles and approaches. Professional updating to underpin ongoing competence, and continuing professional development and the enhancement of potential for career progression, are matters that every health professional should address. In career progression, however, awareness of global political, sociological, economic and technological influences on practice and professional potential tends to become heightened. The complexities of practice across continents and cultures begin to shape thinking in a different way. The efforts therefore to enhance personal potential take a different route.

CRITICAL DISCOURSE WITH PEERS

One of the most rewarding, yet often one of the most demanding ways of enhancing personal capacity is to engage in critical debate with peers through journal clubs, workshops, conferences or other opportunities for semi-formal discourse. Being exposed to other perspectives, having to defend or critique and challenge a position becomes an intellectual challenge in itself. Another way is to use visits or secondments with pre-defined learning intentions to help widen perspectives through discussion with peers. Engaging with peers informally often presents opportunities for mutual learning through networking which, in itself, becomes a means by which like-minded people can keep in touch and provide reciprocal support. These critical debates can often lead to research questions being raised. The critical step forward would be to plan and carry out the research project from the idea that has emerged.

DRAWING ON THE EXPERTISE OF SERVICE USERS

Partnership working with individuals, groups or communities who represent the user population can also be extremely rewarding yet notoriously challenging. Taylor (1997, p. 178) promoted partnership working with service users in the field of education, but warned that if users' contributions to professional education were to avoid accusations of tokenism 'they must be integrated into a coherent framework which reflects user participation in relation to personal, process and propositional knowledge'. Taylor wrote from a position where service users entered the university to contribute to student education as 'experts' in their field. Learning in partnership with service users can, however, operate from many different bases including voluntary organizations, drop-in centres and the community at large. It is really only on the users' ground that new ways of thinking and practising are likely to occur. Here practitioners are likely to come face-to-face with the wider realities affecting the user in their context, which are often infinitely more complex than those presented by a user speaking within the university. It is within the communities that service learning occurs. It derives from collaborative goal-setting and partnership working towards meeting the identified goals. The learning occurs for both parties. As with many learning opportunities that occur with users there can be an emotional side to the learning that, as far as health professionals are concerned, can lead to considerable personal and professional growth. Given the many different perspectives that also emerge through service learning, the collective position lends itself to more systematic methods of learning using the framework of research.

PROFESSIONAL ISOLATION

Taking steps to maintain and develop competence and to advance practice can be challenging and time-consuming, even for the best of occupational therapists and for those working in relatively well-supported and well-resourced environments. For those working in isolation and in areas of significant deprivation, however, engaging in lifelong learning or continuing professional development is nowhere near as easy.

Newton and Fuller (2005) explained some of the challenges for occupational therapists who worked in isolation in rural and remote areas. Limited resources, educational opportunities and professional support were often the norm. Those occupational therapists working in developing countries where the profession is less established are arguably more deprived than their colleagues practising in more developed areas, and this can result in serious professional isolation. The situation could be exacerbated by a political situation that failed to appreciate the role and skills of occupational therapists, who then faced monumental problems in their work as well as in locating professional networks for communication and support.

Watson and Fourie (2004) explained the relationship between history and progress within developing countries, including Africa. They stated that centuries of governance had stripped Africa of all but hope, leaving a legacy of underdevelopment and dependence that, as a trend, was extremely difficult to reverse. They noted that poverty still abounded despite the changes that had taken effect in South Africa since the establishment of the democracy in 1994, and professionals needed to be aware of this. Existing policies required occupational therapists to modify the profession's philosophy to reflect current practice, and to allow it to evolve so as to be continually relevant to the context in which practice took place.

Despite poverty, where a natural focus is likely to be on survival, Watson (2004, p. 62) nevertheless advocated that everyone had the right to be 'occupationally active in health-giving and developmentally enriching pursuits'. This aspiration challenges occupational therapists to work differently and to engage with communities as well as with individuals, groups and organizations to promote the concepts of occupation and skill in realizing human potential. Even though some local initiatives might be successful (Watson & Swartz, 2004), the norm is likely to mean isolation and lack of resources that stretch the imagination in service delivery and restrict opportunity for continuing professional development and growth. Sometimes Action Learning can offer a process for self-development. Reflection on experiences (both positive and negative) can lead to the implementation of new approaches that are informed by the experiential learning (Lorenzo & Cloete, 2004). It is essential, however, that learning in the community becomes a two-way process so as to address the emotional and developmental needs of both parties. Self-care for the occupational therapist and finding appropriate support 'is not an indulgence but an ethical responsibility' (Swartz, 2004, p. 296) that may help counter disillusionment and burn-out. Seeking and using a mentor may be one way forward (Lorenzo & Cloete, 2004).

PROFESSIONAL SUPPORT

Throughout their career, professionals would normally rely on many different individuals for career and psychosocial support (Roth & Esdaile, 2003). Some possibilities for developing informal networks have already been mentioned. More formally, Titchen and McGinley (2004, p. 111) described the concept of a 'critical companion' as 'an experienced facilitator (often, but not necessarily a colleague) who accompanies a practitioner on an experiential learning journey'. McAllister (2003) commented that the relationship allowed for the provision of constructive criticism and support. Additionally, the companion served as a resource and a facilitator to promote learning in order to enhance practice in the workplace. Similarly, McAllister noted the benefits of using critical friends. These were often peers or colleagues who operated within a trusting and open relationship and who were empowered to question critically, but sensitively, each other's practice. This involved reflection, and perhaps the exploration of critical incidents or of a shared story. It could be done face-to-face or on-line, but either way, the relationship provided a medium for professional support and for enhancing individual potential.

Mentorship also offers a facilitative but non-directive relationship with another person that focuses on the employee's needs rather than on the needs of the service or service user. It uses dialogue to facilitate problem-solving and learning, to review strengths, challenge assumptions, and help develop a vision of the future. A mentor can help to explore concerns, serve as a sounding board for ideas and help develop strategies for career development. Mentoring is not a counselling role. It operates within mutually agreed parameters of time, place and purpose, and within a relationship of mutual respect and confidentiality (Alsop, 2000).

Seeking career assistance from a variety of sources could increase the amount of information, resources and opportunities available to support professional growth (Roth & Esdaile, 2003). Building professional networks could result in personal and professional satisfaction and other opportunities for growth. From these networks, mentors might be selected who could help to determine suitable learning and development opportunities. Roth and Esdaile also advocated the benefits for individuals of using peer relationships to discuss thoughts and feelings about life and work.

Professional support may not necessarily be available to everyone. Those working single-handed and in isolation of colleagues do not have ready access to the same kinds of support mechanisms. Those engaging in compulsory community service after graduation may well find themselves in this position. Lone working requires individuals to be self-assured and self-sufficient in their practice. Opportunities for professional updating are likely to be lacking or at least dependent on the initiative and creativity of the individual to ensure that new and relevant learning takes place in different ways. The strategies that are going to enable individuals to survive and thrive in these situations are different. Self-sufficiency and well-developed skills of critical evaluation and reflection will promote personal professional development in a different way. It has to be said, however, that for occupational therapists working in isolation and/or in difficult and challenging circumstances, support mechanisms such as those outlined above are a necessity, not a luxury.

Newton and Fuller (2005) acknowledged the difficulties experienced by occupational therapists working in rural areas, in isolation and with few resources. They described an initiative known as OTION (Occupational Therapy International Outreach Network) that had been developed for the purpose of addressing the needs of isolated occupational therapists. OTION provides a global forum for occupational therapists to communicate with colleagues working in similar circumstances around the world. Not only does it provide a support mechanism, it offers a facility for discussion, debate and for learning from each other. It recognizes the particular issues faced by occupational therapists working often, but not exclusively, in developing countries, without support in challenging and complex situations where socio-political influences and economic constraints are prevalent. Furthermore, the medium provides a forum for emotional support for those exposed to, or withdrawing from, particularly traumatic situations. Occupational therapists can communicate on-line through an internet site linked to the website of the World Federation of Occupational Therapists (www.wfot.org).

CONCLUSION

This chapter has made reference to the speed and nature of change in healthcare systems across the world and to the need for therapists to evaluate the constant flow of emerging new ideas and policies so that they can make informed decisions about progress in practice. Equally, comment has been made about the responsibility of health professionals, not just to engage with change, but also to actively engage with critical thinking and research to inform service delivery and assist the profession and its members to achieve change that leads to growth. This may mean abandoning outdated practices and integrating new modes of working into their practice. The particular needs of occupational therapists working in isolated communities have been addressed and various kinds of support mechanisms have been discussed. The pace of change and the increasingly challenging situations faced by both new and experienced occupational therapists would suggest that all occupational therapists should be seeking and using support from a mentor, critical friend or on-line network. Partnerships for professional development and for the promotion of potential should be seen as an asset and actively sought by everyone.

REFERENCES

Alsop, A. (2000). *Continuing professional development: a guide for therapist.* Oxford: Blackwell Science.

Barnett, R. (1994). *The limits of competence.* Buckingham: Society for Research into Higher Education and Open University Press.

Barnett, R. (1997). *Higher education: a critical business.* Buckingham: Society for Research into Higher Education and Open University Press.

Barnett, R. (2000). *Realizing the university in an age of supercomplexity.* Buckingham: Society for Research into Higher Education and Open University Press.

Brown, G., Esdaile, S. & Ryan, S. (Eds.) (2003). *Becoming an advanced healthcare practitioner.* Oxford: Butterworth Heinemann.

Brownhill, B. (2001). Lifelong learning. In P. Jarvis (Ed.), *The age of learning: education and the knowledge society.* London: Kogan Page, pp. 69–79.

Butler, J. (2004). The Casson Memorial Lecture 2004: The fascination of the difficult. *British Journal of Occupational Therapy, 67*(7), 286–292.

College of Occupational therapists (2002). Position statement on life long learning. *British Journal of Occupational Therapy, 65*(5), 198–200.

College of Occupational Therapists (2004). Strategic vision and action plan for lifelong learning. *British Journal of Occupational Therapy, 67*(1), 20–28.

Creek, J. (2003). *Occupational therapy defined as a complex intervention.* London: College of Occupational Therapists.

Crossley, M. (2000). Bridging cultures and traditions in the reconceptualisation of comparative and international education. *Comparative Education, 36*(3), 319–332.

Dahlgren, M.A., Richardson, B. & Kalman, H. (2004). Redifining the reflective practitioner. In J. Higgs, B. Richardson & M.A. Dahlgren (Eds.), *Developing practice knowledge for health professionals.* Oxford: Butterworth-Heinemann, pp. 15–34.

Eraut, M. (1994). *Developing professional knowledge and competence.* London: The Falmer Press.

Eraut, M. (2005). Continuity of learning. Editorial. *Learning in Health and Social Care, 4*(1), 1–6.

Esdaile, S.A. & Roth, L.M. (2003). Creating scholarly practice: integrating and applying scholarship to practice. In G. Brown, S.A. Esdaile & S.E. Ryan (Eds.), *Becoming an advanced healthcare practitioner.* Oxford: Butterworth-Heinemann, pp. 161–188.

Garbett, R. (2004). The role of practioners in developing professional knowledge and practice. In J. Higgs, B. Richardson & M.A. Dahlgren (Eds.), *Developing practice knowledge for health professionals.* Oxford: Butterworth-Heinemann, pp. 165–180.

Goodfellow, J., McAllister, L., Best, D., Webb, G. & Fredericks, D. (2001). Students and educators learning within relationships. In J. Higgs & A. Titchen (Eds.), *Professional practice in health, education and the creative arts.* Oxford: Blackwell Science, pp. 161–174.

Griffin, C. (2001). From education policy to lifelong learning strategies. In P. Jarvis (Ed.), *The age of learning: education and the knowledge society.* London: Kogan Page, pp. 41–54.

Higgs, J. (2003). Do you reason like a health professional? In G. Brown, S.A. Esdaile & S.E. Ryan (Eds.), *Becoming an advanced healthcare practitioner.* Oxford: Butterworth-Heinemann, pp. 145–160.

Higgs, J., Andresen, L. & Fish, D. (2004a). Practice knowledge – its nature, sources and contexts. In J. Higgs, B. Richardson & M.A. Dahlgren (Eds.), *Developing practice knowledge for health professionals.* Oxford: Butterworth-Heinemann, pp. 51–69.

Higgs, J., Fish, D. & Rothwell, R. (2004b). Practice knowledge – critical appreciation. In J. Higgs, B. Richardson & M.A. Dahlgren (Eds.), *Developing practice knowledge for health professionals.* Oxford: Butterworth-Heinemann, pp. 89–106.

Iwama, M. (2003). Toward culturally relevant epistemologies in occupational therapy. *American Journal of Occupational Therapy, 57*(5), 582–588.

Iwama, M.K. (2005). The Kawa (river) model: nature, life flow and the power of culturally relevant occupational therapy. In F. Kronenberg, S. Simo Algado & N. Pollard (Eds.), *Occupational therapy without borders, learning from the spirit of survivors.* Edinburgh: Elsevier Churchill Livingstone, pp. 213–227.

Jarvis, P. (2001). Questioning the learning society In P. Jarvis (Ed.), *The age of learning: education and the knowledge society.* London: Kogan Page, pp. 195–204.

Joubert, R.W.E. (2003). Are we coming of age or being born again? How does this impact on the education and assessment of competence of occupational therapy students in South Africa? *South African Journal of Occupational Therapy, 33*(3), 2–4.

Longworth, N. & Davies, W.K. (1996). *Lifelong learning.* London: Kogan Page.

Lorenzo, T. & Cloete, L. (2004). Promoting occupations in rural communities. In R. Watson & L. Swartz (Eds.), *Transformation through occupation.* London: Whurr, pp. 268–286.

Madill, H. & Hollis, V. (2003). Developing competencies for advanced practice: how do I get there from here? In G. Brown, S.A. Esdaile & S.E. Ryan (Eds.), *Becoming an advanced healthcare practitioner.* Oxford: Butterworth-Heinemann, pp. 30–63.

McAllister, L. (2003). Using adult education theories: facilitating others' learning in professional practice settings. In G. Brown, S.A. Esdaile & S.E. Ryan (Eds.), *Becoming an advanced healthcare practitioner.* Oxford: Butterworth-Heinemann, pp. 216–238.

Newton, E. & Fuller, B. (2005). The Occupational Therapy International Outreach Network supporting occupational therapists working without borders. In F. Kronenberg, S. Simo Algado & N. Pollard (Eds.), *Occupational therapy without borders, learning from the spirit of survivors.* Edinburgh: Elsevier Churchill Livingstone, pp. 361–373.

Richardson, B., Dahlgren, M.A. & Higgs, J. (2004). Practice epistemology: implications for education, practice and research. In J. Higgs, B. Richardson & M.A. Dahlgren (Eds.), *Developing practice knowledge for health professionals.* Oxford: Butterworth-Heinemann, pp. 201–220.

Roth, L.M. & Esdaile S.A. (2003). Role models and mentors: informal and formal ways to learn from exemplary practice. In G. Brown, S.A. Esdaile & S.E. Ryan (Eds.), *Becoming an advanced healthcare practitioner.* Oxford: Butterworth-Heinemann, pp. 239–259.

Ryan, S., Esdaile, S.A. & Brown, G. (2003). Appreciating the big picture: you are part of it. In G. Brown, S.A. Esdaile & S.E. Ryan (Eds.), *Becoming an advanced healthcare practitioner.* Oxford: Butterworth-Heinemann, pp. 1–29.

Swartz, L. (2004). Rethinking professional ethics. In R. Watson & L. Swartz (Eds.), *Transformation through occupation.* London: Whurr, pp. 289–300.

Taylor, I. (1997). *Developing learning in professional education.* Buckingham: The Society for Research into Higher education and Open University Press.

Titchen, A. & McGinley, M. (2004). Blending self knowledge and professional knowledge in person-centred care. In J. Higgs, B. Richardson & M.A. Dahlgren (Eds.), *Developing practice knowledge for health professionals.* Oxford: Butterworth-Heinemann, pp. 107–126.

Walker, M. (2003). The Casson Memorial Lecture 2003: Past conditional, present indicative, future indefinite. *British Journal of Occupational Therapy, 66*(8), 338–344.

Watson, R. (2004). A population approach to transformation. In R. Watson & L. Swartz (Eds.), *Transformation through occupation*. London: Whurr, pp. 51–66.

Watson, R. & Fourie, M. (2004). International and African influences on occupational therapy. In R. Watson & L. Swartz (Eds.), *Transformation through occupation*. London: Whurr, pp. 33–50.

Watson, R. & Swartz, L. (Eds.) (2004). *Transformation through occupation*. London: Whurr.

18 Looking Ahead: Future Directions in Practice Education and Research

**AULDEEN ALSOP, MADELEINE DUNCAN,
THERESA LORENZO and HELEN BUCHANAN**

OBJECTIVES

This chapter discusses:

- some of the significant drivers that are likely to influence practice learning in the future
- possible curriculum reforms
- the relationship between research and service and practice learning.

INTRODUCTION

Earlier in this book we discussed the calls made by UNESCO for the education of health professionals to be locally tailored in ways that meet prevailing health and social concerns with due consideration of both indigenous and global knowledge developments (UNESCO, 1998). Pressed by these and other deeply systemic and complex local and global demands, such as the rapid pace of technological change and a constantly evolving knowledge economy, universities will have to engage with the demands of society by introducing new modes of curriculum organization (Cloete et al., 2002; Kraak, 2000). Changes may include shifting from

> courses to credits; departments to programmes; subject-based teaching to student-based learning; knowledge to competence; subject based learning to problem-based learning and disciplinary knowledge production to transdisciplinary knowledge production.
>
> (Symes, 2003, p. 4)

Practice and Service Learning in Occupational Therapy. Edited by Theresa Lorenzo, Madeleine Duncan,
Helen Buchanan, Auldeen Alsop
© 2006 John Wiley & Sons Ltd

Universities are undergoing major change anyway because of what Griffin (1997, p. 3) earlier called a 'crisis' related to the legitimacy of higher education that had hitherto been concerned with knowledge but which was becoming increasingly influenced by a consumer society. Instead of continuing to pursue their own agenda, universities were being required to engage with a state agenda and to recognize and adapt to globalization (Barnett, 2003). Many were also being expected to (re)assess their commitment to community development and, in the African context, to ensure the inclusion of African culture in education for sustainable development (Favish, 2003; Mugo, 1999; Ntuli, 1999).

In this respect, universities have to review their position in relation to learning, teaching and research. Historically, universities have had a dual mission related, on the one hand, to knowledge production (research) and, on the other, to teaching (Barnett, 2000). These competing missions must somehow work together, but in redefining their role, Barnett also proposed that universities must increase their 'revolutionary' research output and promote 'increased public understanding for global citizenship' (Barnett, 2000, p. 146). In these times of unpredictability, particularly in the field of health and social care, universities have to work with complexity and uncertainty and must ensure that graduates emerge as critical thinkers able to deal with uncertainty and complexity in a fast changing world (Barnett, 1997; Barnett, 2002; Odora Hoppers, Moja & Mda, 1999). As part of this agenda, those responsible for the education of health professionals could respond in a number of ways such as: adapting curricula to reflect new ways of working in health and social contexts; ensuring that students develop critical thinking skills within and beyond their discipline through multi- and transdiciplinary knowledge generation; being more responsive to student demography; shifting institutional missions to reflect social values and social development agendas; and introducing strategic research directions.

REORIENTATING THE CURRICULUM

Curriculum planning and teaching will continue to be in perpetual flux as faculties and programme coordinators balance the demands of knowledge transfer and the need for practice to be locally relevant yet informed by global developments (Barnett, 2000). Increasingly, curriculum construction will be based on the realization that disciplinary, interdisciplinary and transdisciplinary programmes can co-exist provided that 'each enables wide access to learners, articulates with other kinds and pathways of learning, and facilitates the development of applied competence' (Symes, 2003, p. 10).

MOVING BEYOND DISCIPLINARITY

The days of 'going it alone' are over. One of the critical shifts for all stakeholders in practice education is the development of authentic partnerships, where there is a determined effort to share decision making and responsibility with community members, non-governmental organizations and disabled peoples' organizations. These partnerships would also involve new ways of considering supervision, especially in senior years of study, where supervision may, for example, be done by another health professional or community development worker. The integration of occupational therapy theory and methods would be consolidated through other means, such as tutorials and problem-based learning. Practice education may also shift to include students working with people with different impairments in one placement, rather than having distinct physical, psychiatric and community experiences, as has been the tradition to date. A student may, during one day, see a person with mobility impairment, consult a mother with a child who has learning difficulties and in the afternoon run a group for people with mental illness. The artificial distinction between 'physical'; 'psychiatric' and 'social' or 'community' domains of practice will become blurred as graduates achieve generalist competence in line with the primary healthcare approach and social development goals.

INTERDISCIPLINARITY

Opportunities for new directions in interdisciplinary practice and practice education abound. Interdisciplinarity is concerned with solving complex problems through a parallel analysis (i.e. different disciplines offer their various perspectives) and ultimate synthesis of ideas and solutions (i.e. a unified outcome occurs based on the transfer of knowledge between disciplines) (Macgregor, 2004). In revising the document on community-based rehabilitation (CBR) guidelines, the World Health Organization (WHO, 2004) has identified five strategic components, namely: health, education, livelihood, empowerment, and social inclusion and justice for critical attention in CBR initiatives. These five components suggest that the occupational therapy curriculum may need to consider opportunities for shared learning across disciplines, for example environmental and human geography; politics; anthropology; commerce and law to name a few. New areas of practice may also include bringing an occupational focus to disaster and risk management, as well as social movements that campaign on behalf of different vulnerable groups so that disability and social inclusion issues are mainstreamed (Kronenberg, Simo-Algado & Pollard, 2005).

Another example is the International Classification of Functioning and Health (ICF) (World Health Organization, 2001). The ICF frames, ideologically, the range of comprehensive practice learning pathways that trainee health professionals may be exposed to, including working with impairments, resolving or accommodating activity limitations and addressing the participation restrictions of disabled people. Whilst the ICF provides a unifying frame of reference for a range of disciplines and professions, it also highlights the imminent blurring of professional boundaries and the potential limitations of a narrow, individualistic definition of health. This blurring of disciplinary boundaries has implications for the type of practice learning opportunities that are included in health professional curricula. Practice education is likely to remain within the medical model with a focus on the capacities and needs of individuals unless alternative practice learning approaches that address population health and social development concerns are investigated.

TRANSDISCIPLINARITY

Transdiciplinarity recognizes simultaneous modes of thinking and reasoning using quantum logic in the quest for new knowledge to solve universal problems, such as dwindling natural resources, poverty and violence. It is in essence a new way of seeing the world by attending to both the rational and the relational, the seen and unseen, as well as existential-spiritual dimensions of living in the world (MacGregor, 2004). Transdisciplinarity transcends linear and binary thinking as a means of knowledge generation by transversing (i.e. criss-crossing, zigzagging, moving in and beyond) many disciplines. It involves scientific and non-scientific sources of knowledge and advances new forms of problem solving through cooperation between all sectors of society, including academia (Nicolescu, 1997, 2001).

Transdisciplinarity argues that knowledge, guided by reason, linear logic and science, is only one way or avenue for solving global problems. The other is the way of understanding; the way of intuition, imagination, spirituality and discovering shared truth. Knowing and understanding belong to different realities. By including different realities (for example, indigenous ways of knowing in cultural communities) in the construction of curricula and practice learning opportunities, universities will advance the discovery of new knowledge appropriate for the solution of local and ultimately, global challenges.

Global problems will not be resolved by creating more disciplines or super-specializing within monodisciplines (Max-Neef, 2005; Nicolescu, 2001) or by reinforcing the boundaries that currently exist between various professions. Academia will no longer be the sole prerogative of intellectuals. The academy will move beyond the hallowed halls of universities and the intellectual world of disciplinary knowledge by becoming inclusive of the knowledge of people from all walks of life. This is good news for health professionals committed to health promotion, the prevention of ill-health, the equalization of opportunities for disabled people and the full social inclusion of at-risk and other marginalized people. Health professionals will become co-workers and fellow citizens in the creation of a new, inclusive society.

Transdisciplinary higher education programmes will aim to develop new knowledge that addresses complex, global problems, such as poverty, exploitation of natural resources and social oppression (Gibbons, 1998; McGregor, 2004). Such programmes do not yet exist in universities but the impetus of the global knowledge economy indicates that the time is coming when they will be urgently required because existing solutions to global problems are apparently ineffective. What does this mean on the ground for the future of occupational therapy practice education?

REORIENTATING PRACTICE EDUCATION

In the South African context, Muller and Subotzky (2001) suggest that service learning is a way of giving substance to the notion of the 'engaged university'. They propose that innovative curricula can provide opportunities 'for the academy to break its myopic preoccupation with academic forms of knowledge' and that 'public intellectuals' should place strong emphasis on the social utility of research informed by particularist (*disciplinary*) epistemologies in which truth should not be separated from personal experience' (Muller & Subotzky, 2001, p. 10, italics added). This recommendation also applies to professional practice education. Practice and service learning will increasingly be based on an expanded notion of socially relevant scholarship that rewards not only conventional discipline-based enquiry and action, but also recognizes the validity of experiential, indigenous, tacit and pre-theoretical knowledge. Students and practitioners will have to learn to bridge the gap between the 'meaning of research findings and the meaning(s) constructed by those affected by the results, and between academic and "political" truth' (Muller and Subotzky, 2001, p. 10).

This implied call for social responsiveness has implications for the way in which professional curricula, and practice learning in particular, will be conceptualized, interpreted and implemented in the future. For example, Higgs, Fish and Rothwell (2004) point out that already in the United Kingdom, the Disability Discrimination Act 1995 has influenced thinking regarding the limits and discipline-specificity of competence in professional practice. Creative practice learning pathways are being introduced to prepare professionals with the prerequisite competence, but this is impacting on the way established professional boundaries are being viewed. Professionals are no longer the sole holders of discrete knowledge and expertise.

Horsburgh, Lamdin and Williamson (2001, p. 877) suggest that the increasing overlap of knowledge and skills between health professionals requires 'an educational process through which students are provided with structured learning opportunities for shared learning', a process that is well under way in universities in the UK (Miller, Freeman & Ross, 2001). The educational rationale here is the identification of areas of professional overlap in order to create shared learning opportunities in domains of common interest to the participating professions. Cooperation between professions is seen to contribute to rationalizing educational resources, lessening duplication of training and ultimately, through improved teamwork, to providing a more effective, efficient and integrated service for both users and providers (Leathard, 1994).

If interprofessional learning only exists within the academic environment, however, the students' understanding of teamwork will be limited until it is experienced 'for real' in practice. Jones (2005) suggests that members of teams in today's healthcare environment must be able to understand and respect each other's philosophical views so that they can complement other members' contribution to the team effort. So how can this happen? Interprofessional teams of students who are provided with learning experiences together in practice could provide a way forward. The 'team' in this scenario would include students from a variety of disciplines concerned with universal problems in a local context and not primarily those professions traditionally associated with healthcare. Various initiatives have been tried internationally, such as multi-professional 'training wards' in Sweden and 'team placements' in Canada (personal communication, 2005). Multi-professional teams in a primary healthcare-led society may include legal experts; disability activists; indigenous healers; human geographers; and social developers, as well as occupational therapists and other health professionals.

Multiprofessional education that extends into practice education would extend the core curriculum of each participating discipline and may create further tensions around the maintenance of professional boundaries and ways of working. Each scheme will almost certainly have its strengths, limitations and related challenges, not least in relation to the difficulties experienced in setting it up. Nevertheless, future curricula for the education of health professionals will almost certainly cross the boundaries between professions in order to address complex social problems in new ways.

OPPORTUNITIES AND CONSTRAINTS

Sinclair (2005, p. 123) advocates that professional education needs to undergo 'sweeping change' to embrace enablement, advocacy and social reform. However, statutory regulations for professional registration may curtail the extent to which radically new conceptions of professional education and inter-professional learning may occur. According to Symes (2003, p. 4) 'a general undergraduate education and generic skills within the context of specific disciplinary and/or professional discourse are essential to provide the intellectual tools necessary to span increasingly diverse intellectual fields'. The health professional graduates of the future and particularly those working in highly unstructured, developing contexts require competence in the application of different modes of knowledge. For a significant number of years the education of health professionals has been entrusted to Institutions of Higher Education who devise and approve curricula in association, where appropriate, with relevant professional and statutory bodies. As far as occupational therapy is concerned, there is an internationally recognized curriculum framework that provides minimum standards that can be adapted for cultural and local relevance (Hocking & Ness, 2002). New interpretations of these standards have been possible, allowing for practice-based programmes to emerge in the UK (Alsop & Cooper, 2005) that socialize and educate students from a base in practice rather than from within the university.

Designing service learning to be undertaken with professionals from different disciplines would open up questions around the added value of collaboration between professionals from different disciplines compared with the impact currently of collaborative ventures between students of the same discipline area. The development of shared core curricula for professions goes against the grain of traditional thinking, ways of mono-disciplinary work and established professional accreditation norms and principles. Difficult as it may seem, this approach to curriculum design will increasingly become a major driver in higher education as universities seek to be socially responsive (Favish, 2003). Entirely new conceptions of what it means to be a professional, working in very different sets of arrangements and pressures for new forms of knowledge generation and learning, will be required if systemic social and environmental problems are to be addressed to achieve sustainable human development (Weil, 1999). Since universities are committed to educating professionals who are versatile in their selection and application of knowledge, attention will progressively turn to multi-professional curriculum design. The integration of transdisciplinary epistemology through the co-construction of curriculum content will enable diverse professions to move towards new ways of solving shared concerns (Finch, 2000). Generic, cross-field curriculum content will aim to shape, not only who future health service providers become, but also the way in which they collaborate as agents of change in the communities they serve.

Whilst deconstruction of mono-disciplinary knowledge is a prerequisite for the development of a generic curriculum for multi-professional learning, its impact on intra-professional curriculum development is likely to be profound. As generic content is 'pooled' into core, shared curricula so the unique, defining epistemology and philosophy of each profession will need to be strengthened. Higgs et al. (2004) suggest that knowledge is created from ideas of practice. Practice learning, reflection on practice and documentation of practice outcomes are considered central to the development and maturation of professions. In other words, intra-professional epistemology is most likely to be strengthened through inter- and multi-disciplinary modes of curriculum and research.

THE RESEARCH AGENDA

As with any new educational venture, questions can, and should, be raised about the impact, cost and benefits to the stakeholders, the added value to the curriculum, the practical and emotional implications for participants and the long-term benefits compared with short-term gains for the community and the students. Extending the service learning responsibility beyond practice into the domain of research has to be crucial in order to justify the effect and clarify the future direction of service learning. The growing partnership between higher education institutions and civic society in the area of research and innovation, raises the challenge for university practice educators to explore ways of developing a joint research agenda related to practice learning, where students then develop professional practice skills as well as research skills.

BUILDING RESEARCH AGENDA

Although research into service learning is still at an early stage (Schensul, Berg & Brase, 2001), it can provide opportunities to investigate socio-political action that seeks to improve conditions in local communities (Lagana & Rubin, 2001). These authors proposed a service learning research model that could be integrated into the service learning agenda to facilitate research on any population involved in practice (students, university staff, university, community organization, the clients), although they warned of possible challenges with issues of recruitment and retention of participants. Shumer (2001) not only claimed that service learning and evaluation were inseparable processes, but also suggested that a service learning curriculum tended to follow good qualitative research practice. He noted the apparent relationship between service learning and learning from observation and experience, as in naturalistic enquiry. He further claimed that ethnographic research was firmly in line with the practices of service learning as 'students function like ethnographers, engaging in a process of understanding the places and the people they serve' (Shumer, 2001, p. 186). Reflection was key to students gaining an understanding of their role in service learning. There should be no problem therefore, in determining a methodologically sound approach to research into (and during) service learning although there may be some challenges to overcome with regards to ethics and levels of participation.

As occupational therapy has taken such an important step in engaging with the service learning agenda to the extent that it is now an integral feature of curricula in parts of South Africa, research into its various structures, processes and outcomes would seem an inevitable next step. Any learning from research should, in turn, feed back into the university curriculum. Research should also help inform universities about the wider issues of how quality assurance processes might address service learning, and which features should be reviewed.

Research drives the discovery of new forms of practice and validates exist-ing ways of working. By securing research funding to investigate strategic pro-fessional niche areas within national health and development research priorities, education institutions will ensure a close fit between evolving forms of practice and practice education. Occupational therapy theory can be applied, developed and validated simultaneously. In order to do this, the fol-lowing needs to occur:

- Identification of lead research themes, for example the occupational development of disabled women and children; evidence-based prac-tice; occupation, poverty and disability; economic empowerment and entrepreneurship; indigenous occupational knowledge systems.
- Linking a lead researcher to each lead research theme.
- Building strategic research partnerships across disciplines and local, national and international boundaries.
- Nesting doctoral, masters and undergraduate research projects within a larger research study so as to build systematic, incremental information towards answering lead research questions.
- Building research capacity amongst practitioners and students.
- Equipping practitioners and students with skills in writing for publication.
- Translating research findings into practice through appropriate research methodology, for example, action research or grounded theory.

CONCLUSION

This chapter suggests that practice education in the future will become a new intellectual space that unites and transcends the knowledge that exists in the spaces between different interpretations of reality (Nicolescu, 2001). For occu-pational therapy, the service learning journey has only just begun. The con-tributions in this book have shown how fieldwork has evolved to practice learning. Practice education curricula have been extended to include service learning to reflect the civic responsibility of higher education and to demon-strate the redefinition of occupational therapy as it is now practised. This evo-lutionary process in service learning is one further step for the occupational therapy profession, but of course it will not stop there.

We suggest that the time is right for weak transdisciplinarity (that is, aimed at local problems and achievable goals as opposed to strong transdiciplinarity that focuses on global problems) to guide the construction of professional practice learning curricula (Macgregor, 2004). The voices and knowledge of all stakeholders are needed in the building of a new society. Health professional students, exposed to progressive curricula that encourage the exploration of different levels of reality including learning from and with 'the other' (be they clients, other professionals, community members, representatives of various disciplines, indigenous healers, etc), are likely to contribute substantially to the knowledge economy required for solving the health and development challenges of a developing society and beyond.

REFERENCES

Alsop, A. & Cooper, A. (2005). *Partnership and participation in the workplace: developing the occupational potential of assistants.* Paper presented College of Occupational Therapists 29th Annual Congress, Eastbourne, June.

Barnett, R. (1997). *Higher Education: a critical business.* Buckingham: The Society for Research into Higher Education and Open University Press.

Barnett, R. (2000). *Realising the university in an age of supercomplexity.* Buckingham: The Society for Research into Higher Education and Open University Press.

Barnett, R. (2003). *Beyond all reason: living with ideology in the university.* Buckingham: The Society for Research into Higher Education and Open University Press.

Cloete, N., Fehnel, D., Gibbons, P., Maassen, P., Moja, T. & Perold, H. (Eds.) (2002). *Transformation in higher education: global pressures and local realities in South Africa.* Cape Town: Juta.

Favish, J. (2003). A new contract between higher education and society. *South African Journal of Higher Education, 17*(1), 24–30.

Finch, J. (2000). Interprofessional education and teamworking: a view from the education providers. *British Medical Journal, 321,* 1138–1140.

Gibbons, M. (1998). *Higher education relevance in the 21st century.* Washington: World Bank.

Griffin, A. (1997). Knowledge under attack: consumption, diversity and the need for values. In R. Barnett & A. Griffin (Eds.), *The end of knowledge in higher education.* London: Institute of Education, pp. 2–11.

Higgs, J., Fish, D., & Rothwell, R. (2004). Practice knowledge – critical appreciation. In J. Higgs, B. Richardson & M.A. Dahlgren (Eds.), *Developing practice knowledge for health professionals.* Oxford: Butterworth Heinemann, pp. 89–106.

Hocking, C. & Ness, N.E. (2002). *Revised minimum standards for the education of occupational therapists.* Perth, Western Australia: World Federation of Occupational Therapists.

Horsburgh, M., Lamdin, R. & Williamson, E. (2001). Multi-professional learning: the attitudes of medical, nursing and pharmacy students to shared learning. *Medical Education, 35,* 876–883.

Jones, M. (2005). Cultural power in organisations: the dynamics of interprofessional teams. In G. Whiteford & V. Wright-St Clair (Eds.), *Occupation and practice in context.* Sydney: Elsevier Churchill Livingstone, pp. 179–196.

Kraak, A. (Ed.) (2000). *Changing modes: new knowledge production and its implications for higher education in South Africa.* Pretoria: Human Sciences Research Council.

Kronenberg, F., Simo-Algado, S. & Pollard, N. (Eds.) (2005). *Occupational therapy without borders: learning from the spirit of survivors.* Edinburgh: Elsevier Churchill Livingstone.

Leathard, A. (Ed.) (1994). *Going interprofessional – working together for health and welfare.* London: Routledge.

Lagana, L. & Rubin, M.S. (2001). Methodological challenges and potential solutions for the incorporation of sound community-based research into service-learning. In A. Furco & S.H. Billig (Eds.), *Service learning: the essence of the pedagogy.* Greenwich, CT: Information Age Publishing, pp. 161–182.

Max-Neef, M., & Nicolescu, B. (2005). *Transdisciplinarity workshop.* Sustainability Institute, University of Stellenbosch, South Africa. 12–15 April 2005. Personal communication.

McGregor, S.L.T. (2004). *The nature of transdisciplinary research and practice.* Retrieved 5 May, 2005, from http://www.kon.org/hswp/archive/transdiscipl.html

Miller, C., Freeman, M. & Ross, N. (2001). *Interprofessional practice in health and social care: challenging the shared learning agenda.* London: Arnold.

Mugo, M.G. (1999). African culture in education for sustainable development. In M.W. Makgoba (Ed.), *African Renaissance.* Cape Town: Mafube Publishing, pp. 210–232.

Muller, J. & Subotzky, G. (2001). What knowledge is needed in the new millennium? *Organisation, 8*(2), 163–182.

Nicolescu, B. (1997). *The transdisciplinary evolution of the university condition for sustainable development.* Retrieved 5 May, 2005, from http://perso.club-internet.fr/nicol/ciret/bulletin/b12/b12c8.htm

Nicolescu, B. (2001). *Manifesto of transdisciplinarity.* Albany,NY: State University of New York Press.

Ntuli, P.P. (1999). The missing link between culture and education: are we still chasing gods that are not our own? In M.W. Makgoba (Ed.), *African Renaissance.* Cape Town: Mafube Publishing, pp. 184–199.

Odora Hoppers, C.A., Moja, T. & Mda, T. (1999). Making this our last passive moment: the way forward. In M.W. Makgoba (Ed.), *African Renaissance.* Cape Town: Mafube Publishing, pp. 233–239.

Schensul, J.J., Berg, M. & Brase, M. (2001). Theories guiding outcomes for action research for service learning. In A. Furco & S.H. Billig (Eds.), *Service learning: the essence of the pedagogy.* Greenwich, CT: Information Age Publishing, pp. 125–143.

Shumer, R. (2001). Service-learning as qualitative research: creating curriculum from inquiry. In A. Furco & S.H. Billig (Eds.), *Service learning: the essence of the pedagogy.* Greenwich, CT: Information Age Publishing, pp. 183–197.

Sinclair, K. (2005). World connected: the international context of professional practice. In G. Whiteford & V. Wright-St Clair (Eds.), *Occupation and practice in context.* Sydney: Elsevier Churchill Livingstone, pp. 104–126.

Symes, A. (2003). *University of Cape Town Curriculum Project discussion document: framework for conceptual development and faculty engagement.* Curriculum Project Steering Group. Cape Town: University of Cape Town.

UNESCO (1998). *World declaration on higher education for the twenty-first century: vision and action.* Retrieved 22 August, 2005, from http://www.unesco.org/eduprog/wche/declaration_eng.htm

Weil, S. (1999). Re-creating universities for 'Beyond the Stable State': from 'Dearingesque' systematic control to post-Dearing systemic learning and inquiry. *Systems Research and Behavioural Science*, *16*(2). Available at http://www.nene.ac.uk/solar/dearing.html

World Health Organization (2001). *International Classification of Functioning, Disability and Health: ICF Short version*. Geneva: World Health Organization. Available at http://www.who.int/icidh

World Health Organization (2004) *Meeting report on the development of Guidelines for Strengthening Community-based Rehabilitation Programmes*. Geneva: World Health Organization.

Glossary

The following terms are used in this book.

Clinical practice: learning to treat body function and body structure impairments and associated activity limitations and participation restrictions so as to equalize opportunities for at risk and disabled people.

Community: a body of people with common aspirations in the same locality. In the broadest sense, a community may reside in a geographical area, a district or even a street in a local town. In a narrower sense, a community may exist in an organization or institution, for example a residential facility such as an old age or children's home, a psychiatric unit, or even a prison cell.

Community-based education: a means of achieving educational relevance to community needs (Magzoub, Ahmed & Salih, 1992).

Competence: possession of the necessary skills, knowledge, attitudes, understanding and experience required to perform in professional and occupational roles to a satisfactory standard within the workplace (Day, 1995)

Fieldwork (international definition): is the time students spend: interpreting specific person-occupation-environment relationships and their relationship to health and well-being; establishing and evaluating therapeutic and professional relationships; implementing an occupational therapy process (or some aspect of it); demonstrating professional reasoning and behaviours; and generating or using knowledge of the contexts of professional practice with and for real live people (Hocking & Ness, 2002, p. 31).

Fieldwork (local description): a time-limited, project-based form of experiential learning in the field, for example, factory visits to learn about ergonomics and occupational health; a fieldtrip to different communities to learn about health promotion and poverty alleviation projects; or a period of data collection and implementation of a research project.

Learning site: a place of learning that complies with the minimum standards for the practice development and education of professionals according to professional regulations, through collaboration with individuals, groups and communities.

Practice and Service Learning in Occupational Therapy. Edited by Theresa Lorenzo, Madeleine Duncan, Helen Buchanan, Auldeen Alsop
© 2006 John Wiley & Sons Ltd

Learning facilitator: a person who is responsible for monitoring and assessing the quality of work being done by students and for dealing with practical, emergent issues pertaining to student needs on site. They are also responsible for guiding and enabling the student's learning through role modelling and sharing of knowledge, skills and attitudes in a particular field of expertise.

Population: a proxy descriptor for the epidemiological distribution of people with particular characteristics in a particular geographical region (for example, a health district).

Practice: application and integration of professional attitudes, skills and knowledge in working with individuals, groups and communities.

Practice education: the curriculum (that is the pedagogical outcomes, principles and methods), which guides the application and integration of professional attitudes, skills and knowledge in working with individuals, groups and communities across different sectors such as education, health, agriculture, industry, justice, non-governmental, social services and private sector.

Practice learning: the process of acquiring professional competence by defining the aspirations and addressing the needs of individuals, groups or communities using professional actions with the guidance of a university practice educator and/or site learning facilitator.

Practice learning administrator: administrative assistant who deals with administration of practice learning curriculum such as marks processing, dissemination of information and record keeping.

Practice learning coordinator: an academic staff member responsible for designing, monitoring and ensuring the quality of the undergraduate practice education curriculum, for example documenting learning outcomes and coordinating a professional development programme for site learning facilitators and university practice educators.

Service: to carry out duty; provision of some public need; work done to benefit or be of assistance to someone or to a community; emanating from a moral orientation aimed at equalization of power and opportunities. This orientation is captured in the following quote: 'If you come here to help me then you are wasting my time, but if you come here because your liberation is tied up with mine then let us begin' (Lucy Walker, Australian Aboriginal Activist, source unknown).

Service learning: a strategy through which students engage with a community so they learn and develop together through organized service that meets mutually identified needs. Service learning helps foster civic responsibility through coordinated activity with a higher education institution and a community. It is an integral part of the academic curriculum (which may be credit-bearing) and includes structured time for role-players (students, community, higher education institution and others) to reflect on the service experience and modify actions if indicated (adapted from American Association for Higher Education, 1999; Bringle & Hatcher, 1996).

Site learning facilitator: the site learning facilitator is ultimately responsible for the welfare of the persons with whom the student works, who ensures a functional on-site infrastructure and who monitors ethical, efficient and effective service provision. The site learning facilitator may also liaise with, and mediate between, the student and community as well as guide development of appropriate cultural behaviour through role modelling and coaching. A site learning facilitator may be any one of the following:

- **clinician/health therapist/practitioner:** a registered, qualified occupational therapist or a health trained professional, e.g. nurse, social worker, physiotherapist, psychologist, medical doctor
- **specialized auxilliary services officer (SASO):** a professionally trained assistant or technician
- **health worker:** a person who is trained in health-related service provision, e.g. community rehabilitation worker, home-based carer or health promotion officer
- **complementary health practitioner:** a person who holds indigenous knowledge and complementary health practice expertise and who is registered with a Health Professional Council, e.g. indigenous healers.

Site manager: a person in charge of and/or accountable for the efficiency, effectiveness and quality of services provided at an organization, department, facility, project, programme or learning site. The manager may also be the site learning facilitator if they are in a single-handed position.

Student: an undergraduate (or graduate) adult learner working towards a professional qualification.

Supervision: a continuing dynamic interaction between a senior member of a profession and a junior member or student of the same profession. It is a supportive activity; the purpose of which is to enhance the professional development and functioning of the junior member. Both parties should assume responsibility for the way in which they seek, receive and respond to feedback and for acquiring skills in doing so (Sweeney, Webley & Treacher, 2001).

Tutorial group: a group of approximately five to eight students from various practice learning sites concerned with peer learning about specific or similar domains of professional practice, for example paediatrics, mental health, economic empowerment. Students often refer to these as 'tuts'.

University practice educator: a health practitioner and academic representative employed by the education institution to provide regular on-site academic guidance, support to, and assessment of, a student in collaboration with a site learning facilitator. The practice educator is responsible for monitoring the student's professional development and maintaining academic standards. They may also facilitate tutorial groups for students with the aim of promoting integration of theory with practice.

REFERENCES

American Association for Higher Education (1999). *Writing the community: concepts and models for service learning. Service learning in the disciplines.* American Association for Higher Education Series. Retrieved 10 October, 2005, from http://www.aahe.org

Bringle, R. & Hatcher, J. (1996). Implementing service learning in higher education. *The Journal of Higher Education, 67,* 12–25.

Day, M. (1995). Putting vocational training into practice. *Nursing Standard, 9*(52), 30–32.

Hocking, C. & Ness, N.E. (2002). *Revised minimum standards for the education of occupational therapists.* Perth, Western Australia: World Federation of Occupational Therapists.

Magzoub, M.E., Ahmed, B.O. & Salih, S.T. (1992). Eleven steps of community-based education as applied at Gezira Medical School. *Anals of Community-oriented Education, 5,* 11–17.

Sweeney, G., Webley, P. & Treacher, A. (2001). Supervision in occupational therapy, Part 1: the supervisor's anxieties. *British Journal of Occupational Therapy, 64,* 337–345.

Index

Practice and Service Learning in Occupational Therapy. Edited by Theresa Lorenzo, Madeleine Duncan,
Helen Buchanan, Auldeen Alsop
© 2006 John Wiley & Sons Ltd